INTEGRATED GUIDE
ESSENTIAL OILS
& AROMATHERAPY

SECOND EDITION

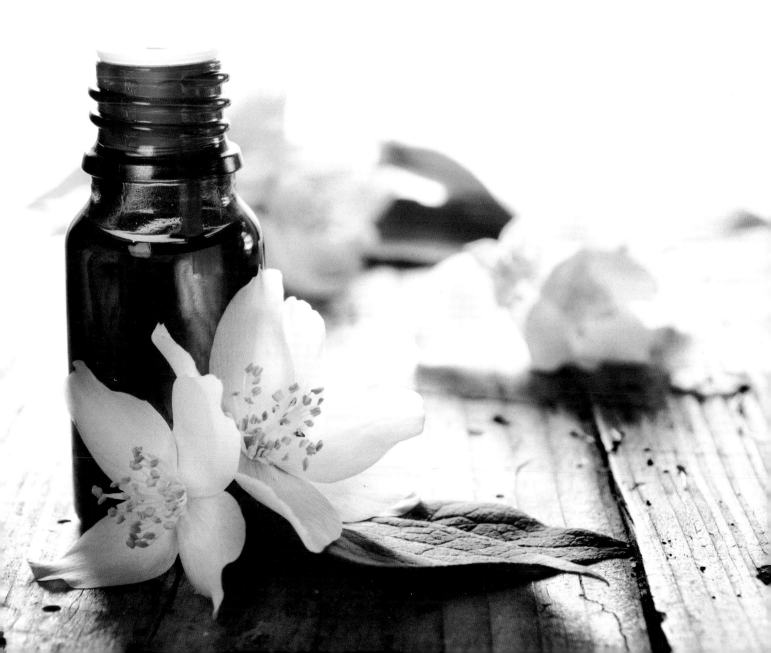

ISBN Number: 978-1-887938-23-5

Disclaimer: This book was written to provide
educational information to help the reader
learn about the subject matter covered.
It is sold with the understanding that the
publisher and authors are not liable for the
misconception or misuse of any information
provided. It is not provided with the intention
to diagnose, prescribe, or treat any disease,
illness or injured condition of the body. The
authors and publisher shall have neither
liability nor responsibility to any person or
entity with respect to any loss, damage,
or injury caused, or alleged to be caused,
directly or indirectly by the information within
this book. The information presented is not
intended as a substitute for medical advice
or counseling. Anyone suffering from any
condition, disease, or injury should consult a
qualified health care professional.

Table of Contents

What are Essential Oils

History of Essential Oils

Chemistry

Essential Oil Quality

How to Use Essential Oils

Singles

Blends

Index of Essential Oils

FOREWORD
By Dr. Daniel Pénoël

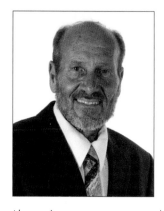

A New Kind of Freedom

Today we are involved in a struggle for freedom—health freedom. Just as the fragile ecosystems of our planet are under attack from greed and industrial exploitation, there is an even more dangerous and hidden attack against the fragile ecosystems deep inside our own bodies. These are the delicate ecosystems that keep us healthy and prevent debilitating disease.

This struggle for freedom from disease began with two contemporaries across the English Channel from each other. In England the discovery of antibiotics took place in 1928 by Sir Alexander Fleming. It spread to Germany with the discovery of sulfa drugs 1935. At the same time, a French chemist, René-Maurice Gattefossé, created a concept and coined the word "aromathérapie." At that same time, in Australia, doctors, surgeons, and pharmacists were showing interest in antimicrobial essential oils. There were two paths to freedom from disease: patentable synthetic drugs and natural, multi-constituent essential oils.

The first path has seen spectacular success but also alarming danger to the delicate ecosystems of the body as costly synthetic drugs have proliferated and grown enormous industries throughout the world.

In countries other than France, aromatherapy took on a new meaning—recreational fragrances, ceramic diffusers, aromatic candles, massage with a drop or two of a fragrant synthetic or natural oil in a relaxing massage oil. But when French doctors use the word, "aromathérapie," we think of medical and surgical procedures and pharmaceutical applications of natural essential oils. We are delving into the field of medicine and surgery with biochemical and pharmacological research, studying and using the tens of thousands of bioactive molecular components.

Such research has been conducted for decades and is fully recognized by the research communities of almost all universities worldwide. Thousands of papers and articles have been published in the most respected, peer-reviewed scientific journals regarding essential oils. The goal of this book is to expand your definition of aromatherapy far beyond the aromatic hobbies and pot pourris ("rotten pots" in French). Here you will discover simple, practical actions you can take to free yourself and your family from bondage to a health care system that is becoming financially out of reach for more and more people.

You are beginning an adventure that will restore your **freedom** from disease and from a lot of *synthetic, chemical molecules that have no place at all in the complex and delicate ecosystems of your body or our living planet.*

I am a medical doctor and I respect medicine as a science, as an art, and as a technical discipline. But I want you to have *an intelligent and respectful medicine*, a medicine independent from the relentless pressure exerted by the all-powerful pharmaceutical lobbies.

I simply wish that my medical colleagues all over the world might accept that there are ways for creating true, deep, and sustainable health outside of the synthetic/chemical/pharmaceutical industries. And this applies to animals and plants as well. I call it *Life Helping Life*, and it applies to every living creature.

Don't get me wrong. I am not saying that pharmacies must be totally excluded from our health-care systems. I am simply saying that, for hundreds of millions of people and for thousands of years, we have turned to the natural properties found in plants, and especially in aromatic plants and their powerful molecules. They should be our first choice in trying to stay healthy and eliminate diseases.

This book was born out of a close relationship with an American disciple of mine, Bill Fifield, who not only studied under my supervision, but has also lived the aromatic lifestyle for many years. I have carefully proofread the text for accuracy and safety from a scientific and medical perspective. I am grateful to Bill for keeping my teachings simple, practical, and understandable because I have a natural tendency to delve too deep and make things too complex. This book was also a perfect way to introduce other interesting, efficient, and simple ways of applying essential oils, like the "M" technique invented by Jane Buckle.

The medical use of essential oils is at the core of my daily medical practice. I have a deep interest in all forms of natural medicine, but essential oils remain at the top. They represent the ultimate power of nature. They also represent **the ultimate way to empower each person on this planet to become responsible for his/her own health and the health of their loved ones.**

This book will give you the intensive procedures and powerful techniques that have been implemented in France by medical doctors for decades. I like to compare the timid, aroma and massage-style aromatherapy to using a pocket knife that is kept in its leather pouch and never opened!

If you suffer from sinusitis, whether acute or chronic, you cannot expect significant results from a few drops of essential oils evaporating from a warm ceramic. You need to learn safe, clinical techniques.

Ingesting essential oils has always been "strictly forbidden" in the soft, massage approach. But culinary spices and aromatic herbs have been used all over the planet for thousands of years. These contain exactly the same molecules that penetrate from essential oils into our digestive system! Our digestive systems, and our bacterial flora, have lived with aromatic molecules from the very beginning. You don't get a prescription to buy a "tabasco" bottle! You don't need a pharmacist to press a clove of garlic into your favorite sauce, sprinkle curry powder on your rice, or use pungent oregano on your pizza!

In these chapters, you will learn to use essential oils in a natural and easy way in your beverages and your foods. You will also learn when larger amounts are needed. When the taste is not too pleasant, you will learn how to prepare aromatic capsules. My tens of thousands of patients in France are trained to do exactly what you will learn here. And, guess what? They love it! Being your own pharmacist makes a huge difference. You're not only being independent but also frugal!

Let me briefly tell you why so much research and medical aromatherapy took place in France in the last century. You will learn in this book how, in the 1950s, Dr. Jean Valnet had a strong desire to launch medical and pharmaceutical phytotherapy (plant therapy), and aromatherapy in France. His work was highly respected in France. In those early decades, whenever a French M.D. wrote a prescription using plants, plants extracts, or clinical grade essential oils, it was given to a pharmacist who would then manufacture what is called "une préparation magistrale." It was a custom prescription made for each patient. The pharmacist would make complex herbal teas, aromatic creams or lotions, aromatic suppositories and capsules, aromatic blends for inhalations or aerosols, etc.

It may seem hard to believe, but the French welfare system ("La Sécurité Sociale") would pay 90% of the cost. Complementary insurance would pay the other 10%. The patient would pay nothing and would receive a complete natural-based treatment! During these years we performed hundreds of thousands of laboratory tests (aromatograms) using essential oils on bacteria and fungi. We could clearly see their inhibiting power on numerous kinds of strains. The amount of knowledge and practical experience in France, Belgium, and French-speaking Switzerland was unique and huge.

This financially favorable situation, where thousands of French M.D.s were working hand-in-hand with thousands of pharmacists, lasted for about forty years. In 1990, in the year Pierre Franchomme and I published our scientific and medical book on essential oils, *l'aromathérapie exactement* (*Precise Aromatherpy*), the French parliament issued a law stopping reimbursements for all plant and essential oil preparations from the welfare system.

Everything had to be totally reorganized. I wanted my patients to continue taking care of their health in a natural way at an affordable cost. We began offering clinical grade essential oils at an affordable price, and began training our patients to be their own "pharmacists." The research has never stopped. For nearly a quarter of a century, we have seen extensive proof of the effectiveness of clinical-grade essential oils and their affordability. Our patients appreciate receiving an education that opens the way to freedom from disease and pharmaceutical bondage.

This book is the first step in offering you, and all those who you will influence, the health freedom my patients enjoy. Even as the number of natural health products grows, the role and potential of clinical grade essential oils, **used with relevant and appropriate training**, will always set them above whatever has existed or will yet exist in the field of complementary medicine.

Yes, I am convinced that you will love learning so many ways to improve your health, vitality, and inner strength, "***from the life of your cells to the power of your mind.***" Here is my motto and my commitment to myself:

"I will use clinical grade essential oils to support the life force inside me, and I will use them every day of my life until my last day on this planet."

Once you truly understand the life-enhancing power of clinical grade essential oils and how easy they are to use, you will not be able to imagine even one day without their active and synergistic support.

With my best wishes for your personal quest for health-freedom.

Dr. Daniel Pénoël
Vallée de la Drôme

August 15, 2014

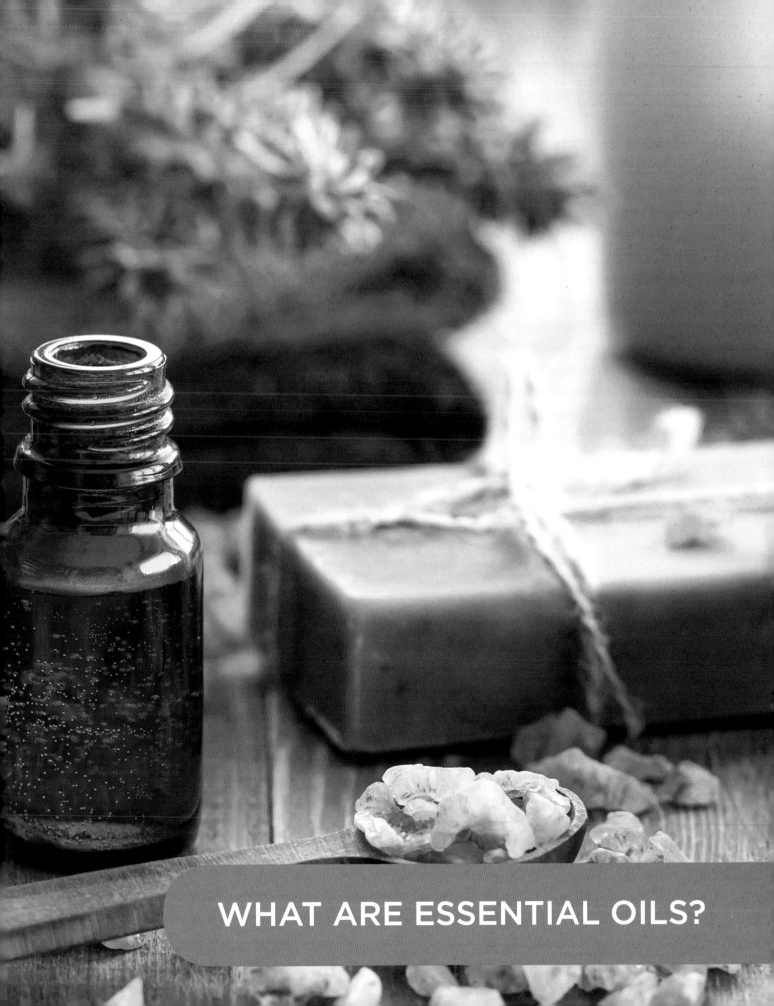

WHAT ARE ESSENTIAL OILS?

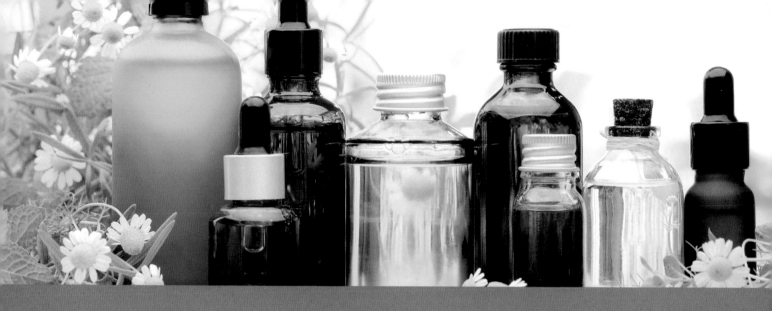

WHAT ARE ESSENTIAL OILS?

Essential oils are highly penetrating aromatic extracts from many kinds of plant material—seeds, rind, bark, leaves, twigs, flowers, nuts, etc. Unlike the more familiar vegetable oils, the highest quality essential oils have the potential to penetrate quickly through the skin, the lungs, the olfactory organs, and the digestive tract. They travel throughout the body, cleansing, repairing, and bringing vitality where it is most needed. They are only soluble in alcohol or other essential oils or vegetable oils. Essential oils have an amazing potential to perform many powerful functions in the body, but only when true clinical grade essential oils are applied. (See Chapter 3 for ways to identify clinical grade essential oils.)

Like salt, essential oils are highly concentrated. A little goes a long way. A drop or two can represent the distillation of pounds of plant material. A small number of essential oils can replace hundreds of dollars-worth of supplies in the most complete medicine cabinet.

Essential oils are most effective when used on a daily basis in dilution for massage, diffused into the air, a drop at a time in drinks and recipes, in dilution in a capsule, or dispersed in bath water or the shower.

They can also be used "neat," meaning undiluted, straight from the bottle for many applications like diffusing or applying to a cut or a scrape.

They are powerfully anti-infectious, yet safe to use as you follow the simple guidelines in this book.

3 Things That Essential Oils Do

1. They bring vitality. They bring life into your body. Unlike synthetic molecules that can only block certain body functions or kill microbes, essential oils actually vitalize and restore health.

2. They lower body toxicity. They have an extremely important and safe cleansing function that respects the beneficial flora ecosystem of the body.

3. They allow for a free flow of energy throughout the body.

The dead, lifeless, synthetic substances promoted by the pharmaceutical industry can't restore vitality and health. They're the antis—antibiotic, anti-inflammatory, anti-fungal, anti-depressant, anti-histamine, etc. They're lifeless. They have only two functions—to kill and block. While essential oils are also antibiotic, anti-inflammatory, etc., they also bring life-giving, restorative benefits. For example, using marjoram, lavender, or sweet basil on a cut or a scrape not only sterilizes, but you can also experience faster healing and closing everything up.

Essential oils are versatile. They follow four main pathways to enter your body with many beneficial functions. They are applied topically, ingested, used aromatically, and absorbed through respiration.

Aromatic Influence of Essential Oils

Our sense of smell influences many physical functions, including stimulating your hormones, influencing your emotions, and helping regulate various metabolic processes. They influence the emotions because the delicate sensory nerves associated with smell communicate instantly with the limbic system of the brain—the seat of the emotions.

That's why certain aromas can trigger instant emotional reactions, like your old girlfriend's favorite perfume or your grandfather's aftershave. Those limbic emotions and feelings come up even after many years have passed.

Aromas can be calming, relaxing, refreshing, uplifting, and inviting. They can create and reinforce important memories and thus strengthen relationships. They can improve memory and concentration.

You can use essential oils in household products to replace the toxic, synthetic fragrances. We call this household aromatherapy. Create an aromatic spray to disinfect and deodorize countertops, cutting boards, refrigerators, microwaves, trash cans, bathroom surfaces, etc. They can be used in the wash water to disinfect and freshen clothes. The spray can even repel insects.

Use them on a small piece of fabric or rag in the dryer to freshen instead of toxic dryer sheets. Essential oils will stop mildew, germs, and viruses. Use a few drops of an essential oil on your dust cloth. Use them on pads, cotton, or string near air vents to purify the air and repel bugs. Tuck aromatic cotton balls in car air vents and between the tubes of a radiator.

Reduce the toxicity of paint fumes by adding 5 to 15 ml of your favorite essential oil to a 5-gallon bucket of paint.

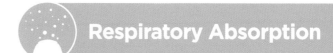

Respiratory Absorption

Essential oil molecules enter the lungs, and through the lungs, the bloodstream. With all their tiny sacs, your lungs have the surface area of a tennis court. Microscopic diffused molecules of essential oils landing on this surface enter the bloodstream quickly.

Certain essential oils, when diffused into the air you breathe, can be very stimulating, while others can be calming and soothing. Diffusing essential oils can purify the air from odors and some infectious microbes. They can dissolve hardened, glue-like mucous and open up the air passages so we breathe more freely for more efficient oxygen exchange and increased energy.

We recommend cold-air, nebulizing diffusers because they don't alter the chemical structure of the oil being diffused and they deliver the maximum amount of aromatic molecules into the room for therapeutic purposes. Different types of diffusers will be discussed in Chapter 3.

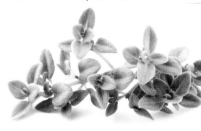

Topical Uses

Complex but tiny essential oil molecules are easily absorbed into the skin and can be safely applied topically. They not only help the immediate area of application as in a burn or a scrape, but they can travel quickly throughout the body to give relief wherever it is needed. They can be cooling, calming, warming, or stimulating depending on the oil and the need.

When you combine different methods of absorption, you can experience significant synergistic benefits that compound the power of the oil. Dr. Daniel Pénoël teaches that using multiple means of absorption doesn't just add a benefit but actually compounds the benefits exponentially.

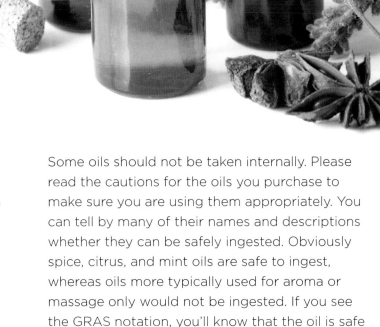

When speaking of topical application of essential oils, it's important to understand that while many oils can be applied undiluted (often referred to as "neat"), some oils require dilution with a carrier oil (such as coconut oil or sweet almond oil) because of their unusual potency. Simply follow directions on the bottle label whether the oil can be applied neat (undiluted") or should be diluted with a carrier oil.

Internal Uses

Essential oils are also used as "dietary supplements" by ingestion—capsules; a drop in a tea, water, or juice; or a drop or two in a recipe; etc. Many essential oils are Generally Regarded As Safe (GRAS) for ingestion like those used in flavorings lemon, eucalyptus, basil, wintergreen, peppermint, etc. GRAS is a designation of the U.S. Food and Drug Administration (FDA) that an oil is safe for human consumption as a food additive or flavoring agent.

Some oils should not be taken internally. Please read the cautions for the oils you purchase to make sure you are using them appropriately. You can tell by many of their names and descriptions whether they can be safely ingested. Obviously spice, citrus, and mint oils are safe to ingest, whereas oils more typically used for aroma or massage only would not be ingested. If you see the GRAS notation, you'll know that the oil is safe to ingest within the safety guidelines.

Extraction Method

Most clinical-grade essential oils are distilled with steam according to exact heat, timing, and pressure parameters for each plant species and sub-species as well as the part of the plant being distilled. Steam is circulated under low pressure through plant material, liberating the essential oil molecules. As the steam cools and condenses, the water and oils separate, and the oil is collected and filtered.

To guarantee the highest quality and most dependable chemical composition for consistent therapeutic benefits, timing, temperature, and pressure must be closely regulated. Too little or too much heat and pressure will not release the finest quality clinical-grade oil. The extraction method that may be fine for spearmint used for chewing gum will not be right for clinical use.

The selection of medicinal or clinical-grade oils depends on a complex network of individual botanists, growers, distillers, and chemists from all around the world working to gather an array of quality products you can depend upon. These networks are developed over years of association.

While most oils are extracted by steam distillation, some are distilled in water. Others, like citrus oils, are extracted by mashing and pressing the aromatic peels to release the oils. A few delicate aromatic oils can only be extracted using solvents that bind with the oils and are later removed from the final product. You will see CO_2 extraction, absolutes, enfleurage, and other names, typically on perfume oils. There are many methods that have been used through the centuries, but these are the most common.

Will every batch of oil smell exactly the same?

No. These differences are, in fact, a sign that the oils are clinical grade and natural products. Synthetic ingredients will be standardized and uniform. Natural substances grown under varying climate conditions in differing soil will change slightly from batch to batch. Quality suppliers monitor and label each batch so they can identify differences. Just

as with different years of fine wines, growers and suppliers are aware of the slight changes. The best companies will maintain a wide range of suppliers in different countries and regions around the world in order to provide their customers with the finest batches from year to year. If one company claims that their lavender always smells "crystal clean," it may be a signal that they are tampering with the product or do not recognize the best, most therapeutic, natural ingredients. The "crystal clean" ingredients could contain simple synthetic compounds instead of natural ingredients. Your body will recognize the difference.

Over time as you compare the nutritionally dead, synthetic fragrances with the more full-bodied, complex, natural fragrances, you'll come to tell the difference by smell alone.

Clinical Quality Essential Oils Versus Synthetics

You can replace many things you now use from your medicine cabinet with safer and more effective essential oils. There are 9 reasons why high-quality essential oils are superior to those patented and pricey drugs and over-the-counter products that so many unfortunate people depend on to control their chronic conditions.

1. Essential Oils Have a Longer, More Complex and Proven History

For many millennia, aromatic molecules from plants have been adapting, protecting, energizing, and working synergistically with the world of beneficial and toxic bacteria, fungi and viruses. Humans have used aromatic plants for thousands of years and have, at first pragmatically and later scientifically, verified their safety and functions. The cells of your body recognize a natural aromatic substance and know what to do with it. Your body may not recognize or be able to effectively use a synthetic one. Nature's purpose in giving us aromatic molecules is to bring us vitality, harmonious balance, and protection. Dr. Daniel Pénoël teaches that "synthetic substances have only two functions—to block and to kill." Essential oils, on the other hand, "help regenerate, balance, calm, bring energy, and many more functions too numerous to mention" (Daniel Pénoël, *Guide to Home Use of Essential Oils*, 10).

2. Essential Oils Will Not Encourage "Superbugs"

Bacteria can mutate to form resistant strains of "superbugs" to outwit the toxic, synthetic, antibiotic drugs. **Living, un-patentable, aromatic oils have never created a superbug.** Scientists are now turning to essential oils to fight these fierce invaders because they realize that only nature can win the antimicrobial war with nature. Dr. Pénoël has stated, "In all my experience with bacteria and essential oils, I have never seen strains mutate and develop resistance. There are no superbugs created by essential oils" (Dr. Daniel Pénoël. *Guide to Home Use of Essential Oils,* p. 9).

3. Essential Oils Will Not Produce Side Effects

You've seen the pages of horrible-sounding side effects that follow every pharmaceutical advertisement. You know the extreme dangers of drug reactions. You've heard of the drug recalls that occur each year. Would you prefer using nature's complex essential oils with multiple health benefits and virtually no side effects?

4. Essential Oils Bring Vitality to Your Body

Would you prefer using simple, man-made synthetic drugs whose only function is to block and kill? Or would you prefer complex, natural substances designed by nature and proven safe through centuries of use? Dr. Pénoël says, "My patients who complete the sometimes slower but more complete treatments I conduct, do not end their treatment ready to return home and begin the slow recuperation back to health. They are full of life. They are energized. Synthetic drugs lower your energy (entropy) while essential oils raise your energy (reverse entropy)" (Pénoël, p. 10). Have you ever felt mentally and physically exhausted after taking a round of synthetic antibiotics or other drugs? You won't feel that way after completing a protocol of essential oils.

5. Essential Oils Work in Many Ways All at Once

The complex synergies of essential oils improve your mood, strengthen multiple systems of your body, and do not disrupt the delicate balance of your beneficial bacteria. They can stop pain, reduce inflammation, stop muscle spasms, decongest, destroy microbes, and calm anxiety—all at the same time. They spread throughout the body bringing vitality and life. Synthetics only block body functions and kill pathogens, leaving their toxic waste behind. Synthetics are like a hammer hitting a single nail and often missing and hitting your thumb. Essential oils are like engineers, constructing and restoring health and vitality.

6. Essential Oils Can Enter The Body by Many Avenues

What do you have in your medicine cabinet now that can be diffused, added to your food, inhaled, added to bath water, added to your tea, and applied in a massage or under your nose? Essential oils are more complex and creative than synthetics. They can work on all these interfaces

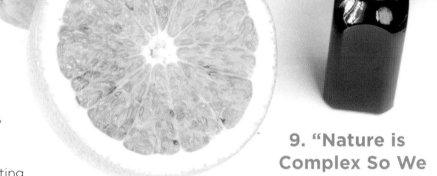

at once. If for some reason one doesn't work for you, there's always another one that can be used. And these different therapies work synergistically with each other multiplying their effectiveness.

7. Aromatic Plants Tell Us by Their Aroma What They're Good for

We are familiar with the toxic, disgusting smells of decaying, rotting foods that make us want to avoid them and discard them. The alluring aromas created by nature in spices, mints, citrus, and evergreen forests tell us that these substances are designed by nature to combat the bad microbes that cause decay and spoilage. Synthetics don't offer these natural signals. In fact, they're more often synthesized from fungus and disgusting-smelling petrochemicals. What does that instinctively tell you about the safety of their long-term use?

8. The Pleasure of Essential Oils Makes Us Want to Use Them Continually

What pleasure is there in taking a synthetic drug? You would never want to use one when you're well. But as Dr. Pénoël says, "My patients, once they have completed the therapies I recommend, are always eager to continue using the essential oils on a daily basis throughout their lives. And the ones that are most pleasurable are typically the ones that are best for daily use" (Pénoël, Guide, p. 11).

9. "Nature is Complex So We Don't Have to Be"

This quote by Dr. Pénoël gives us perhaps the most compelling reason to use essential oils in our daily lives (*Pénoël Guide* p. 12). Aromatic plants produce hundreds of thousands of complex aromatic molecules. Mortals struggle to classify and put to use this vast complexity. Without even knowing how they are functioning in your body or all the different things they may be doing, you can be confident, knowing that they are doing their magnificent work, restoring what is injured and bringing life and health. What simplistic synthetic can do that?

Most essential oils are perfectly safe for daily use in moderation. The most important function for optimal health is daily use. Prevention is our most effective health practice. We can modify the old sayings to read, "a drop of prevention is worth a gallon of cure" or "a few drops a day keeps the doctor away."

Dr. Pénoël offers this remarkable promise: "I can safely make you a promise that if you will use essential oils on a daily basis ... you will have no need to return to medicine cabinet remedies. Your life will be simpler, and you will find greater sensory and emotional pleasure in staying healthy" (*Pénoël Guide* p. 12).

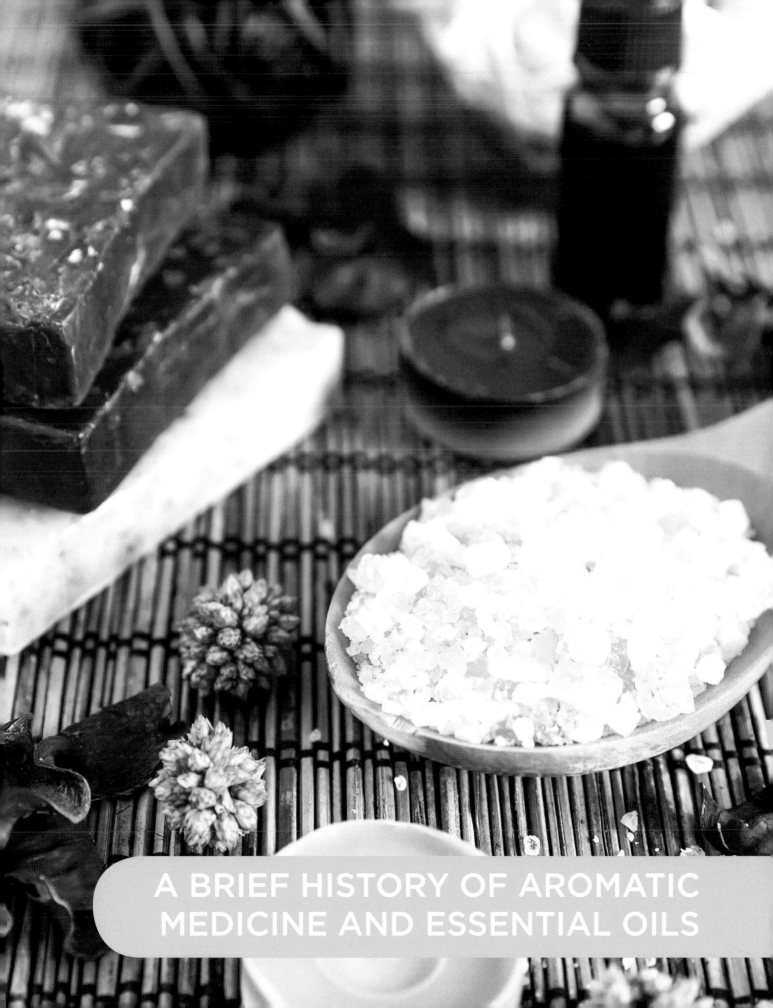

A BRIEF HISTORY OF AROMATIC MEDICINE AND ESSENTIAL OILS

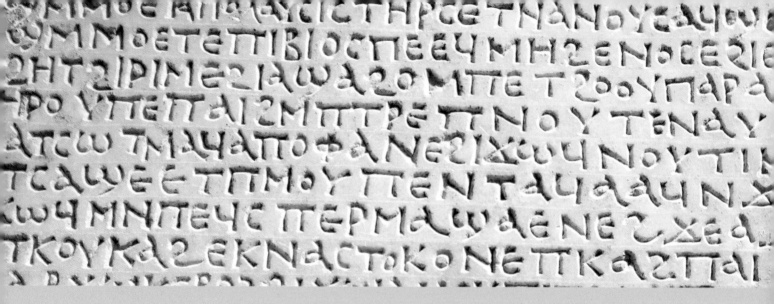

A BRIEF HISTORY OF AROMATIC MEDICINE AND ESSENTIAL OILS

What we know about the use of aromatic plants for therapeutic and religious purposes began possibly 6,000 years ago with the dawn of recorded civilization in Egypt, where religious and healing rituals, along with skin therapy, involved aromatic plants. Primitive extraction methods like cold pressing, boiling plants in water, and extracting their essences into animal fats, vegetable oils, or alcohol resulted in pomades, tinctures, and oils. These uses were chronicled in many early writings and suggested in art.

During the third Egyptian dynasty (2650 – 2575 B.C.) the process of embalming and mummification was developed. Frankincense, myrrh, galbanum, cinnamon, cedarwood, juniper berry and spikenard were all used to preserve the dead. The famed incense trail transported precious frankincense and myrrh across the desert. Because the demand for these precious resins outstripped supplies, they were at times traded as currency and comparative in value to precious gems and metals.

Marcel Lavabre recounts the story of a Queen of the land called Sheba [modern-day Ethiopia and Somalia] whose fabulous wealth was built on the trade in frankincense and myrrh. Legend has it that *"The Egyptians took personal hygiene seriously, as shown by the earliest recorded recipe for body deodorant in the Papyrus Ebers of 1500 B.C."* (Valerie Ann Worwood, The Complete Book of Essential Oils and Aromatherapy, p. 8).

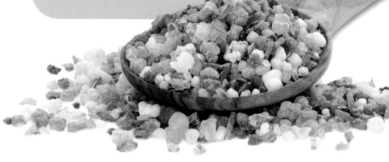

Between 1,359 and 657 B.C. the Egyptians became masters of the perfume trade to the point that when Julius Caesar returned to Rome with

Cleopatra, he tossed bottles of perfume to the crowds to symbolize his total conquest of Egypt. Cleopatra's use of perfumed cosmetics are legendary. On meeting Marc Anthony, the sails of her ship were said to be soaked in jasmine, and he gave up his chance at the empire to follow her.

"The Greeks believed that after death they went to Elysium where the air was permanently filled with a sweet-smelling aroma which rose from perfumed rivers." (Worwood, p. 9).

Hippocrates (circa 460 – 377 B.C.) dismissed the traditional Egyptian view of disease caused by supernatural causes and substituted natural explanations. We give him credit for introducing a more holistic view of health and medicine. He is reported to have studied over 200 herbs for healing.

Worwood quotes Hippocrates instruction: "The way to health is to have an aromatic bath and scented massage every day" (Worwood, p. 8). He taught that burning aromatic substances offered protection from some infectious diseases.

After Alexander invaded Egypt in the third century B.C., the Greeks expanded the use of aromatic herbs and perfumes. Theophrastus of Athens, a student of Aristotle, even studied how aromas affect the emotions. His books on the healing properties of herbs became one of the three most important references for centuries of physicians to study.

"The ancient Greeks had a very high opinion of aromatics, attributing sweet smells to divine origin. In ancient myths, gods descended to earth on scented clouds, wearing robes drenched in aromatic essences" - (Worwood, p.9).

"The Egyptian priests used aromatic substances not only for embalming their pharaoh but also in their role as 'psychiatrists' for treating manias, depression, and nervousness" - (Worwood, p.8).

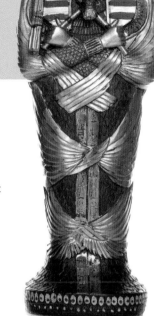

India has the distinction of carrying the most longstanding tradition for aromatic herbal remedies; the practices of Ayurvedic medicine were never discontinued and were codified in their sacred volume, The Vedas, one of the oldest books on record (1500–1000 B.C.). The volume codified over 700 products, including many aromatics for religious and therapeutic use, such as cinnamon, spikenard, coriander, ginger, myrrh, and sandalwood.

With the fall of Rome, the center for aromatic medical knowledge moved to Arabic countries. The celebrated philosopher Avicenna (A.D. 980 – 1037) is credited with perfecting the art of distillation of essential oils, though others may have used crude forms of distillation prior to his time. He became the most famous and greatest of the Islamic physicians. At age 16 he began the study of medicine and at the young age of 20 was appointed as a court physician eventually earning the title "Prince of Physicians."

He authored 20 books and 100 treatises on medicine. His epic encyclopedia, Al-Qanun fi al-Tibb, translated as The Canon of Medicine, was over a million words long and contained all the known medical knowledge of the day, including the traditions of Hippocrates, Galen, and the physicians in India. It became the definitive medical textbook for over 700 years.

In Europe during the fourteenth to sixteenth centuries, many herbals books were published. Many included recipes for making essential oils. "Glove-makers used aromatic oils, and it is reported that these and others who used aromatics of various sorts were the only people to survive the ravages of the plagues that struck Europe during these centuries" (Worwood, p. 9).

The Birth of Modern Medical Aromatherapy

In the 20th century the medical benefits of essential oils were recognized by a French chemist, Rene-Maurice Gattefossé (1881-1950), who is considered the "father of aromatherapy." He "suffered serious burns to the hands in a laboratory explosion, and the wounds soon became gangrenous; he was able to effect a perfect cure using essence of lavender" (Jean Valnet M.D., The Practice of Aromatherapy, p. 66).

In 1928 when Alexander Fleming began his work on penicillin—the origins of modern antibiotics—Gattefossé in France was doing his serious investigative research into the therapeutic properties of essential oils. It is interesting that both of these famous pioneers were born in 1881 and died in the 1950s. Gattefossé coined the term "aromathérapie" and is now considered the "father of modern aromatherapy."

Pharmacists in France were quick to recommend eucalyptus and tea tree essential oils for things that were being treated elsewhere in the world with penicillin. Oil of oregano and penicillin have relatively equivalent strength against harmful bacteria.

The big difference is that penicillin and all the subsequent strong, pharmaceutical antibiotics could make a fortune for their manufacturers because they could be standardized, synthesized, and patented, while essential oils were natural substances. So essential oils were largely ignored by the medical establishment except in France and elsewhere in Europe where there was already significant published research.

Gattefossee incorporated a blend of essential oils used in treating the Spanish flu epidemic of 1918. His successor in the practice of aromatherapy, a French medical doctor and surgeon, Jean Valnet, "made use of the healing properties of essences in wartime surgery on some of [his] patients in Tonkin, and though having only a very limited quantity of [his] own aromatic essences [he] was able to treat as many patients at [he] … liked, the results … were consistent" (Valnet p. 66). When he returned to Paris, he continued his great work with plant extracts and devoted his life to the research and development of therapeutic plant medicines.

In 1971 Dr. Maurice Girault coined the term "aromatogram" for antimicrobial therapy involving essential oils. Doctors would take microbial cultures and use various essential oils in vitro to recognize which oil or blend would be best to treat the disease. Dr. Valnet helped to spread this concept to the general public.

Valnet also published the book The Practice of Aromatherapy in 1978, which became the first training for Dr. Pénoël and Pierre Franchomme on essential oils therapy.

The modern use of essential oils has continued to grow rapidly as chemists like Pierre Franchomme and medical doctors like Daniel Pénoël conducted research in the laboratory and medical clinic to validate the numerous health and wellness benefits of clinical-grade essential oils. Their book, L'Aromathérapie Exactement [Precise Aromatherapy], published in 1990, became the "bible" of aromatherapy at the time. And everyone who was to be trained in the use of therapeutic essential oils after 1990 had to understand its contents.

Essential Oils for the Common Man

These pioneers could see that they needed to do worldwide training to avoid serious problems for their new industry. Essential oils would be severely restricted in some countries; others would use them in ways that were unsafe. So there began extensive training.

The English-speaking countries were already doing what the French medical doctors called "timid" aromatherapy with too many restrictions and rules. In these countries the oils were greatly diluted and only applied topically.

"You can't really accomplish anything significant with microbes and many health issues with that timid approach," says Dr. Pénoël. "It's like having a wonderful pocket knife without ever opening the blade." You have no real therapeutic value when all you can do is use a two percent essential oils solution in a carrier oil for topical massage.

While medical doctors in France were prescribing essential oils for internal and external use, the English and American schools of aromatherapy allowed for no ingestion and no undiluted application. According to Dr. Pénoël, "they were missing most of the power of true medical aromatherapy. And that's why we see in the USA and the UK mostly recreational fragrances and dead, synthetic essential oils in most shops."

The pharmaceutical establishment has always tried to instill fear about essential oil safety even though they are used extensively in the food industry and animal husbandry. The English-speaking aromatherapy establishment seems to want to keep the information so complicated that all medical decisions have to be kept away from ordinary people and only in the hands of trained professionals certified to practice aromatic medicine.

You Can Care for Yourself Affordably, Safely, and Effectively

Because of the simplicity and safety of essential oils, the mission of Dr. Pénoël and the companies he has worked with has been to empower people to care for themselves safely, affordably, and effectively using the most beneficial oils and blends. Because essential oils are so multifunctional, powerful, and effective, a large body of training literature is available online. It can seem overwhelming to the newcomer, but you don't need a medical degree or even a certification to use them effectively. Here are Dr. Pénoël's instructions for our training:

"We need to distill all the complicated training into its essential simplicity. What you will find in my training is profound in its background and depth of knowledge and research, yet simple in its teachings and habits. I advocate fundamental habits using ... essential oils that will restore health in a deep way. My training is not about the quick cure. A quick cure is like a mirage—all show but no permanent health" (Pénoël, notes from online training, not in print).

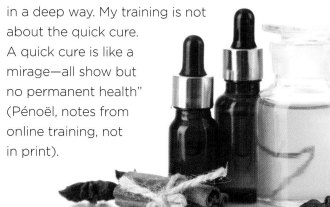

Historical Times

4,000 B.C. Primitive extractions from aromatic plants using water, alcohol, fat, and oil

2650 – 2575 B.C. Mummification begins in Egypt

1500–1000 B.C. In India The Vedas codifies over 700 products including aromatics for religious and therapeutic use

970 – 931 B.C. King Solomon & the Queen of Sheba meet because of the trade in incense

460 – 377 B.C. Hippocrates studies over 200 herbs for natural, holistic healing

371 – 287 B.C. Theophrastus of Athens, a student of Aristotle studies how aromas affect the emotions

A.D. 980 – 1037 Islamic philosopher Avicenna perfects the art of distillation of essential oils and authors The *Canon of Medicine*, the definitive medical textbook for over 700 years

A.D. 1346 – 1353 During the Black Plague those in trades involving aromatic oils were spared

1910 René-Maurice Gattefossé heals a serious burn with lavender oil and begins his lifetime study of essential oils. He coins the word "aromatherapy."

1928 Alexander Fleming discovers the effectiveness of penicillin, which begins the development of modern-day antibiotics

1945 – 1978 Dr. Jean Valnet treats patients using essential oils in Southeast Asia. He authors The Practice of Aromatherapy, published in 1978

1977 Robert Tisserand authors The Art of Aromatherapy, the first major work on aromatherapy in the English language

1990 Pierre Franchomme and Dr. Daniel Pénoël publish *L'aromathérapie Exactement* [Precise Aromatherapy], considered the bible of the chemistry and clinical practice of aromatherapy

Biographies

The following individuals are renowned experts and pioneers in the field of aromatherapy. Each has contributed either directly or indirectly to this book through his or her research, clinical work and decades of experience with essential oils.

Dr. Daniel Pénoël, M.D.

is one of the foremost authorities in the world on essential oils. He has worked with essential oils in his medical clinic since 1977. He is a world-renowned medical doctor, researcher, educator, and author. With his wife Rose-Marie, Dr. Pénoël has authored three books in English: *Life Helping Life: Unleash Your Mind/Body Potential with Essential Oils, Natural Home Health Care Using Essential Oils,* and *Guide to Home Use of Essential Oils.* He has authored several books in French, his most notable being *L'aromatherapie Exactement,* considered by many professionals to be "the encyclopedia of essential oils" when it was published in 1990. It was written with Pierre Franchomme, a chemist, who is credited with laying the foundation for the practical study of essential oil chemistry. Dr. Pénoël's role in the book was to provide the practical, clinical foundation.

Dr. Pénoël has lectured to, encouraged, and trained most of the foremost professional aromatherapists in the world. He has either personally or through his students and books trained virtually all well-respected aromatherapists worldwide. Most English authors reference *l'aromatherapie exactement* frequently even though the book has never been translated into English.

The Pénoëls have lived in France and Australia and have traveled the world lecturing and training. Dr. Pénoël is considered by many to be the world's leading medical authority on newly discovered essential oils. He analyzes and certifies them as therapeutically valid for clinical use.

Shirley Price

is one of the world's leading aromatherapists and the founder of the Shirley Price School of Aromatherapy, which offers accreditation through distance learning. There are branches worldwide. She is the author of many well-respected books including *Aromatherapy for Health Professionals, Aromatherapy for Common Ailments, Aromatherapy for Women, Aromatherapy for Babies and Children, Aromatherapy Workbook, Practical Aromatherapy, Aromatherapy and Your Emotions, Aromatherapy: a Step-by-step Guide,* and more.

Jane Buckle, PhD, RN

has over 25 years of background in critical care nursing. She is trained in massage therapy, clinical aromatherapy, and herbal and aromatic medicine. She has an MA in Clinical Aromatherapy (Middlesex Univ., London) and a PhD in Health Service Management (Columbus University, USA). She was an NIH-funded post-doctoral Complementary and Alternative Medicine Research Fellow at the Centre for Clinical Epidemiology and Biostatistics (CCEB) within the School of Medicine, University of Pennsylvania, Philadelphia. Before joining the CCEB, Dr. Buckle was faculty at University of Minnesota, and adjunct faculty at New York University, Bastyr University, WA and The College of New Rochelle NY.

Her first book, *Clinical Aromatherapy in Nursing*, was published in 1997 and was accepted as the text for aromatherapy in nursing. Her second book, *Clinical Aromatherapy: Essential Oils in Practice,* was published in 2003, has been reprinted 9 times and has been called "the evidence-based text for clinical aromatherapy".

Dr. Buckle is the director of R J Buckle Associates, an educational consultancy dedicated to integrating clinical aromatherapy and the "M" technique® into mainstream medicine. She created a certification course for health professionals in clinical aromatherapy that was the 1st to be endorsed by National Nursing Organization.

Dr. Buckle is published widely in medical and nursing journals. She lectures and presents internationally and was a guest speaker at the World Economic Forum in Davos, Switzerland in 1999. In the USA, she was a board member of ARC (Aromatherapy Registration Council) and has been an advisor to NAHA's education committee. She is a reviewer for several peer-reviewed journals and has been a reviewer for NIH and NHS grants.

Dr. Buckle pioneered a method of touch for the critically ill or fragile called the 'M' technique®. It is a registered method of structured touch suitable for those too fragile to receive massage, or when the giver is not trained in massage. Simple to do and easy to learn, the 'M' technique® has measurable effects within 5 minutes and has been taught in universities, hospitals, hospices and long-term care facilities in the USA since 1999.

Kurt Schnaubelt

holds a PhD in chemistry and is the founder and scientific director of the Pacific Institute of Aromatherapy in San Francisco. He is a Munich-born chemist who left his native land in his 30s to spread the science of aromatherapy in California. He became interested in aromatherapy in 1978 when he contracted hepatitis and began looking for alternatives to the prescribed medicines he was given. As a chemist he knew his molecules and recognized that the drugs he had been prescribed were potentially harmful. He discovered The *Art of Aromatherapy* by Robert Tisserand and *The Practice of Aromatherapy* by Dr. Jean Valnet, two of the leading books in the field at that time. He sourced the finest oils he could find and began sharing. He is the author of 7 books on aromatherapy and many articles on the subject.

Dr. Jean Valnet, M.D.

(1920 – 1995) was a French physician and military surgeon who was one of the foremost pioneers in modern medical aromatherapy. He received his Doctor of Medicine degree in 1945 as a surgeon. During the war he served in hospitals in Germany and France.

From 1950 to 1953 he was appointed surgeon to the advanced surgical unit in Tonkin, the northern area of Vietnam that borders China. Being low on medical supplies, he bandaged the wounded with aromatic solutions that delivered results well above average.

From 1953 to 1959 he became Chief of the Secretariat of State for War, and in 1959 he left the army to continue his research in herbal medicine and aromatherapy in Paris.

As early as 1948 he began to publish articles on herbal medicine and aromatherapy in many medical journals.

In 1981 he founded the College of Phyto-aromatherapy and Medicine to pursue research on herbal medicine and aromatherapy, establish criteria for quality, and educate practitioners and users of essential oils. He gave lectures on phytotherapy on television and the radio. He popularized the "aromatogram," a method of identifying the best essential oils to combat microbes in individual patients.

His best known book, *The Practice of Aromatherapy,* was translated into English and published in 1982

Julia Lawless

became interested in aromatic oils as a child when her mother, who was a biochemist, began research on essential oils. In 1983 she became responsible for creating products for the family business, Aqua Oleum, using essential oils as ingredients. She studied Western and Tibetan herbal medicine and became a qualified aromatherapist and member of the International Federation of Aromatherapists. She is well known for her numerous books on aromatherapy including *The Encyclopedia of Essential Oils.*

Valerie Ann Worwood

is an aromatherapist, a reflexologist, and a member of the International Federation of Aromatherapists. She founded her own clinic in Romford, England where she conducts research on aromatherapy and its effects on various diseases and medical conditions. She consults and lectures all over the world on the benefits of aromatherapy. She is the author of several books including the *Complete Book of Essential Oils and Aromatherapy.*

Marcel Lavabre

was born in the lavender-growing region of southern France and since 1974 has been studying every aspect of essential oil production and aromatherapy. He is cofounder of the American Aromatherapy Association and is the founder and president of a company that sells essential oils. He is the author of *Aromatherapy Workbook*, a best-selling classic in American aromatherapy.

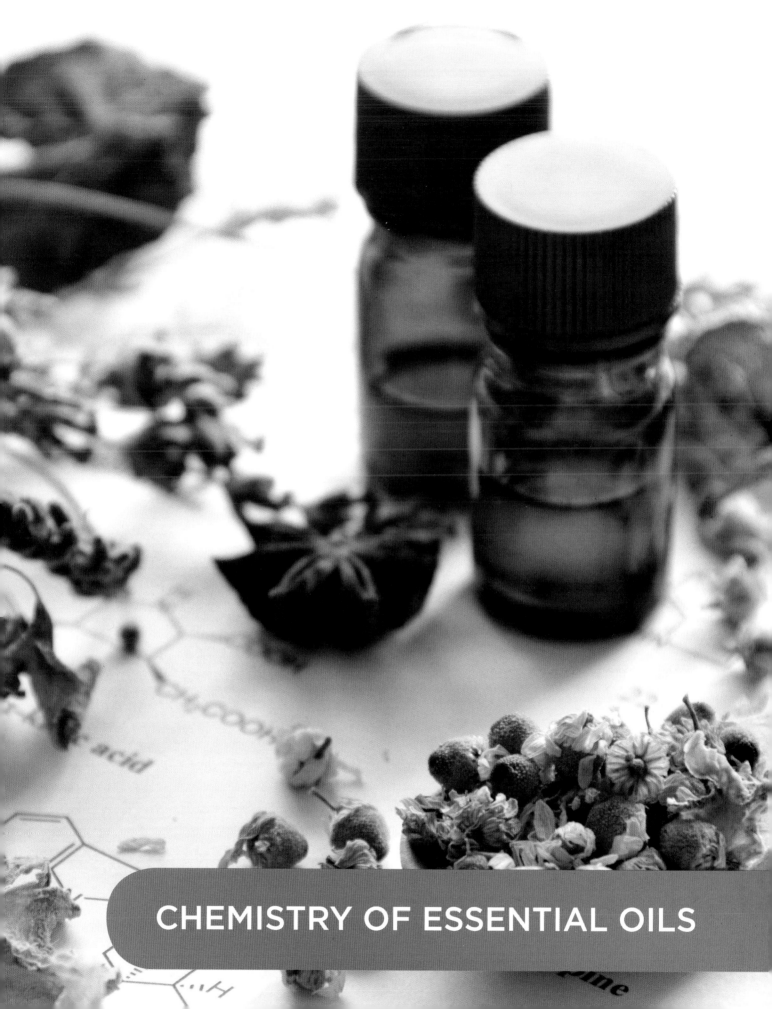

CHEMISTRY OF ESSENTIAL OILS

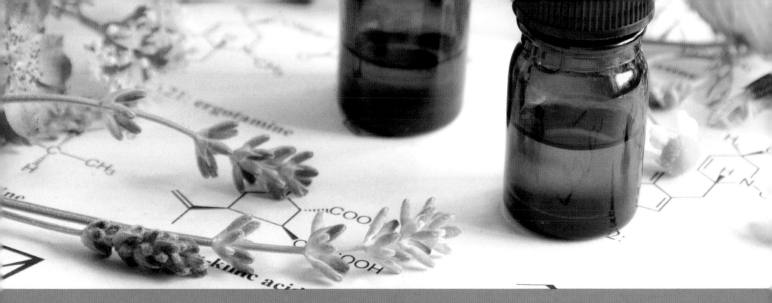

CHEMISTRY OF ESSENTIAL OILS

Useful Chemical Classification For Understanding Essential Oils

Pierre Franchomme was Dr. Daniel Pénoël's partner for 13 years and co-author of the landmark book in French, *L'Aromatherapie Exactement*, or Precise Aromatherapy. In this volume, Franchomme taught us a very useful molecular approach to chemical classification of essential oils. Instead of studying isolated individual molecules, he taught us to classify them by groups, then families, and ultimately by individual molecules.

In classifying aromatic molecules and their families, Franchomme used a double frame of reference:

- From left-to-right he used the behaviour of molecules toward water (hydrophilic or hydrophobic). Franchomme called it the "polar left" and the "non-polar right."

- From top-to-bottom he considered the electrical charges of the molecules (negative or positive)

Electric relationships: Location of family and chemical groups

Negative Molecules (anions)
They Give electrons

Aldehydes	Esters
Cetones	
	Polyunsaturated Sequiterpenes
Coumarines & Lactones	
	Oxydes
Alcohols C_{15} & C_{20}	Terpenes C_{10}
	Phenols
Acids Aromatic adehydes	
Alcohols C_{10}	Hydrocarbons
Phenols	

Positive Molecules (cations)
They capture electrons

Electric relationships: General properties related to the electric class

Calming & Relaxing

Toning & Stimulating

Electric relationships: Location of family and chemical groups

Anti-Infectous
Litholytic

Antispasmodic

Mucolytic
Lipolytic
Cicatrisant

Antiparasitic
Expectorant

Estrogen-Like

Cortisone-Like
Antispetic

Anti-infectious
Immune
stimulating

Anti-infectious
Antispasmodic

Lytholitic: Prevents stones
Lipolytic: Helps break down fats
Mucolytic: Dissolves & breaks down mucous
Cicatrisant: Helps promote healing
Antispasmodic: Prevents or eases spasms or convulsions
Antiparasitic: Prevents & destroys parasites
Expectorant: Helps reduce & remove mucous
Cortisone-like: Helps treat arthritis

This made it easy to establish relevant relationships with Oriental or Energy medicine. It also helped establish relationships with pathological conditions, with diseases, and even with individual temperaments. Thus, starting with an objective, scientific approach, we were able to incorporate both traditional allopathic medicine and also holistic energy medicine.

In Eastern Energy Medicine they speak of the "wet" and the "dry" on the one hand, and the "hot" and the "cold" on the other. The quadrants become "wet and warm," "wet and cold," "dry and warm" and "dry and cold." Or you could explain it according to yang-yin harmony:

- The strong yang molecular families: the phenols (plus cinnamic aldehyde) and the monoterpenols are both warm and wet—the sanguine temperament.

- The less yang molecular family: hydrocarbonated monoterpenes are warm and dry—the bilious temperament.

- The extremely yin molecular families: hydrocarbonated sesquiterpenes (especially the polyunsaturated ones like azulene) and esters are cold and dry—the nervous temperament.

- The less yin molecular families: ketons and terpenic aldehydes are cold and wet—the lymphatic temperament.

Electric & hyrdic relationships: Temperament quadrants

Lymphatic temperament
(soft, round, languid, congestive issues)

Nervous temperament
(emotional & Kidney ailments)

Aldehydes

Esters

Cetones

Polyunsaturated
Sequiterpenes

Coumarines
& Lactones

Oxydes

Alcohols C_{15} & C_{20}

Terpenes C_{10}

Phenols

Acids   Aromatic adehydes
Alcohols C_{10}

Hydrocarbons

Phenols

Sanguine temperament
(outgoing, cardiovascular issues)

Bilious temperament
(ill-tempered, energetic hormonal & Liver ailments)

This chemical organization helped Dr. Pénoël create blends for individual clients. If a client was of the nervous temperament and was prone to catching infections, he would create a strong anti-infectious, yang blend made of phenols and other strong constituents. He was thus able to integrate both his holistic naturopathic training with his traditional medical training.

Each chemical constituent has a range of functions indicated by the size of the circle or the oval in the diagram. An individual oil also contains a variety of constituents. This makes blending oils for different therapeutic effects a little like playing Sudoku. Fortunately, as Dr. Pénoël teaches, the oils themselves are complex so we don't have to be. They tend to find their way to the problems in our bodies that need to be remedied, helping the body to heal itself. So armed with the general direction you want a therapy to go, and a few specifics you'll learn in this book, you'll be armed with a lot of oils, blends and specific ways of using them that are based on the real science of molecules that have proven physiological functions in the body.

For those of you who are comfortable with the language of chemistry, here are the most common molecular families of compounds found in the essential oils discussed in this book along with their typical physiological functions.

Please don't feel that you need to understand the chemistry of essential oils before you start using them. It's just comforting to know that well-qualified chemists throughout the supply chain have dissected and analyzed essential oils for their safety and effectiveness and identified the best sources for clinically effective oils. The advice in this book is built on their understanding plus decades of practice among medical professionals in the safe and beneficial use of essential oils

Group		Example Diagram	Properties	Therapeutic Properties
Terpenes	Monoterpenes 10 carbon atoms	alpha pinene	High volatility, Low boiling point, Oxidation-prone, Weak aromas	Antiseptic, Antiviral, Mucous cleansing ,Cleansing action, Drying action
	Sesquiterpenes 15 atoms of carbon and no oxygen	Chamazulene	Make up the largest group of terpenes in the plant world, Less volatile than monoterpenes, Stronger aromas	Antiseptic, Antiviral, Immunomodulation, Anti-inflammatory, Calming, Some may be analgesic & antispasmodic
	Diterpenes 10 atoms of carbon and no oxygen	diterpene	Higher boiling point & oxidation level	Antiviral, Antifungal, May be endocrine balancing

Oxygenated Compounds	Alcohols 10 atoms of carbon and one oxygen	Linalool	These are most, therapeutically, beneficial of the oils, Low toxicity, Pleasant fragrances	Antiviral, Antibacterial, Immune-stimulating, Uplifting, Warming, Hydrophilic (dissolve in water), Antifungal
	Phenols and Phenolic aldehydes	eugenol	Slightly acidic, Strong action, Found in: cinnamon, clove oregano, thyme. Dilute well	Antiseptic, Bactericidal Antiviral, Antifungal Immune-stimulating Stimulating to the nervous system
	Phenolic ethers	thymol	Found in sweet basil	Antispasmotic, Mucolytic, Antiviral
	Aldehydes and Terpanic Aldehydes	Geranial	May become irritating if not stored correctly Contained in: lemongrass, lime, lemon	Anti-infectious, Calming to the nerves, Temperature reducing, Anti-inflammatory
	Ketones	alpha thujone	Found in: sage, rosemary, peppermint, spearmint, dill. Many ketones are neurotoxic	Calming, sedative, Mucolytic, Analgesic, Digestive, Encourage wound healing
	Esters	linalool acetate	Generally safe, low toxicity Exception: Methyl salicylate Found in wintergreen & birch. Dilute	Gentle in action, Sweet, fruity aromas, Antifungal, Anti-inflammatory, Antispasmodic, Calming, Effective for rashes
	Lactones & coumarins	coumarin	One of these is bergaptene, found in bergamot and other citrus oils. Phototoxic. Stay out of direct sunlight.	Lactones break down mucous in lungs, Temperature-reducing, Coumarins lower blood pressure and are uplifting and sedative.
	Oxides	Use 1,8-Cineol (Eucalyptol)	Found in eucalyptus, rosemary	Break down mucous in lungs and make it thinner in the respiratory system Stimulating for digestion & respiratory system

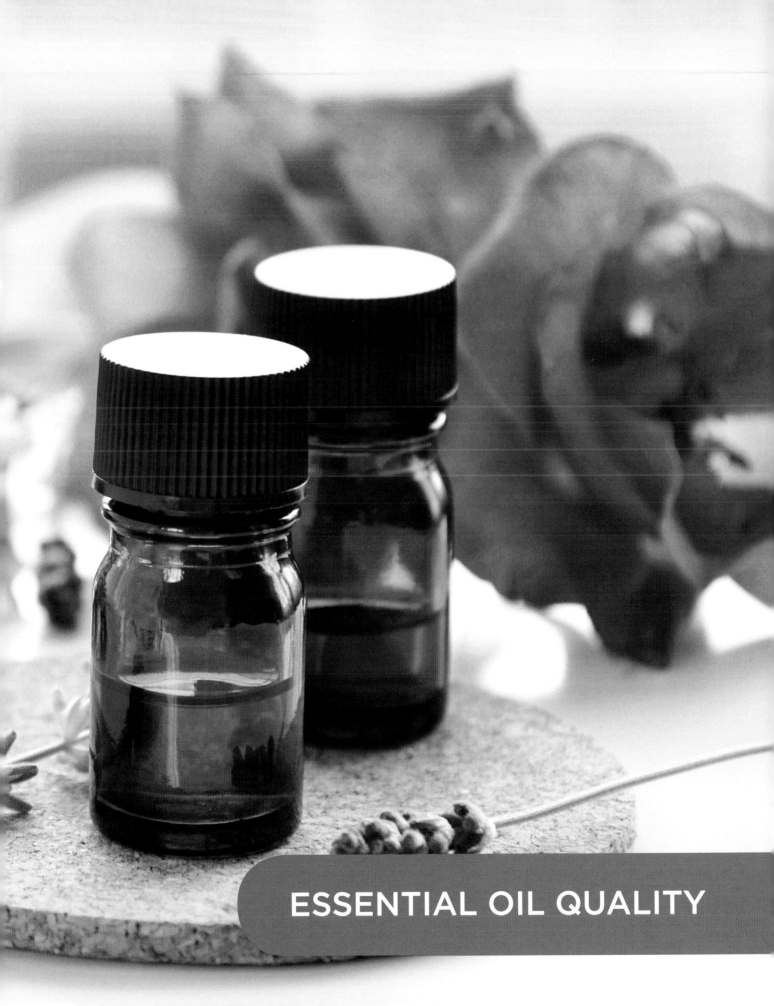

ESSENTIAL OIL QUALITY

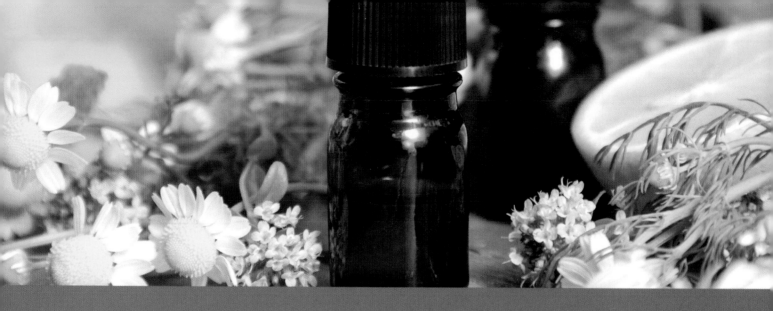

ESSENTIAL OIL QUALITY

How to Recognize and Work with Clinical Quality Essential Oils

There was a time not long ago when buying essential oils for dependable clinical use was remarkably difficult, especially outside of France where essential oils have been used for medical purposes for decades. There were plenty of less expensive oils created for the recreational fragrance and flavoring industries where consistency, flavor, and pleasing smell were king. But for clinical, medical uses, health care professionals required the natural, complex qualities of the aromatic plants farmed and extracted according to exacting standards.

There are four general types of essential oils:

1. Recreational fragrance oils for things like candles, perfume, household products, personal-care products, and potpourri

2. Food flavoring oils for things like chewing gum, sodas, and toothpaste

3. So-called "certified oils" from various marketing companies that claim therapeutic value but may not provide consistent quality

4. Essential oils consistently suited for professional, medicinal, and clinical use

The first two can be synthetic, natural, or mixtures of the two. Consistent, pleasing flavor or aroma are more important than medical or clinical value. Cheap, synthetic, aromatic oils work for candle, fragrance, or chewing gum companies. Even if these oils come from natural sources, they can be distilled or extracted in a way that doesn't preserve their clinical, medicinal qualities. They typically lack the botanical and chemical precision to work effectively, safely, and consistently in clinical practice.

In the earliest years of medical aromatherapy, doctors and researchers discovered that they got better and more consistent results when plants were grown in a certain way, on the correct kinds of soil under the right climate conditions. The plants also had to be handled and extracted according to exacting standards. Through the years health care professionals have continued to experiment and have developed increasing trust in certain suppliers who deliver dependable, clinical-quality oils.

Because there has been no mutually-agreed-upon clinical standard, individual companies in the third category have felt the need to invent their own "certification." Here is the problem. When marketing companies create their own certification rules, they can compromise quality in many ways for many reasons and still pass their own "certification." A company-defined certification can be a meaningless marketing system that does not guarantee quality. But here is another standard.

Follow these standards for a "Clinical-Grade Oil"

As the industry has evolved and devoted essential oil users are experiencing consistent results in their homes, there is an increasing demand for quality standards. There are three areas that clinical-grade essential oil users need to consider: quality and development.

Quality

#1: The sourcing standard: soil, botany, organic certification, climate, harvest, distillation practices, and handling procedures

These are complex issues because with oils coming to us from all over the planet, there are a multitude of things that could go wrong. Botanical precision is extremely important because in some cases even different chemotypes within a species of plants can yield dramatically different clinical results. Chemotypes are like sub-species where a particular constituent or group of constituents dominates. Even when two oils are called the same name, the chemistry of an oil can be different because of inaccurate botanical precision. You need a company who understands and respects these critical factors.

The climate can change dramatically from place to place and season to season, yielding remarkably different oils from the exact same

species and chemotype. The same is true of the soil. A bergamot orange tree grown in Italian soil will yield a different oil—even from starts from the exact same tree—than one grown in West Africa under similar climate conditions but in different soil.

Organic certification is a popular but surprisingly complicated standard that many people like to use to simplify their purchases. It is not as simple as it seems, however. Over the last decade organic certification has become a platform for a lot of unnecessary greed and corruption. We can all see when we shop that there is sometimes spoiled or damaged organic fruit being sold for twice the price of higher quality, ripe, and nutritious fruit.

However, there are many sources from around the world where organic certification is used as merely a way to fleece the buyer. In many cases the certification is unreliable. Even the most precise chemical analysis cannot identify the slightest difference between organic and non-organic. Many crops, especially wildcrafted ones, cannot post organic certification.

In this area it is extremely important to have skilled chemists and buyers who understand where organic certification is vital and where it is merely a way to make everyone pay more. A reliable company will have purchasing staff that understands these challenges and works

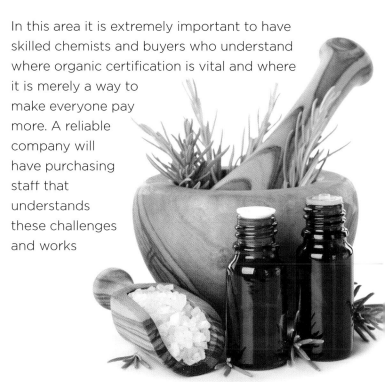

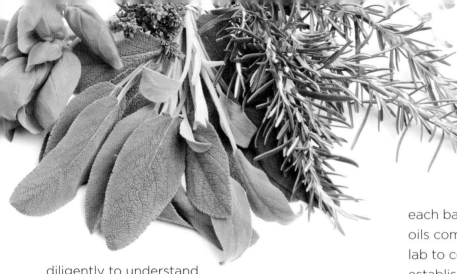

diligently to understand the market and not gouge the customer with unnecessary costs due to corrupt certification and pricing practices.

Then there's the precision required for growing, harvesting, handling, and distilling the crops. Dr. Pénoël has personally visited farms and distillers all over the world, because it has been extremely important to his medical practice to know the care that farmers and distillers take to create a clinical quality oil. For many years he felt he could only trust small boutique farmers and distillers that he personally knew in Southern France. They exacted a high price from him for the highest quality oils, but he has said again and again, "I would rather have a single drop of a high quality oil than a whole drum of junk product." The industry has become so large now that we must purchase oils from larger farms all over the planet, and we must be able to certify that they practice the same farming, harvesting, and distilling procedures as those small farmers Dr. Pénoël came to know personally in the early days of the industry. Once again, buyers must be trained and know what they are looking for.

#2: The Chemistry Standard—Gas Chromatograph/Mass Spectrometer (GCMS)

One universal standard that suppliers and retailers agree to use is a chemical analysis of oils using the mass spectrometer and the gas chromatograph (GCMS). Every batch of oil comes with data from these two analyses. But every batch isn't always analyzed. Because these tests are often done by independent labs, they are expensive, and suppliers and wholesalers may choose to not pay for a new test with each batch of oils. A well-established essential oils company will commission an independent lab to conduct these analyses with each batch to establish a consistent level of quality.

There are ways to verify a quality oil from these two tests, but they are not foolproof. There are many ways to adulterate an expensive oil with cheaper oils or oils that have not been extracted properly, and still pass this test. So we still need other checks on quality.

In addition to the GCMS testing, there are tests that identify other impurities in an essential oil, ensuring, for example, that there are no heavy metals, no pesticide residues, no foreign substances that don't belong in the oil, etc.

It goes without saying that a reliable company supplying essential oils for clinical use will not only have these tests done independently on each batch of oils, but they may also do these tests themselves, just to make sure that all tests from (1) the supplier, (2) the independent lab, and (3) the company match with each other.

#3: Full disclosure standard

Health care professionals need to be able to rely on a consistent high quality of essential oils for their clinical use. However, the essential oils industry has been troubled by loose quality standards.

Companies have been known to claim internal certification of purity, yet deliver adulterated oils. A company focused on quality will create reliable systems of full disclosure where professionals who can read the GCMS charts can recognize the key constituents on each batch of essential oils and certify their purity to their patients.

Not only will the company disclose the GCMS charts and purity certifications for each batch of oils, but they will also identify the region of the world the oil came from and any sensitive growing or distilling practices that produced the oil. This can be important because, just as professional wine tasters can identify better years in the wines they sample, so professionals in our industry all recognize that essential oils are natural plant substances. Climate, harvesting, and distilling conditions can change from year to year, and a high quality oil from a supplier one year may not be as high the next. Buyers in a company with expert quality control will be trained and skilled at identifying the very best oils from around the world in every season.

#4: The government test: Is the oil Generally Recognized as Safe (GRAS) for ingestion?

Because the flavoring industry has certain standards for a "food grade" essential oil, the government has established what it calls the GRAS list for oils that are "Generally Recognized as Safe." This is not a clinical standard. However, these oils are used for all kinds of foods and beverages where there is no call for therapeutic or clinical use to help with any ailment. The government just wants them to be safe for toothpaste, mouthwash, peppermint candy, Coca Cola, and alcoholic beverages. They can be adulterated. They don't even have to be natural.

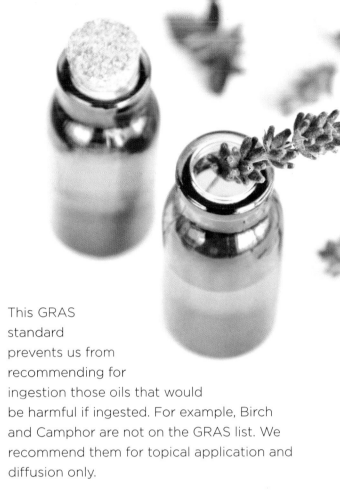

This GRAS standard prevents us from recommending for ingestion those oils that would be harmful if ingested. For example, Birch and Camphor are not on the GRAS list. We recommend them for topical application and diffusion only.

#5: Organoleptic and physical tests

The standards of visual, texture, smell, and taste

An experienced analysis will include evaluation by each of the senses: the distinctive color of the oil, how it feels, its thickness, its smell, and even its taste. These evaluations require long experience with adulterated and low-quality oils, but they are one of the most vital test for quality assurance. A company must use someone qualified to recognize authentic oils by each of their senses. This is called organoleptic evaluation.

The standard of density

The specific chemical weight, or density of an oil can be measured to spot adulteration. There is also a test for authenticity that measures the time it takes for the oil to pass through a specific calibrated channel. This will help indicate the quality of the oil as well.

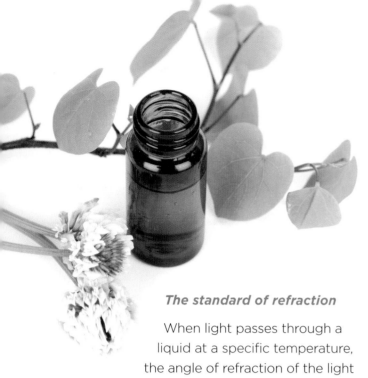

The standard of refraction

When light passes through a liquid at a specific temperature, the angle of refraction of the light can be measured to give a consistent figure for each individual oil. This is another useful measurement that can help identify adulterated oils.

The standard of optical rotation

A beam of polarized light is used to identify oils that could be adulterated with synthetic substances. An authentic oil will cause the light to rotate in a specific direction, whereas the synthetic version of the same or a similar chemical will not. The rotating angle of polarized light will show a specific movement to the right or the left. If the light rotates to the left it is called levogyre. If it rotates to the right it's called dextrogyre. The more active this rotation, the more pharmacologically active the oil will be.

The standard of solubility in 70% alcohol

We can also calculate the amount of 70% alcohol it will take to create a solution. This measurement is specific for each essential oil. The test is performed at 20 degrees centigrade.

Many of these measurements and standards are not expensive to do, but they are too often neglected by companies that do not adequately test their oils.

#6: The research-quality standard

The most well respected scientific and medical journals also recognize that studies must be done using the most scientifically pure, high quality, standardized, natural products. This is critical to their unbiased scientific reputation and repeatable results. They maintain a carefully guarded list of suppliers of products that can be used in their research. These suppliers use chemists, botanists, and biologists who collectively vet (evaluate and approve) the oils using the most advanced technologies in their respective industries ensuring their overall reproducible quality. When research is done on products not on this exclusive list of scientifically vetted quality oils, the findings are usually not published in journals that are considered unbiased and clinically sound.

That is one of the major reasons why research done on products from some essential oil marketing companies are rarely found in the most respected journals.

A clinical-grade oil will conform to this high quality standard, a standard the scientific community trusts for consistent quality they can recommend to health care professionals and serve as a basis for medicinal advancements.

#7: The human cell test

How does an essential oil interact with actual human cells? Health care professionals have used various inexpensive ways of testing the quality of the oils they purchase. Many practitioners use muscle testing. They claim that the muscle cells of the body respond with greater strength to higher quality oils. They will hold a bottle of oil in one hand, raise the other hand and have someone push down on it. If the natural force is weaker for one oil than another, these professionals claim that the oil is less therapeutic or fit for therapeutic use. While this test is widely used, it can be subjective and influenced by individual bias.

There is a unique test developed by Dr. Joshua Plant for identifying a grade of essential oils that will more effectively penetrate the human cell. He uses a unique, patented process developed while he was studying at Harvard Medical School to test the cell activity and permeability of an essential oil, thereby giving the essential oil powerful clinical benefit that functions at the cellular level. With a unique labeling process, Dr. Plant developed a mechanism to track the molecular movement of the specific constituents in a complex essential oil. The patented labeling system allows Dr. Plant in combination with the most advanced fluorescent confocal microscopy technologies the ability to track in real time the molecular movement of oils interacting with living cells. This process has been applied to epithelial cells, fibroblast cells, cancer cells, kidney cells, and dozens of other types of living human cells. Ultimately, this process allows one to qualify essential oils for their efficacy of working at the origin of all human health, namely the cell.

Oversight

Science and professional expertise

This is a team of research scientists, chemists, and medical and health care professionals who are skilled in many disciplines. They will work synergistically with the company to verify and constantly seek to improve the clinical quality of the products. They will offer their collective expertise to bring forward the latest research and clinical practices available

throughout the world. They will apply their expertise gathered through decades of clinical practice oil to eliminate any possibility of adulterated oils. This professional expertise is called in the industry a "nose," or someone who has developed a professional aptitude in identifying any degree of adulteration. They will also suggest the introduction of new products, new blends, training procedures, and tools for use with essential oils.

Development

The delivery standard

As a final step after passing all other tests, a company must bottle the oils in a lab that meets every standard for clinical-grade products and ship them to your door in a way that preserves every constituent you are counting on. You will want to know that the company can pass the highest standards for processing and shipping medical-quality products. There may be companion products like lotions, capsules, and other related products they are offering, so you will want to receive clear certification for the highest quality and manufacturing standards for all the products they carry. For a company to meet the highest expectations of the most discerning consumers and health care professionals, they cannot compromise quality. They must control for such elements as temperature, humidity and air quality. Similarly, they must develop a lean manufacturing

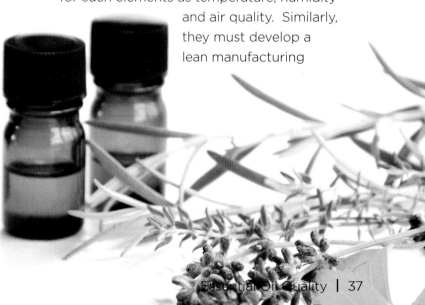

system where the oils are assembled in a rapid, reproducible, and error-free way ensuring that no adulterations or degradations are introduced during the manufacturing process.

The problem with the word "pure"

Will only pure essential oils be clinically effective? The word "pure" used in marketing does not necessary mean that an oil is of clinical quality. A pure oil can be distilled incorrectly or can come from a species that is not ideal. Pure can mean that all the complex components of the extracted oil are intact. But it can also mean that some important components have been subtracted to make the oil smell better to boost sales. Both of these definitions can claim ownership of the word "pure".

Don't be misled. "Pure" can be a marketing word, much like the word "natural," with multiple meanings. The purest possible oils that someone in marketing might call "crystal clean" could well be synthetic or of the lowest possible quality where health-care professionals are concerned. Synthetic oils are always consistent in smell and taste. For anyone using oils for clinical use, a "pure" oil should mean one that has no synthetic components at all. It is extracted according to medicinal, clinical, and scientific standards, and not just fragrance-and-flavor standards.

Can "therapeutic grade" also be a marketing term?

As natural substances, essential oils are not patented or standardized. Calling a company's oils "certified" or "therapeutic grade" can be misleading. Several companies have promoted the misconception that there is some kind of independent body that certifies oils as "therapeutic grade." There is no such body, at least not a widely recognized one.

This doesn't mean that "therapeutic grade" couldn't have real meaning to health care

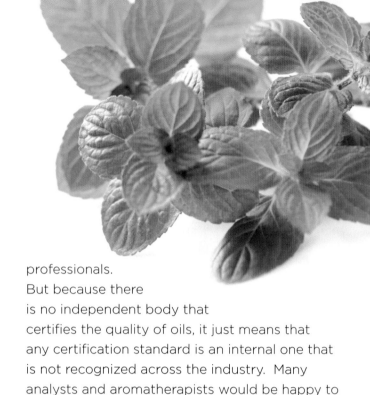

professionals.
But because there is no independent body that certifies the quality of oils, it just means that any certification standard is an internal one that is not recognized across the industry. Many analysts and aromatherapists would be happy to find an independent, trustworthy standard.

We recommend the standards given above.

Do companies have to own their own farms and extract the oils themselves to guarantee quality?

No single supplier could maintain farms and extract oils from where they are best grown all over the globe. A single supplier may grow and distill a small selection of aromatic plants on large farms and gain a deeper understanding of the farming and distillation process, but most of their oils will come from a large number of growers all over the world. A broad pharmacopeia of therapeutic aromatic plants requires many different types of soils in many different countries and climates.

Maintaining farms and distillation factories all over the world is costly and does not make economic sense if a company is trying to keep their oils as affordable as possible.

Instead, look for a company who uses qualified independent experts to guarantee the quality of the oils they purchase. Find a company willing to be flexible in purchasing their oils from different parts of the world as climate conditions shift from growing season to growing season. Find a company whose single oils are slightly different from batch to batch, because that signals attention to a complete, natural oil with all its constituents kept intact. Choose a company whose peppermint smells more like a field of plants than a candy store.

Must essential oils be certified organic?

Organic certification is certainly important, but it is far from being the only qualification for clinically powerful oils.

There is a test that is essential to be applied for citrus oils to avoid pesticides that could be especially harmful. This is an absolutely critical test for all citrus oils. In addition, we believe a company should choose organic sources wherever possible.

It's also important to note that the global supply of truly "organic" oils is very limited. In truth the classification of "organic" is largely misleading. In most countries, companies can still use the "organic" label with products that have been cultivated, grown and harvested while using pesticides, herbicides and other chemical agents. Ultimately, the quality of an essential oil is determined by specific quality control measures, purity tests and complete constituent profiles—not a nebulous "organic" classification.

So who can you trust?

Choose a company that uses all the points of quality listed earlier—botanical accuracy, farming and distilling standards, chemical accuracy using scientific charts, government food-grade certification, sources used by the scientific research community, a test for how the oils react as they actually come in contact with human cells, an expert, "nose" and quality delivery standards.

Choose a company committed to science and the research community that supports it. A trustworthy company will use evidence based research to promote those oils with the most well-established clinical track records. It will promote those uses and therapies that science has proven to be most consistently effective.

Essential oils are not cure-alls. They have safety issues that must be addressed. They are highly effective for certain uses but less effective for others. A trustworthy company will work hard to promote what consistently works to keep you healthy. They will not attempt to oversell, and will be transparent about the relative power of each oil and each therapy.

The company you can trust will not try to sell a novice more than they need for convenient, in-home use. They will offer blends that combine therapeutic amounts of rare and expensive ingredients so you don't have to purchase the whole pharmacopeia and learn to blend them yourself. Again, leave the blending to the experts who understand the clinical uses of these complex aromatic tools.

How can oils be adulterated?

There are many and diverse ways to adulterate essential oils. It's a bit like asking how thieves steal or how forgers forge. The minute you think you have an exhaustive list of ways, someone invents a sneaky new way.

Enterprising suppliers have, from the beginning, looked for ways to cut quality and charge more. The more expensive the oil, and the more money to be made on the oil, the more

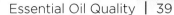

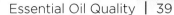

ways there will be to adulterate and cover up the adulteration. Here are a few.

Early on, suppliers found ways to dilute expensive oils with less expensive ingredients—synthetic, natural, or mixed. Enterprising suppliers even found ways to modify cheap oils like orange and mix them with expensive oils in ways that would not make the gas chromatograms and mass spectrometer readings disqualify the oil. The smell could even be a bit more pleasant, so no uninformed consumer would complain. The oil seemed more "pure" to them. There were the same high prices with more sales and more profits. More oils were being shared and becoming popular. Would it matter if the therapeutic results were a bit lower? There is some therapeutic value in all oils if only for the placebo effect.

Deceptive subtraction

Some suppliers have learned that by subtracting certain slightly disagreeable components from a popular oil, they will sell more. Their peppermint will smell a bit more like a candy store and their lavender more like a beauty boutique. The slightly meadow-like aroma is missing, and only an expert can smell the deception. But what about the lost medical value from those less aromatically pleasing components?

Essential oils can have hundreds of constituents, each of which performs its unique medical function in the oil. There is plenty of scientific evidence that when you isolate the individual chemical components you miss the buffering and synergistic effects of the combination nature has given us in having all the components together.

A trustworthy company will not claim to give you all the components of a clinically complex oil and yet subtract ingredients without disclosing the subtractions.

The "nose" knows

Just as we need experts in forgery to catch the craftiest crooks, we sometimes need experts with significant practical clinical experience to spot the craftiest adulterations. Dr. Pénoël has been used for decades to identify fraudulent oils. He knows the "noses" in the industry – the experts whose experience and integrity can be trusted. He knows when a poor quality oil will not help his patients.

It's interesting to watch his ritual as he evaluates an assortment of oils. He will carefully experience and evaluate the range of constituents in each oil, remembering the vast numbers of oils sent to him from every corner of the world for his evaluation. When he finds a fraudulent oil, he will exclaim like a banker who has

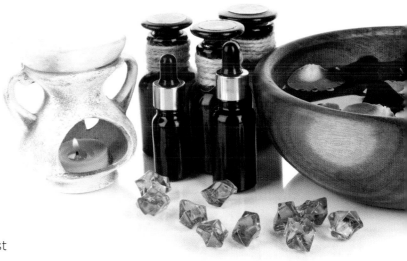

spotted a forged check, "Just smell that oil! It is dead. Can't you smell it? It is therapeutically dead!" The amazed onlooker attempts without success to smell and feel the difference. But the nose knows. And the nose knows other noses he can trust to know.

So does your nose know? With plenty of clinical experience comparing effective and less effective essential oils, we can all educate our noses. Until then, we will need to trust the trained "noses" on the medical advisory boards of the most reliable companies.

How to certify to your health care provider that you are using the highest quality essential oils and following recommendations from trustworthy health care professionals

We believe in science-based, alternative and complementary medicine. We want you to be knowledgeable enough about essential oils to help identify those medical doctors, naturopathic doctors and other health care professionals who will be happy to take advantage of the amazing benefits of clinical-quality essential oils. Then we want to assure them of the quality of the oils you will be using and the advice you will be following. In France there is certification training for medical professionals in the use of essential oils and other plant extracts. There is a need in the English-speaking world for such training.

Here are some questions Dr. Pénoël suggests that we could ask our health care providers to recognize if they are receptive to working with clinical-quality essential oils. We are not trying to disqualify them, but we want to learn how much experience they have with clinical aromatic therapies and how open they are to integrating them.

- What training or certification, if any, have you had in plant-based medicine, alternative medicine, naturopathic medicine, or more specifically, essential oils?

- Is your practice integrated with alternative therapies or are these kinds of clinical practices only recommended occasionally?

- Can you refer me to patients who have worked with you in alternative medicine?

- If you have worked with essential oils, do you recommend them for dermal absorption, olfaction and ingestion; all three, or just the first two?

How essential oils are different from prescription medications?

Essential oils are deeper, typically slower, and definitely safer. They offer more complete restoration of health, but they take time. Dr. Pénoël says, "I always tell my patients that they are beginning a program of at least one year of combining essential oils with balanced whole food nutrition. In most cases, even after my patients are completely healed, they continue using essential oils and healthy nutrition" (Pénoël, Guide, p. 14).

Those who take many synthetic medications, especially elderly people, need to work with knowledgeable health-care professionals and should never discontinue medications without consulting with them. Drug interactions are complex and dangerous with significant risk.

Essential oils are like concentrated foods, and like wheat, dairy, or nuts, some may cause allergic reactions, especially in those who are not accustomed to a largely plant-based diet. And some essential oils will help overcome allergies or their symptoms.

Even though our internal organs may look the same, they can function very differently from person to person. Essential oils may not work for you exactly as stated in this book in every case.

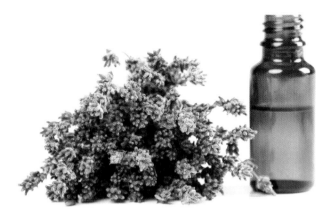

That is true for pharmaceutical medications as well as essential oils.

In France medical doctors exchange essential oils frequently in an attempt to identify the perfect oil or blend for each patient and each disease. They will take a swab of a microbe that seems to be causing the disease and measure the sensitivity to 30 or more essential oils. They will measure the size of the circle created when the oil is applied to the microbial culture. This is the very same test that is used to identify the specific antibiotic that should be used to combat a particular bacteria.

We encourage you to exchange oils and blends as well, and try different ones until you find those that work exceptionally well for the concerns that you have. For example, if peppermint is too strong for you, try spearmint. Rosemary may not be as effective as sweet basil for your body. Your body will tell you as you try different oils and blends. There are always multiple options.

This is not a fix-the-symptom, fight-disease program

This book was created to help you embrace health and prevent illness by helping you adjust your lifestyle and form new, healthy habits involving essential oils. Most serious illness has been developing in the body for 20 to 50 years. Dr. Pénoël teaches that however serious a disease may be, all disease is a result of only three things: (1) poor vitality, (2) toxic buildup,

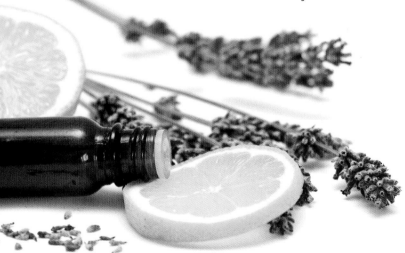

and (3) blocked energy flow. All three can be helped safely and effectively over time by using essential oils.

Science-based allopathic medical professionals are usually extremely good at diagnosis. All serious conditions require professional diagnosis. This book is not designed for diagnosis. Serious medical conditions like cancer and other degenerative diseases that have been forming in the body for decades require treatment beyond the scope of this book. Essential oils can greatly enhance such treatment, especially under the supervision of trained and certified professionals in complementary medicine. They will become more open to complementary medicine if you assure them that your use of essential oils is not an attempt to replace their professional guidance.

A professional who works with serious illnesses is like a pilot trained to fly a commercial jet. You wouldn't expect a teenager new from drivers training to pilot the jet. The conditions you can work with from home using essential oils are like learning to drive a car. When we mention serious illnesses, we do not imply that our treatment is the only thing that can work. It will be complementary to the treatment offered by trained professionals. We will not attempt to oversell or over-recommend essential oils. They can stand alone for many in-home uses, but for serious illness, you will want to work with a trained expert. Please don't attempt to diagnose or prescribe essential oils for anything that requires professional attention. Our recommendations later in the book will attempt to guide you in these decisions.

The challenges of essential oil research

How is research on the medicinal value of essential oils different from research on synthetic pharmaceutical products? The research process, as Dr. Kurt Schnaubelt describes it, is typically "reductionist,"

meaning that the medical value of an oil must be researched as the sum of its chemical constituents. As Schnaubelt explains it, "In a reductionist experiment only one of all possible variables is allowed to change. All others have to be kept at a constant value (Kurt Schnaubelt, The Healing Intelligence of Essential Oils. p. 12). This type of research works well for single-component drugs like aspirin. But with essential oils, "there is a potentially very large number of components contributing to the curative effect—this process is elusive, as the same experiment would then have to be repeated for each component of the essential oil. While this might then be a proper reductionist procedure, it is neither practically possible nor would it describe a meaningful reality" (Schnaubelt, Intelligence, p. 12).

"Using Lavender as a remedy for burns is ... highly effective, but only within the aromatherapy community. Pharmacology does not recommend the use of Lavender, since it cannot find an active ingredient that mimics the effect of the whole oil" (Schnaubelt, Intelligence, p. 12). And, therefore, because it can't be researched in a traditional way, it isn't typically recommended by the scientific community no matter how effective it is shown to be in actual clinical practice.

Dr. Pénoël also explains that essential oils are difficult to test using typical double-blind studies because of the telltale aromas involved. These constraints, along with the obvious lack of funding, keep the research on essential oils relatively limited. All pharmaceutical companies are looking to earn huge profits from patentable, standardized, synthetic ingredients. They can afford expensive tests. Essential oils are natural and do not have huge pharmaceutical profits to promote their research.

Is there solid scientific research on the medicinal uses of essential oils?

Absolutely. You have only to type "essential oils" into www.pubmed.gov to see at least 12,891 items of published research, most of them in well-respected scientific journals. In several sections of this book, we will list some of the studies.

Because these products work and are being used in millions of homes all over the world as well as by medical professionals in clinics and hospitals all over the world, they cannot be ignored by the scientific community. Because of the dangers of overprescribing antibiotics, essential oils are also becoming the best alternative for use in veterinary medicine and agriculture.

In the European Union, laws have recently been established to phase out half of the antibiotics in the food given to livestock and replace them with essential oils. This is a huge effort that will require the production of much larger quantities of essential oils. This is encouraging news for the entire essential oils industry.

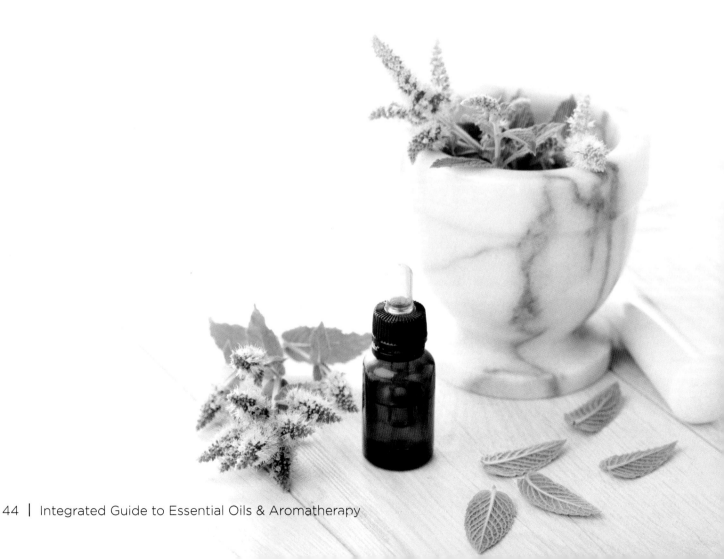

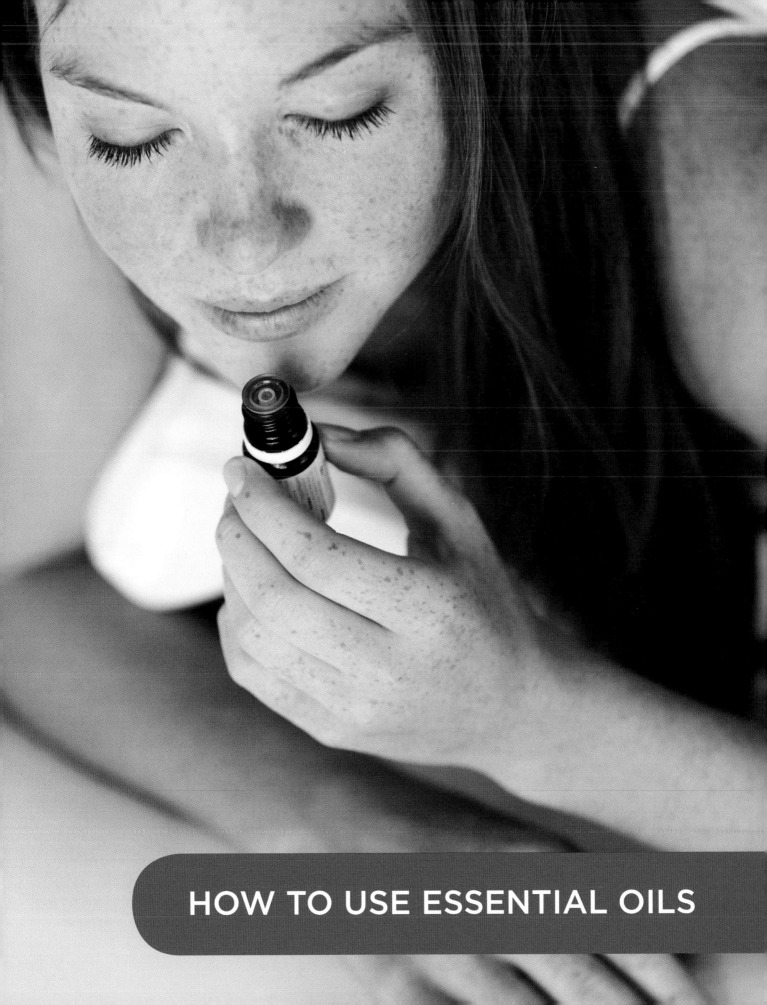

HOW TO USE ESSENTIAL OILS

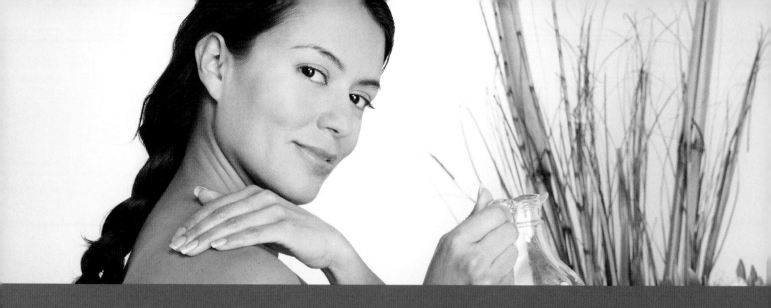

HOW TO USE ESSENTIAL OILS

 Internal　　 Topical　　 Inhalation

We've learned in previous chapters that essential oils contain an extremely complex assortment of chemical constituents. For thousands of years, natural aromatic substances have worked in harmony with the human body. Essential oils are merely the distillation of these aromatic substances. Your body recognizes the oils as safe and natural. Even your cells respond to them and know what to do with them. It's amazing to think that with every drop, the intricate metabolizing and healing systems inside your body are interfacing with complex, natural, molecular combinations to bring you optimal health and deep healing. Those of us who have used them for decades can assure you that they work amazingly well for what they're intended. And they deliver many beneficial surprises as well.

In this chapter we'll explore many ways to use essential oils not only topically and aromatically but also through respiration and ingestion. These therapies are not only effective in a medical, clinical way, but they're also full of unexpected pleasure and delight. They're also safe and convenient.

One of the great advantages of essential oils is their versatility. If you can't ingest them, you can apply them topically. If you can't use them topically, you can inhale them. Or you can do it all and compound their effectiveness.

 TOPICAL APPLICATIONS

General Massage Therapy

Healing touch is the most natural of instincts. We massage the back of our neck when we feel tense. We massage our toe when we stub it.

Essential oils enhance massage. And the more regularly we use them the more effective they become. We feel it's counterproductive to suggest overly complicated ways of using essential oils. There's no need for elaborate application systems or complicated massage movements. We are more likely to use essential oils regularly if we can quickly master safe, simple, convenient, and pleasant ways of using them.

Mothers have been instinctively massaging their babies for millennia with a caring touch that has just the right pressure. So go with your instincts about massaging yourself and your loved ones.

If you feel insecure, watch a few basic YouTube massage videos, and incorporate essential oils into your massage oils, lotions, liniments, and creams according to the following guidelines.

How to create a simple massage oil blend

Depending on the specific therapy outlined later in this book, you'll want to blend a carrier (mixing) oil such as grapeseed, jojoba, rosehips, or coconut (fractionated) oil with a few drops of essential oils or blends. Be sure to mix well.

Oil Strength	Carrier Oil	Essential Oil
Strong oils like oregano, thyme, cinnamon, lemongrass,and clove	8 teaspoons	1 drop for a mild, aromatic massage application
	1 teaspoon	15 drops for a stronger therapeutic massage application
Milder Oils	1 teaspoon	5 drops for a stronger therapeutic massage application
	1/8 cup	30 drops for a stronger therapeutic massage application

To decide how much oil to use per massage, according to Valerie Ann Worwood, you will simply "cup your hand and pour the oil into it but not so much that it pours into the finger creases or over the edge of your hand. One teaspoon is adequate for most bodies" (Worwood, p. 12). You can mix the oil in a small bowl if you feel you need more. Keep it simple.

The most common, convenient, and effective carrier oils for use with essential oils are jojoba, grapeseed, rosehips, and coconut (fractionated). There are many other vegetable oils that can be used as well.

Rosehip oil is a rich, amber, organic oil that is high in essential fatty acids. It is a wonderful mixing oil for preparations that treat dry, weathered skin. It works wonders on scars and is the premier oil for wrinkles and premature aging. Use it in all your finest skin care blends.

Grapeseed oil is a light, silky, easily-absorbed oil that is used in many light creams and lotions. It doesn't leave a greasy feeling on the skin. It is the oil of choice for those with any type of skin sensitivities.

Jojoba oil is actually a plant wax that is liquid at room temperature. It is favored because of its stability. It is wonderful for the skin because it is so similar to the skin's own sebum. It has a rich golden color.

Fractionated coconut oil is odorless and colorless. It doesn't stain and easily washes out of clothing and sheets. It has a long shelf life. It absorbs quickly into the skin and at the same time reduces essential oil evaporation so the essential oils have a better chance of penetrating. It is a digestible and healthy cooking oil and can be used in capsules.

Be sure to keep your blends in dark amber or dark blue bottles and store them away from heat and sunlight.

Sensitivity

The likelihood of an allergic reaction to a natural substance like an essential oil is much more remote than an allergic reaction to synthetic substances in typical massage lotions. But, if you have any hint that you may be allergic to any topically applied substance (hair dye, lotions, acetone, etc.) or if you get hay fever, asthma, or other allergic reactions, it may be wise to try a patch test.

Dr. Jane Buckle suggests that you double the strength of the dilution you will use for massage and put it on an adhesive bandage applied to the inside of your arm for up to 24 hours. If the area becomes red and inflamed, you may want to dilute a little more than recommended or even restrict your topical use to the bottoms of your feet only. Dr. Pénoël claims that he's never seen an allergic reaction from applying essential oils only to the bottoms of the feet. However, it is possible, because anyone can have an allergic reaction to any number of things that would be safe for the vast majority of us.

Fragrance allergy affects only about 1% of the population and most of it is attributed to synthetic fragrances. Natural essential oils have been used in soaps and lotions for hundreds of years without significant allergic concern (Buckle, pp 84-85).

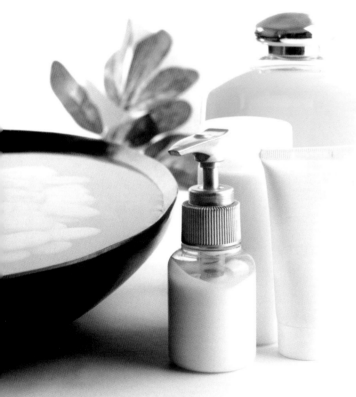

Body lotions and creams

It's difficult to create body lotions and creams from scratch using raw materials from home, so it's best to find an un-fragranced body lotion you like and add essential oils in ratios similar to those you would use for massage oils (about 10 drops of essential oil per ounce of lotion or cream). Be sure to mix well or you may get too much or too little essential oil in some applications.

Reflexology of Hands, Feet, and Ears

When Dr. Daniel Pénoël was receiving his medical training in Paris, he also trained as a professional acupuncturist and has practiced Energy Medicine in his clinic for decades. Thus he understands the amazing benefits of daily aromatic massage of the parts of the body that most easily release stress and blockage of energy. It is remarkable how a simple, daily foot massage can relieve pain, stress, and discomfort all over the body. The same is true of hand massage, and even ear massage.

There are elaborate charts you can find online showing on each extremity the precise points for inserting acupuncture needles. But for simple reflexology massage, following these complex charts is not necessary. A simple diagram of the areas of the feet corresponding to the parts of the body will do. In Dr. Pénoël's training, he simply uses an eyeliner pencil and draws the organs of the body on someone's feet—no obsessive precision, just general understanding. Then a simple two-minute self-massage of the feet with essential oils every day will make sure that energy is flowing throughout your body.

After a few weeks of regular foot massage, you will not only experience changes in overall body functions, but you'll notice that you are calmer and less stressed.

When you understand the remarkable range of benefits of consistent reflexology massage and how quickly it can be done, you'll want to commit to doing it daily, and you'll become skilled at doing it quickly so you never need to miss a day even on your busiest days.

Many physical disorders have psychological roots. Regular massage, especially on the feet, in the way Dr. Pénoël teaches, can release deeply hidden blockages.

Dr. Pénoël uses reflexology to check his patients for problems and weaknesses in various systems of their bodies. Then he trains them to do simple daily foot reflexology at home, focusing on those areas of greatest concern. He teaches that daily attention to the feet is indispensable for the deep healing he offers his patients.

Why reflex therapy?

If we have a bump or a pain, we instinctively massage the area. Over the ages, especially in the Orient, therapists have discovered that it can help a painful or distressed area of the body even more if you massage areas other than the painful spot itself. Archaeologists have found ancient foot massage charts in Greece, Rome, Egypt, Arabic countries, and India. In China acupuncture successfully uses hair-thin needles and massage to relieve pain in places not even being touched by the massage or needles. In Cook County Hospital in Chicago, medical professionals trained in acupuncture are training patients to deal with their pain drug-free by using techniques similar to acupuncture, acupressure, and reflexology.

Eunice Ingham (1889–1974), the author of *Stories the Feet Can Tell*, is considered the mother of modern foot reflexology. Dr. Paul Nogier was a pioneer in the French study of auriculotherapy using the picture of the body on the ear through massaging points on the ear—ear reflexology. Dr. Pénoël received his training in reflexology from Nogier. Throughout this book you will see many simple therapies you can use that were discovered and initially taught by Ingham, Nogier, and Dr. Pénoël. When you learn to massage these areas on a regular

basis using clinical-grade essential oils, you will experience remarkable health benefits.

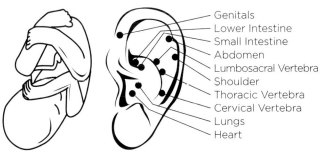

Genitals
Lower Intestine
Small Intestine
Abdomen
Lumbosacral Vertebra
Shoulder
Thoracic Vertebra
Cervical Vertebra
Lungs
Heart

Others have developed a variety of therapies, sometimes a bit different from each other, for the areas of the body corresponding to healing points on hands, ears, face, feet, etc. Combining these therapies with the use of essential oils greatly enhances their effectiveness.

When you see the relative emphasis given the various parts of your body by your brain, you can see that your hands and feet are far more important than the larger areas of your body. Your thumb, for example, takes up a much larger area of your brain than your thigh. Your hands, feet, and face are rich in nerve receptors and motor fibers, so your brain focuses a disproportionate amount of attention on them.

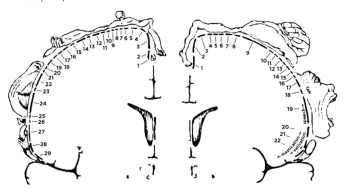

Representation of sensory functions of the body in the postcentral gyrus (a) and of the motor functions in the precentral gyrus (b). Sensory: (1) gonads, (2) toes, (3) foot, (4) leg, (5) thigh, (6) trunk, (7) neck, (8) head, (9) shoulder, (10) upper arm, (11) elbow, (12) forearm, (13) wrist, (14) hand, (15) little finger, (16) ring finger, (17) middle finger, (18) index finger, (19) thumb, (20) eye, (21) nose, (22) face, (23) upper lip, (24) lips, (25) lower lip, (26) teeth, gums, jaw, (27) tongue, (28) throat, (29) viscera. Motor: (1) toes, (2) ankle, (3) knee, (4) thigh, (5) trunk, (6) shoulder, (7) elbow, (8) wrist, (9) hand, (10) little finger, (11) ring finger, (12) middle finger, (13) index finger, (14) thumb, (15) neck, (16) eyebrow, (17) eyelid and eyeball, (18) face, (19) lips, (20) jaw, (21) tongue, (22) swallowing. The dimensions of the parts of the body represented in the figure correspond to the representation of the body's motor and sensory functions in the anterior and posterior central gyri of the cortex

Acupuncture is a complex and involved science that charts a system of channels of energy called meridians. It teaches that a balanced and even flow of energy throughout your body keeps you healthy. This is especially important in the hands and feet where the brain focuses so much attention. Any blockage in these important areas will eventually lead to poor health and disease. To use the power of reflexology to keep yourself optimally healthy, you simply need to visualize the image of your body on the feet and understand the following four main points:

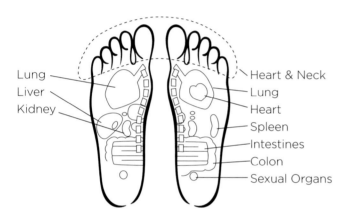

- Whenever an organ or a function is weak or impaired, a sore or tender spot will often appear on the corresponding area of the foot.

- Likewise, a traumatized area on the foot, such as a stubbed toe or an ingrown toenail, may affect a corresponding organ or function of the body.

- As you massage your feet and notice sore or tender areas, you can identify blockages or weak areas in the corresponding areas of your body. This by itself doesn't diagnose a disease, but when you identify a blocked or painful zone of the foot, you can recognize a weakness and take measures to heal it or strengthen it.

- By massaging a little more aggressively and consistently the painful area of your foot, you can effect, at a distance, the health of the corresponding area of your body. This is not directly treating a disease, but it allows a better flow of energy. By itself this can greatly help the healing process and enhance other treatments.

Why the feet?

Our feet carry the weight of our body much of the day. They are imprisoned in socks and shoes for many hours without any healing touch or spontaneous massage. Because of this, energy blockages are far more common and obvious on the feet than on other reflex areas of the body. Foot massage using essential oils can produce far better results than massage on any other area of the body.

Picture your body on your feet

Visualizing the bottoms of your feet together, you'll see that your head is on the toes, your rib cage is on the balls of the feet, your abdomen is on the arch, and the sexual organs are on the heel and on the sides of the heel (on the ankle). The spine is located along the insides of both feet. Except for the organs that don't come in pairs such as the heart, the liver and the gall bladder, what you find on one foot you also find on the other. The colon begins on your right foot and goes up and toward the inside. On the left foot, it moves across the top of the arch, toward the outside, and downward. It then turns toward the inside of the left foot. When massaging the colon area, you need to follow a clockwise direction on each foot because that is the direction food passes through the colon at the final stage of digestion and elimination.

Toes are extremely important. They correspond to the head and the brain. Working on specific areas on your toes can produce remarkable results. In reflexology spending time on your toes is like working directly on the command center of your entire body. The center of the big toe corresponds to the pituitary gland with the hypothalamus above it. These are extremely important points.

Dr. Pénoël has found that each toe seems connected to a particular emotion:
- The big toe with stress and sorrow
- The second toe with desires
- The third toe with anger and frustration
- The fourth toe with attachment
- The fifth toe with fear

Essential oils for foot massage

In massaging the reflex points of the feet, it's helpful to select essential oils with low notes that are grounding like frankincense and sandalwood. On the feet you can use single oils or blends undiluted (neat) or add a carrier oil. You are free to use an undiluted essential oil when you want to work in a deep way on a specific point. For example, if you want to unblock the pituitary gland, which is the command center for all the hormones of your body, or what we call the hypothalamus-pituitary axis, you would use a drop of frankincense undiluted and massage ten to thirty times down the bottom center of each big toe.

When you massage the whole foot, you may want to dilute 4 or 5 drops of essential oil in less than a teaspoon of carrier oil.

Before the massage, both the person giving and the person receiving the massage should take a moment to enjoy the aroma they will be using. The aromas of myrrh and frankincense alone can call up wonderful images of ancient origins that may make the massage more effective for you.

Sandlewood and frankincense help activate the immune system, heal wounds, and decongest the respiratory system. Some books recommend frankincense for treating various cancers, but from his vast experience with essential oils and cancer, Dr. Pénoël feels essential oils are only complementary to a more aggressive program, including conventional medical care. He recommends frankincense for anxiety, stress, depression (especially after childbirth), and fears of all sorts.

A nightly foot rub helps my asthmatic son

When I learned about the benefits of frankincense for respiratory situations and that it makes a great foot massage, I decided to try it by massaging my asthmatic 5-year-old son's feet every night. It really helps him relax and sleep through the night, which he rarely did before because of his asthma.

Step 1: General massage

Mothers calm their babies with massage. Think of massage within a family as an extension of something natural, loving, healing, and intimate.

Even if you did nothing specific to identify and work on specific reflex points on the feet, you would see wonderful benefits from a generalized foot massage using essential oils. If you're ever on your feet all day, you deserve this daily treat for your feet.

- It's great to begin with a shower, a bath, or merely soaking your feet. You could even use bath salts with essential oils or an aromatic bath oil with one of your favorite essential oil blends added.

- It's a special treat to receive a foot massage from a partner. But it's better to do it on yourself than to not do it at all. Obviously for consistent daily foot massage you will want to learn to give yourself a quick foot massage.

- Start by mixing four or five drops of your essential oil in less than a teaspoon of mixing oil.

- If you are massaging your own feet, bring your right foot comfortably on your left thigh and apply about half of the oil, then put the other half on the other foot.

- If there are two of you, make sure both of you are comfortable. If the one receiving the massage is in an armchair or on a bed, the other should be on a lower stool or chair so he or she isn't forced to bend forward in an awkward position and block the full flow of energy.

- Gently apply the diluted blend all over each foot, massaging gently toward the heart. Start at the toes and move upward onto the ankle.

- Start gently but increase pressure progressively. The pressure must always be acceptable to the person receiving the massage.

- As we begin using true reflex procedures, we will apply even more intense pressure to specific areas of the foot using the knuckles. If you find a sore area, you can work a little bit on it, turning clockwise, but a more focused, aggressive phase normally comes later.

- Massage each foot for up to five minutes if you have time. Your entire body will become more relaxed, even though you're only touching your feet.

Step 2: Reflex massage of the feet

We are not training you to become a professional reflexologist or therapist but rather giving you a practical and simple habit you can use on a regular basis. It is ideal for spouses or older children to give the massage. When you perform the treatment on yourself, you will not receive the same benefit as when someone does it on you, but it will still be very beneficial.

- Beginning with the right foot, start by massaging clockwise on the center of the foot, enlarging the circles and pressure progressively and following the pathway of the large intestine on right side of the foot— following the ascending colon up the outside of the foot, angling right and moving across the transverse colon.

- Do the same on the left foot. If you finish the entire treatment on one foot and then do the other, it creates an imbalance, so if you have the time, go back and forth between the feet.

- Then work on the center small intestine area, massaging the lower arch strongly with your knuckles in the middle part of the foot.

- Massage the liver area on the right foot and the spleen area on the left foot.

- Work hard on the arch of both feet, especially on the pancreas area. Use your knuckles if it is tolerable.

- When it becomes painful, decrease the pressure. Progressively the pain will taper off, if not in one session, generally over several sessions, and you'll be able to apply more pressure each time.

- Next focus on the balls of the feet, corresponding to the area of the torso under the rib cage. Use your thumbs and knuckles

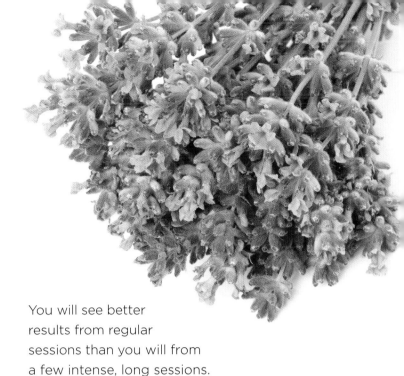

with enough pressure to release any blockages. As you work on yourself, you will begin to recognize how much pressure it takes to bring relief to someone else.

- Next work on the **toes,** beginning with the big toe. It's most important to unblock the hypothalamus-pituitary axis at the middle of the bottom of the big toe. Use a downward stroke toward the foot. This balances the endocrine (hormonal) system, the nervous system, and the immune system. For many women the big toe of the left foot is more tender than the right.

- Work aggressively on the base and inside neck of the big toe where many stresses accumulate. Dr. Pénoël's patients have experienced many remarkable recoveries after repeated massage of this "psi" point.

- Work on each toe to help unblock other hidden emotions. Think of or talk about any emotion you are helping to release. This gets your mind involved in the therapy.

- Finally, work the sexual area at the center of the heel and just under the large bones on each side of the foot called the malleolus, where many sore points are often found.

- Close the session with an overall massage, stimulating the top of the feet with your knuckles. Mobilize the foot by turning it gently in all directions. Massage the leg up to the knee to help the flow of energy.

- Allow a little time to relax. When you stand up, you may feel a new sense of balance.

- It is helpful to receive this deep, longer reflex treatment once a week. In between the longer treatments, it's important to work on a few important areas of the feet each day.

You will see better results from regular sessions than you will from a few intense, long sessions.

Your daily two-minute reflexology treat

Keep your reflexology supplies handy just as you exit your bath or shower every day, and while your feet are still damp, take 2 minutes for a quick reflexology massage. Then slip on your socks or shoes for the day.

Try different oils according to whatever emotional or physical goals you have. This treatment won't solve all your problems, but you will experience much better and deeper results from whatever other healing modality you are using.

If you look at foot reflexology charts online or read different books on foot zoning or reflexology, you'll be surprised to see some extreme variations among the different charts. Don't let this bother you, simply work on the whole foot and focus on the points that feel sensitive or sore: the body will take care of the rest for you.

Reflexology on the ears

Now that you understand the principles behind reflexology, it will be easy for you to recognize the easy and convenient benefits of massaging your ears. It can happen discreetly anywhere at any time. All you have to do is think to do it. Use a dab of essential oil and maybe a little carrier oil and massage your whole ear. Remove earrings of course. You can visualize the whole body on the ear if you think of a baby in a fetal position, head down.

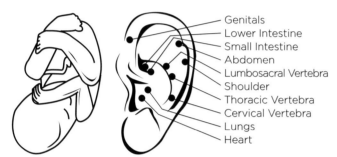

Genitals
Lower Intestine
Small Intestine
Abdomen
Lumbosacral Vertebra
Shoulder
Thoracic Vertebra
Cervical Vertebra
Lungs
Heart

Here again, with frequent massage, you may become aware of specific points and relief in those areas of the body, but if you massage the whole ear, you'll touch all of them. If there are particularly sensitive areas, focus on them, and massage them to release blockages just as you would on your feet.

Here is a chart indicating areas on the ear that release emotional blockages. Don't worry about where one reflex point ends or another begins. You'll feel those sensitive areas. The ears are small and you are sure to press and massage the correct reflex spot if you perform an overall massage.

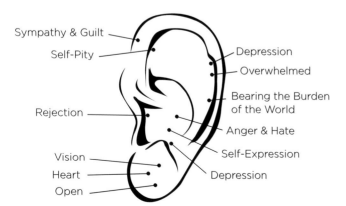

Sympathy & Guilt
Self-Pity
Depression
Overwhelmed
Bearing the Burden of the World
Rejection
Anger & Hate
Self-Expression
Vision
Heart
Depression
Open

Reflexology for the hands

Like the ears, the hands can be conveniently and discreetly massaged at any time of the day. You can use acupressure with a press-and-release action or simple massage as you would on your feet. Again, do not be too concerned about specific points. There is plenty of disagreement among professionals as to the exact points for specific organs. Just use the general diagram as a guide and massage your hands using your favorite essential oils.

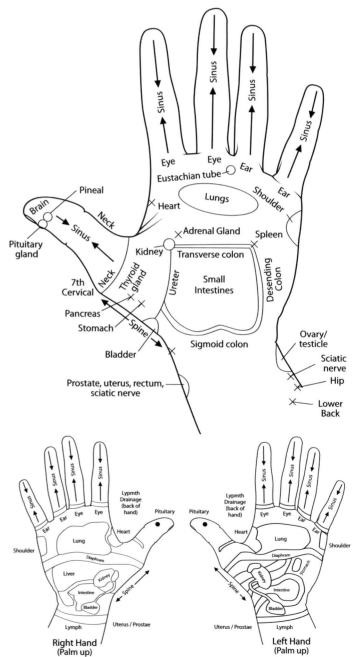

This is an acupuncture chart for the back of the hands indicating points along the spine, legs, and arms that correspond to the fingers and the hand. It can be useful for helping you overcome headaches and joint pain.

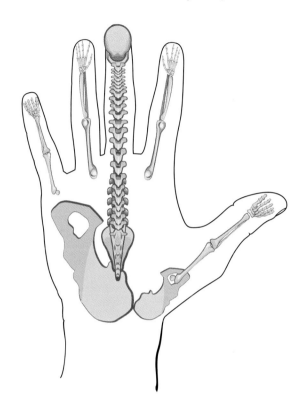

The "M" Technique® developed by Dr. Jane Buckle

This hand massage was developed to provide a rapid relaxation response in nursing patients in the least invasive way possible. It is safe, easy to learn and helpful for anyone caring for a person who needs to relax. You can watch a quick YouTube video of this technique by searching "The 'M' Technique®".

Make sure there are no open wounds or traumatized areas on the hands and arms being massaged. It is given at a pressure of 3 (if 10 is crushing and zero is no pressure at all). The receiver is in charge of telling the giver what a "3" feels like to them. Each movement is done slowly 3 times so there are no surprises and the movements stay

relaxing and predictable. Make sure both the giver and receiver are comfortable with no uncomfortable leaning, twisting, or stretching. The massage oil/essential oil blend should be chosen for the least likelihood of an allergic reaction. Grapeseed oil with a little lavender in it is ideal. Pour less than a teaspoon into your palms and rub your palms together to warm it up. Then rub it on the top and bottom of the hands up and back down the forearm 3 times. Then supporting the hand with both hands stroke from the center to the outside of the hand three times. Start from the wrist area and move to the knuckles. Then use your thumb to circle each knuckle three times starting with the little finger. Hold the finger between your first and second fingers and press the pressure point at the tip of each finger and you finish that finger. Use one of your hands for some of the fingers and the other for the others so you balance the action. Your aim is to relax the patient and move as slowly as you need to for relaxation. Don't forget the thumb.

Then turn the hand over and massage the palm from the wrist to the fingers. People who are in pain often clench their fists, so this palm massage is highly beneficial for them. Then, holding the hand in a handshake with one hand, finish off the massage by going up and down the arm 3 times. (Buckle, Clinical Aromatherapy, pp. 152-154).

Application of essential oils on affected areas

On a minor scrape, cut, bruise, or cold sore, dab a small amount of one of the more mild essential oils or blends neat (undiluted). If you are using a stronger oil like oregano, thyme, birch, wintergreen, cinnamon, or clove, be sure to dilute (25% essential oil to 75% carrier oil).

For larger areas such as joints, abdomen, or larger muscles, dilute the oils before applying.

Always apply digestive oils on the abdomen in a clockwise direction following the direction food flows through the colon.

Liniments

A liniment rub can be convenient, refreshing, invigorating and useful for sore muscles. You can use up to 10 drops to a teaspoon of water, apple cider vinegar, witch hazel, floral water (hydrosol), or even rubbing alcohol. If you are mixing a larger quantity of any of these, be sure to shake the mixture well before each application so the oils are evenly distributed (Schnaubelt, Intelligence, p. 121).

Even though water-based ingredients don't mix well with oils, the moisture will help the oil to penetrate, and it will also dilute the oil for fast and even application. Liniments are preferred over carrier oil blends for athlete's foot.

Mix essential oils in water and use in a spray bottle for things like chicken pox, shingles, boils, and scrapes over larger areas of the body. Be sure to shake contents before each use to disperse the ingredients together as much as possible.

Use essential oils as perfumes to replace toxic, synthetic fragrances

"In the nineteenth century, a Frenchman called Piesse instigated a new approach to perfumery work by classifying odours according

to the notes in a musical scale. He transposed the idea of musical harmony into the realm of fragrances where the corresponding notes to teach scent formed perfectly balanced chords or harmonies when they were combined together" (Lawless p. 32).

Fragrances are still divided into "top", "middle" and "low" notes.

The top notes have a fresh, light quality which is immediately recognized because of its quick evaporation rate.

The middle notes are the heart of the fragrance. They usually make up most of the blend. This scent emerges sometime after the first impression.

The base notes are richer and heavier. They appear more slowly and linger longer than the middle notes. They can also act somewhat like a fixative to keep the lighter oils from dispersing too quickly.

Ylang ylang is said to be a well-balanced perfume oil in its own right. It could be described as having a very powerful sweet, floral top note; a creamy-rich middle note; and a soft floral, slightly spicy base note.

Essential oils are classified in this way according to their dominant

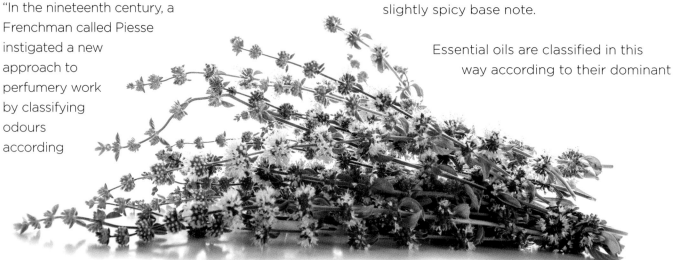

note. This is useful information for those who are blending oils for perfumery, but it's also important to know how long the strong aroma you are using will be staying around. For example, because tea tree has a rather high top note, you won't have to worry about a lingering aroma of tea tree throughout the day if you apply it in the morning. The pleasant aroma of geranium, on the other hand, applied to the pad of a bandage is a middle note and could be with you all day.

There are different opinions about which oils have predominant top, middle, or base notes. This list from Julia Lawless provides a general frame of reference. We will provide a general guideline in the upcoming pages focusing on each oil and each blend. In the Blends chapter, we will go into the topic in greater depth and teach you more about blending oils for both therapy and pleasure.

The following are examples of the 3 level of notes:

Top notes: may include tea tree, eucalyptus, mandarin, lemon, and basil.

Middle notes: may include geranium, lavender, marjoram, rosewood, and rosemary.

Base notes: may include patchouli, rose, jasmine, benzoin, frankincense, and myrrh (Lawless p. 32).

Hot and cold compresses

"Make a hot compress by filling a bowl with very hot water and adding 4 – 5 drops of essential oil. Dip a folded piece of cotton cloth or flannel into the bowl, squeeze out excess water and place the cloth on the affected area until it has cooled to body temperature, then repeat" (Lawless p. 27).

Cold compresses are used in a similar way except that you will use ice cold water.

You can also apply the oil directly to the body then put a hot or cold, wet towel or dressing over the oil to help it penetrate.

Make your own floral water or hydrosol

A hydrosol or floral water is a natural byproduct of distillation, but you can approximate it by adding 20 to 30 drops of your favorite essential oil to 100ml of spring or de-ionized water. Leave it for a few days in the dark, then filter it through a coffee filter paper. While essential oils won't dissolve in the water, they will add a scent to the water and the properties of the essential oil will be infused into the water. You can create all kinds of safe misting products using this method for spraying on the face and other delicate and sensitive tissue (Lawless p. 28). If you are creating a product for use on the face, Dr. Pénoël recommends using only 5 drops of essential oils for every half cup (4 oz.) of water.

Take aromatic showers for natural cleansing and disease prevention

"A shower with just soap and water cannot provide the deep cleaning your body requires, but using essential oils will help to eliminate

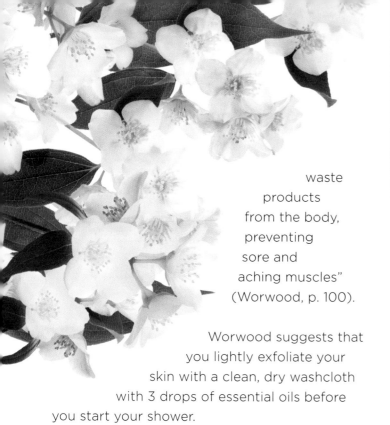

waste products from the body, preventing sore and aching muscles" (Worwood, p. 100).

Worwood suggests that you lightly exfoliate your skin with a clean, dry washcloth with 3 drops of essential oils before you start your shower.

Kurt Schnaubelt describes a remarkably beneficial way to incorporate essential oils safely and quickly into your daily regimen by showering with them. His suggestion gives you 3 important benefits: (1) safe, diluted distribution over your entire body, (2) aromatic benefits mixed with steam for wonderful respiratory benefits, and (3) remarkable disease prevention benefits, particularly over the lymph nodes of your body.

Here's how:

After soaping and rinsing, turn the water off and apply a few drops of essential oils on your hands. Rub your hands together and distribute the oils lightly to your wet skin, focusing on the areas of lymph nodes at your neck, under arms, and groin. Without adding more drops of oils to your hands you can sweep your hand across your face. They will not mix with water but the warm water will help them absorb quickly into your skin. "Every square inch of skin can be used as an absorbing surface" (Schnaubelt, Intelligence,

p 123). Afterwards you can rinse and towel dry or simply towel dry. If you feel timid about applying oils over your whole body, start with your legs and feet one day and see what it's like. Then progress up your torso on subsequent days.

Start by using light and safe oils like lavender, then try fir, pine, rosemary, tea tree, or your favorite blend. Simply use the ones that feel most attractive to you each day. Variety offers lots of extra health benefits (Schnaubelt, Intelligence, pp. 123-125).

Aromatic baths and foot baths

There are three ways to use essential oils in the bath.

1. Take a 20 minute aromatic bath with 10 to 15 drops of an essential oil mixed with a dispersing agent like a capful of bath gel, shampoo, or a cup of Epsom Salts.

2. Add essential oils to a carrier oil and pour a tablespoon of the mixture into the bath. The oils will float on the top of the bath but then cling to your body when you get out. This can be stronger mixtures of oils than typical massage oils—up to 50:50.

3. Apply massage oils before getting in the bath. The oils will become heated in the hot water and absorb quickly and easily. This method is especially helpful for aches and pains (Worwood p. 141).

Back & Spinal Therapy (Layer Therapy)

Chiropractors have taught us that the proper alignment and health of the spine as well as all the muscles and nerves radiating from the spine are critical keys to overall health. Essential oils are particularly useful in chiropractic care, and can be safely used in home applications for the following reasons and many more:

1. You can ease back and neck pain, including pain that radiates out from the spine down the leg or into various organs of the chest, head, arms, and abdomen.

2. Essential oils will relax the tiny muscles, ligaments, and tendons along the spine so the spine will more easily align with proper posture and correct stretching and exercise. You can use this benefit with or without the help of a chiropractor.

3. Essential oils will quickly penetrate along the spine and radiate throughout the body, quickly supplying all of their natural benefits including their powerful antimicrobial action. This can benefit you for almost any ailment.

As in reflexology, there are multiple complex ways and techniques for applying oils to the back and the spine. You can watch and try various hand movements shown on YouTube videos if you wish, but we have found that the best way to apply the oils is often the easiest way without much fuss or concern over technique. Focus on the true purpose of this therapy, and you will find it to be extremely beneficial.

What makes spinal therapy work so well?

1. The slow, relaxing application of the oils using healing and comforting touch.

2. The careful layering of strong oils and what you learn about how much to dilute with a carrier oil to regulate the warming effect of each oil.

3. The radiating effect of the oils facilitated by various hand movements.

4. The relaxing, comforting warmth and penetration of the compress at the end of the treatment.

Step 1

Start by selecting four to eight oils according to the health goals you want to achieve. In later chapters you will read recommendations for oils to use for various goals like respiratory, digestive, pain, emotional calming, etc.

Step 2

You can perform this therapy on a high bed or a massage table. Just make sure both the person giving the massage and the one receiving it are comfortable and the bed covers or sheets are protected appropriately with towels or separate sheets.

Step 3

Start with the person receiving the therapy lying on their back. Simply apply a relaxing blend to the feet and massage them to prepare the mood, release tension, and reassure the one receiving the massage that you will only be using gentle and safe strokes.

Tip: Be sure he or she experiences each oil by inhaling it before you apply it.

Step 4

Have the one receiving the massage then turn over to expose the back. Lower the trousers a little so the whole length of the spine is exposed. Protect the trousers with a cloth.

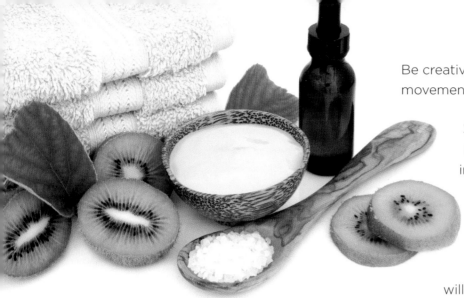

Step 5

Apply three to six drops of the first oil along the spine. This should be an oil for relaxing and aligning the spine in preparation for receiving the subsequent oils. Gently spread the oils along the spine, always keeping one hand touching the back to maintain constant contact.

Step 6

Help the oils spread, radiate, and penetrate by working them in. You can use various hand movements. Here are three suggestions.

1. Try rocking your knuckles along each side of the spine from the base to the skull. Do each procedure three times so the one receiving the therapy can relax and predict what will happen next.

2. Try moving your first and second fingers on each side of the spine from top to bottom and gently applying intermittent pressure with your other hand.

3. Try using the nail side of your fingers to feather the oils, first of all up the spine, and then from the spine outward onto the back. This will encourage the nerves to help the aromatic molecules to radiate by nerve passageways throughout the body

Be creative. Try various other massage movements of your own moving up the spine.

Step 7

In Step 7: "Add 3 to 8 drops of each oil in its turn and massage the oils into the back along the spine. Use whatever variations of these techniques you like."

If you use strong oils like oregano, thyme, wintergreen, or birch you will want to talk with the one receiving the massage to make sure you are using sufficient carrier oil so the chemical action doesn't become too hot.

If you are using these hot oils, please do not use spinal therapy too frequently (more than once or twice a week) because so much of these strong oils can build up in the system and not be released through perspiration or through the kidneys fast enough. Drinking extra water and taking hot baths will speed the flow of the oils through the system and prevent any uncomfortable detoxification.

Step 8

Apply a hot (or warm), damp towel compress along the spine after the last oil has absorbed into the skin. Place a dry towel over the compress to hold in the heat. Replace the warm compress each time it cools to body temperature.

For muscle tension, bone pain, or tendon or cartilage inflammation, apply a cool compress at first, then rotate between cool and warm compresses as they adjust to body temperature. Apply a warm compress only for all other needs.

Step 9

While the body is relaxed you may wish to apply gentle stretching exercises to the feet and head according to instructions given by your chiropractor or health care professional, but leave any manipulation of the spine, the legs, or the head to the professionals.

This whole procedure should take no longer than 30 to 45 minutes. The one receiving the massage may become so relaxed that they will fall asleep. Let them. They will wake up refreshed and rejuvenated by the experience.

Ways to increase absorption

Because essential oils are so volatile, many of their molecules disperse into the air without penetrating your skin. You can increase absorption into the skin by covering a compress with something impermeable or semi-permeable. A simple drop of oil on the pad of an adhesive bandage will focus the therapeutic energy of the oil directly on a scrape or cut much longer than merely dropping the oil on the cut.

Dr. Pénoël suggests mixing a few drops of an essential oil in a green clay compress and wrapping the area with a cling bandage (Pénoël, Guide, p. 86).

It may seem counterintuitive, but mixing water and essential oils actually increases absorption into the skin. The moisture opens a pathway for the oil to absorb. This is why compresses and lotions work well, and aromatic baths and showers allow the oils to penetrate very quickly—100 times faster than water penetrates the skin (Price, p. 88).

This is also why you don't want to add water if an essential oil starts to sting. You want to dilute with a vegetable oil rather than water because water will only increase penetration. If no vegetable oil is readily available, soap and water can dissolve the essential oil and stop the stinging.

Heat will also help essential oils absorb better. For example, Dr. Pénoël suggests using a hair dryer to help oils penetrate on the feet (Pénoël, Guide, p. 43). A heating pad, hot water bottle, or a warm cloth over a compress can also increase penetration. Beware of too high a heat, however, because perspiration, as after a sauna, can drive oils out of the skin rather than into it.

Covering the application of an essential oil with a bandage or a compress keeps the oils from evaporating and aids absorption and the natural warming action of the oils themselves. Applying a lotion or carrier oil over a neat application of oil also helps prevent some evaporation. Even covering the skin with clothing will prevent some of the molecules from dispersing.

Aromatic body wraps

Marcel Lavabre recommends creating a warming aromatic body wrap by placing a plastic/foil sheet on a warm blanket, then a large towel with a hot essential oil-and-water mixture. You can spray the towel with the mixture or dip it in the mixture and wring it out. Most of the oil will remain in the towel. Lay the towel on the plastic/foil sheet, then lie down on the towel and wrap the towel, the plastic/foil sheet, and the blanket around yourself and relax. The ratio Lavabre suggests is 8 to 12 oz. of water to 10 to 50 drops of essential oil (Lavabre pp. 57-59).

Similar wraps and bandages can be used to help with sores and wound healing. Bed sores are an especially challenging problem in elderly care where healing can be slow. Compresses with a mild solution of essential oils and rosehips oil as a carrier have proven to be highly effective (Buckle, Clinical Aromatherapy, pp. 267-269).

Dr. Pénoël's "Live Embalming" Therapy

In ancient Egypt various aromatic extracts were used for embalming mummies (preventing corpses from rotting and disintegrating). It's far better to use essential oils while you're alive than after it's too late!

Here's how ...

There are times when you have an urgent need to get a large amount of essential oil to penetrate into the body quickly through the skin. You can use this therapy at the outset of a flu virus.

A flu virus is extremely aggressive in the lungs. One hundred viral particles can quickly duplicate themselves in a single cell. The cell explodes and each of those particles can begin invading another cell, creating 100 new particles each. Each of those cells explodes and the infection spreads rapidly. A war is quickly waging with your immune system. Who will win the war? The speed of this initial multiplication is far too rapid for your immune system to control at first, as the flu takes over your body. You need enough essential oil molecules in your lungs to quickly control the invasion of this aggressive virus.

Start with the 1,8 cineole molecule found in Eucalyptus radiata and ravintsara, among others. This molecule can penetrate into your body quickly, especially when it is helped in with this therapy. When this molecule is applied to the skin undiluted as it should be in this extremely infectious situation, the cineole molecule will create a strong cooling sensation when used in large amounts (which you need to apply). This cooling sensation needs to be overcome

because the flu virus is most often caught in wintertime. So you use a hair dryer to warm the area to accelerate the penetration. Dr. Pénoël has used this therapy for over 35 years to win battles against respiratory winter viruses.

Hold the hair dryer and a 6-inch pipette filled with the essential oil in one hand. Use your other hand to massage where the oil is being applied. You use a quick rotating movement from the hair dryer directed at the drops on the warmed area. When using a hair dryer, it only takes few seconds for the drops to be totally absorbed into the skin. Without a hair dryer it takes much longer for the oils to penetrate, and much of their benefit is lost due to evaporation rather than penetration. But with a hair dryer, you will be amazed at how much oil the skin can take in.

Another secret to the effectiveness of this technique is changing locations on the body each time the oil is applied and heated. This helps prevent any allergic reaction to the oils by those who may be marginally sensitive.

Begin the series of applications with each foot at a separate treatment. Then move to each ankle, each knee, the sides of the abdomen, and then the sides of the chest. You can also apply it to the breast plate (sternum) area.

If your nose feels blocked with mucous, apply three drops on the top of the head (the anterior fontanel) where your "soft spot" had been when you were a baby. Point the hair dryer at this area as you apply a few drops of Eucalyptus radiata, and you will be surprised at how easily and quickly your nasal passages will clear.

When you're doing the therapy on someone else, apply it first to the lower back, then the middle of the back, and then the upper back with each successive treatment.

When using the hair dryer in a back massage, invite an assistant to hold the hair dryer and the dropper while you massage the back. This procedure works wonders in wintertime. Those receiving the therapy love it for its relaxing warmth on cold winter days.

Here is a story of a "live embalming" therapy from Dr. Pénoël. "I have a good friend who is a veterinary doctor. One evening he called because he had a relative who was dying at the nearby hospital. She was in the terminal stages of cancer. He didn't call me to try to cure the cancer, because that would have been impossible at that stage. But she had developed a severe systemic infection (as often happens in terminal cancers). All antibiotics had failed and the infection was about to take her life before her time. I made sure that the doctors at the hospital would accept a treatment involving the intensive use of clinical-grade essential oils. The situation was totally hopeless from their allopathic perspective. I had almost 200 ml of an undiluted blend of clinical-grade essential oils that would have to be applied. Her husband agreed to perform the therapy throughout the night. Every five minutes a few drops were applied on a specific area of the body. With each application the area would change. The therapy started at the feet and progressed, step by step, up the entire body (except, of course, the most sensitive parts of the body). Throughout the night, the procedure was carefully followed, and when morning arrived, the high fever had gone away and the severe infection appeared to have vanished. The body had accepted the intensive live embalming procedure under warm air flow

and the massive and accelerated penetration of essential oils. This allowed the patient to live the rest of her life in a peaceful way and to welcome her departure with serenity."

 ## Inhalation

There is a significant difference between how essential oils enter the body by inhalation and how they enter by smell or olfaction. When you smell an aroma the molecules move along specialized sensors and nerve passageways on a very tiny area near your eyes called the "olfactory bulb." Only a relatively few molecules reach this tiny area, and yet their effects are remarkable because they ignite impulses in the limbic brain that accomplish great wonders.

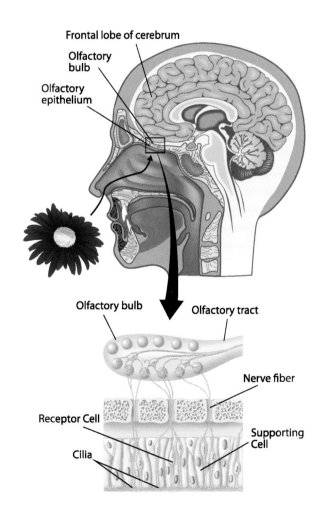

Frontal lobe of cerebrum
Olfactory bulb
Olfactory epithelium

Olfactory bulb
Olfactory tract
Nerve fiber
Receptor Cell
Supporting Cell
Cilia

They instantly affect the limbic brain, the emotional control center of the brain and greatly influence taste of foods. Did you know that your tongue alone can only experience four tastes—sweet, sour, salty, and bitter? It's your sense of smell that provides all the nuances in the flavors you enjoy as you experience exquisite gourmet foods. Olfaction also influences heart rate, blood pressure, breathing, memory, stress levels, and hormone balance. Aromas can produce profound psychological and physiological results. They can affect sex drive, energy levels, the production of hormones that influence our longevity, and levels of serotonin. Aromas can have a great influence on our appetite, both to our advantage and disadvantage.

Ways to simply smell essential oils

Open the bottle and wave it under your nose—not too close. Close your eyes. Allow the aroma to instantly trigger all the functions of your brain. Just smelling an oil from the bottle may send your olfactory nerves into overload. To get a more accurate aromatic impression as you choose among several oils, you may want to use a strip of blotting paper or a toothpick.

Once you've made your choice, put a drop or two of your essential oil on a cotton ball, a tissue, a pillowcase, a handkerchief, a clay pendant, or your stationery. You can carry it around with you and experience it throughout the day or night. Enclose it in a plastic bag, and it will evaporate less quickly so you can experience it whenever you wish. There are multiple therapeutic and emotional uses for this technique.

Recommendations

1. Stroke a few drops between your palms, cup them over your nose and mouth and inhale.

2. Stroke them into your hair.

3. Wear them for perfume. Apply a drop to your wrists, behind your ears, to your temples, along the back of your neck, wherever they can slowly evaporate and release their aromatic magic throughout the day to calm you, make you more alert, energize you, or release wonderful memories too long forgotten.

There are interesting diffusers for deodorizing your car. There are nasal inhalers with little felt pads you can saturate with oils and use to discreetly inhale important aromas throughout the day. There are many other interesting tools to help us enjoy these wonderful aromas more conveniently

Mix inhalation with olfaction

For centuries people have burned incense for religious ceremonies, to dispel unpleasant odors, and to eradicate microbes. Essential oils can accomplish these and many more functions all at the same time.

When you take a trace of an essential oil like tea tree on your tongue and mix it with saliva in your mouth, some if it makes its way to your olfactory bulb. But most of it makes its way into your

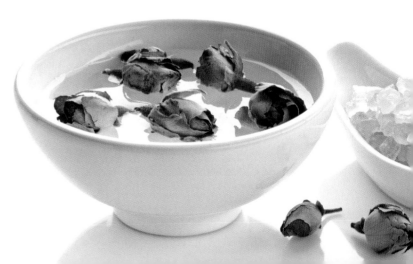

bloodstream through the "buccal" walls of your mouth and throat, disinfecting your mouth, tongue, throat, and gums. Some of it is also absorbed through the lining of your sinuses and even down into your lungs.

Hot water vapor

When you heat an essential oil in hot or boiling water it evaporates quickly and the combination of steam and oil is highly therapeutic. But it dissipates quickly and some of the constituents may be lost because of the heat. You can capture the aromatic blend of oil and steam by placing a towel over your head and inhaling. Blow into the water to stir up the mixture. Heat the water again and add more oils as needed.

Oils in candles, on light bulb rings, in small bowls on radiators, and on heated diffusers also help deodorize and disinfect. But they also alter the chemical structure of the oils so they lose some of their therapeutic value with the heat.

What is a diffuser?

A diffuser is a device that allows an oil to evaporate and disperse an aroma into the air. If all you are after is a pleasing aroma, there is a large variety of affordable ways to disperse oils—in candles, on light bulb rings, in small bowls on radiators, and on heated diffusers. But there are many more choices. There are four categories of diffusers, ranging from the most therapeutic and clinical to the more aromatic and recreational with limited therapeutic benefits. They include (1) nebulizing diffusers, (2) ultrasonic or humidifying diffusers, (3) evaporative diffusers, and (4) heat diffusers.

To keep your diffuser in tip top shape, read and follow the manufacturer's cleaning and maintenance recommendations.

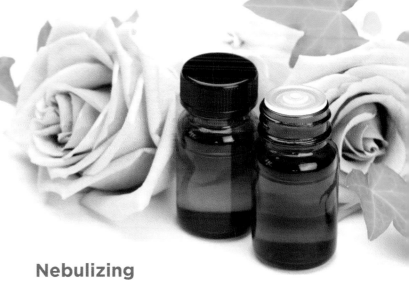

Nebulizing Diffuser (also called an atomizing diffuser)

A nebulizing diffuser is capable of dispersing the greatest amount of essential oil into the air and into the lungs. This type may be the best choice for most clinical purposes. It uses a jet of cold air blowing across a small tube, pulling a fine mist of droplets of pure essential oil up through the tube. The continual flow of air disperses these fine droplets into the room, where they can remain suspended for an extended period of time. It disperses the complete, unaltered oil with all its complex, therapeutic constituents into the air.

The particle size is small enough for the lungs to absorb rapidly and transfer molecules efficiently into the blood stream. The surface area of your lungs is equivalent to the surface of a tennis court. Each lung sack has capillaries that carry aromatic molecules directly to the heart and throughout your body.

While this technology can be relatively quiet, because of the air jet, it is not as whisper quiet or as completely silent as other types of diffusers. This type of diffuser will use your essential oil at a faster rate than other diffusers. It is often equipped with a timer and ways to regulate the air pressure so you don't get too much oil in too short a time. But you need to monitor and regulate the timing and the air pressure. You can set the timer at 15-minute intervals for a steady, slow stream of aromatic molecules over a two-hour period.

If you have your diffuser on too long at a high output in a small room, you may begin to become light headed within 10 to 20 minutes.

Ultrasonic Diffuser

These diffusers create a fine mist of aromatic oils in a different way. The essential oils are added to another liquid, usually water. And the device uses electronic frequencies to break the essential oil into tiny microdroplets. The oil is dispersed, mixed with the water in a fine mist. Because these tiny particles are mixed with water, they can be more quickly absorbed by the lungs, just like oils mixed with water are more quickly absorbed by the skin. It normally takes heat to transform liquids into vapor, but the ultrasonic vibrations do it without heat.

The fine mist humidifies the air and is quieter than the nebulizing diffuser, with only a slight sound much like trickling water. Only a small percentage of the mist is from the essential oil, however. The ratio, for example, might be a teaspoon of essential oil for every two quarts of water dispersed into the air.

Choose this type of diffuser if you only want a small amount of oil in the room at a time. Some models have timers that will disperse an oil for up to 9 hours. This type of diffuser can be beneficial in a dry climate or when humidity is important for a respiratory issue.

Some come with light, sounds, and even music.

Features in both the nebulizing diffuser and the ultrasonic diffuser make it easy and convenient to experience all the benefits of every constituent of each essential oil through your olfactory nerves to your brain and through your mouth, sinuses, trachea, bronchioles, and lungs.

A well-placed diffuser supplied with a few selected essential oils or a blend can add remarkable immunity to your life. It can purify the air, lift your spirits, create all the marvels of olfaction, and pass molecules throughout your body detoxifying and bringing life-giving vitality.

You can put your diffuser on a timer to gently wake you up each morning like an aromatic alarm clock with oils that give you energy and keep you alert. You can use your diffuser in the evening with oils to calm you into a profound sleep. Use a unit in the kitchen or bathroom to dispel disagreeable aromas and purify the air. Use it to greet invited guests into your warm and welcoming home. Use it to repel insects.

Use your diffuser every day and you will more easily make it through cold and flu season without incident.

Evaporation Diffusers

These diffusers use a fan to blow air through various types of pads or filters that have essential oils dropped into them. This causes the oil to evaporate more quickly than usual, as the air containing the evaporated oil is blown throughout the room. This is an inexpensive way to get the aroma of an oil into a room or into your car if you're using the air vent. But it isn't effective at getting the therapeutic value of the whole essential oil into your lungs. The lighter,

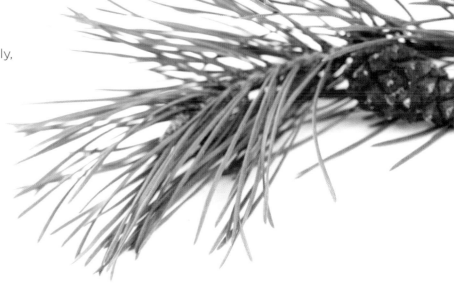

more volatile parts of the oil flash off quickly, leaving the heavier constituents for later.

Some evaporation diffusers use no fan. They simply use the movement of air in the room to disperse the aroma as the oils evaporate. There are clay pendants, air fresheners with pads containing oils, and small personal inhalers with essential oils on a pad.

Heat Diffusers

Heat makes essential oils evaporate quicker than simple evaporation diffusers: the hotter the heat source, the stronger the smell; the lower the heat source the more subtle the smell. Higher heat also alters the chemical constituents of the oil, making it less beneficial from a therapeutic point of view.

Dr. Pénoël's therapy for treating sinus conditions

As you may remember from Dr. Pénoël's experience in South Australia with Abby Bean, or "little Abby," as he calls her, one of his special areas of expertise is respiratory diseases, which comprises the lower respiratory system (lungs) and the upper respiratory system (called ENT, or ear, nose, and throat). Infectious conditions of the nose the sinuses are extremely widespread. Millions of sufferers receive large amounts of synthetic drugs and undergo painful surgeries, but do not get rid of their infections.

He insists that we always start with a healthy diet, a 2-mile walk, and using clinical-grade essential oils in a systemic way (by taking capsules). In addition, he developed a therapy for sinus infections that works extremely well, is safe, and simple to understand. He calls it Post Inhalation Apnea Aerosol (PIAA).

He uses a cold-air atomizing diffuser with a pump blowing molecules of oil through a glass tube called a nebulizer. The diffuser must have a regulator to control the output of molecules generally set to its minimum level, especially at the beginning of the therapy. Between the minimum and maximum output, there is a multiplication factor of 10! So each person has to find the right setting, but he recommends starting at the lowest setting.

When you inhale, most of the air goes into your lungs. But when you have a sinus infection, the problem is in your sinus cavities—maxillary, frontal, ethmoidal, or even the sphenoidal (inside the skull itself)—and when you inhale aromatic molecules they go into your lungs and miss the sinuses. You need also the tiny aromatic particles to penetrate up into the sinuses. The only way to make this happen is to hold your breath as long as you can to allow the particles move upward into the sinuses. Because each particle is so small (a micron in size), if you are breathing normally, they will automatically go into the lungs and miss the sinuses entirely.

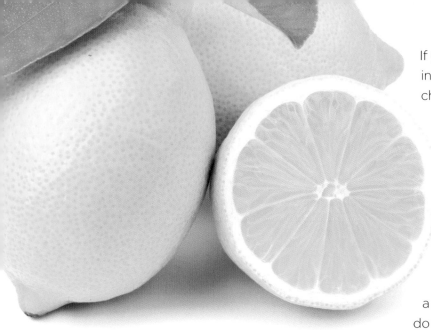

If you have acute sinusitis, repeat the sessions in an intensive way, once every hour. If you have chronic sinusitis, do a session in the morning, a session when you return home from your work, and a session before bed. Make adjustments according to what you feel your body is telling you.

Which oil do you use?

Tea tree is perfect for this therapy. It is easily tolerated at a low power. It offers the powerful yet gentle molecule of terpineol-4 in a sufficient quantity. It is affordable. What more do you need? Use no more than 20 or 30 drops at a time. When the oil runs out, simply add 20 more drops and continue with the therapy.

Here is one more piece of advice from Dr. Pénoël regarding sinus conditions whether chronic or acute. Try giving up dairy products and see if that doesn't help. Here's his story, "I suffered from sinus infections many years ago, and finally realized that I had to give up white cheese made from cow's milk. When I made this change the sinus problems disappeared. That was the root of my problem."

A Personal Experience:

Here's another story from Dr. Pénoël about using a diffuser: "I had undergone an extensive dental surgery with several extractions. My dentist insisted that I take the antibiotics he felt compelled to prescribe. He knew that I would not use them because I had essential oil alternatives. When I went home I used my nebulizing diffuser aimed at my mouth where the surgery had left open wounds. Even though I was used to seeing many wonderful cures, to experience the healing in my own bleeding gums was fantastic. My dentist expected it to take 10 days for the gums to heal, but within three to four days, the tissues had repaired themselves and no antibiotic had been used. I

Recommendations:

Step 1. Take a deep breath and keep your lungs filled with air.

Step 2. Turn on the diffuser, keeping it at the minimum output.

Step 3. Place your left nostril right where the molecules are headed. You can even place your nostril over the opening a little. You will feel the aerosol particles performing their therapeutic action right where they are needed in your sinuses.

Step 4. At this step you can either let the particles penetrate into the left side until you need to exhale and then do the same for the right nostril. Or, if you prefer, take 5 seconds on the left nostril and then five seconds on the right side, alternating every five seconds, until you can no longer hold your breath and you exhale.

Step 5: Take a few normal breaths, turn off the diffuser, then take a deep breath, turn the diffuser on again and repeat the procedure between five and seven times. The whole process only takes a few minutes.

took my capsules of a protecting blend in a more intensive way during these few days. I have my second homeland, Australia, to thank for the gift of tea tree essential oil!"

Ingestion

There has been a barrage of false and misleading information about how unsafe it is to ingest essential oils, while we consume them constantly in highly processed food and drink flavorings. Kurt Schaubelt debunked many of these foolish attempts to frighten us in his book, "Aromatherapy Safety in the Information Age." Here are a few of his arguments.

The fragrance industry in the 1970s and 1980s promoted the misleading idea that essential oils are merely "random mixtures of potentially unknown and treacherous chemicals" (Schnaubelt, Intelligence, p. 72). Scientists at the time asserted that we could only guarantee the safety of any natural product if we could isolate each of its components and test it independently. The reasoning was that "there is no difference between natural and so-called nature identical substances (synthesized in the laboratory and considered identical to those that occur in nature, because superficially they have the same structural formula as their natural counterparts..." (Schnaubelt, Intelligence, p. 74).

Solid science has proven that they are simply not the same even though they share the same molecular structure. Plus all the separate components in an essential oil affect and moderate the others, working together to make them safer and more effective. A single synthetic constituent standing alone doesn't have that synergistic benefit of a blend of a hundred or more separate chemical constituents.

The synthetic chemical proponents also assert that synthetics are somehow more pure, when in actuality their impurities are merely different than those found in nature and clearly much more harmful. "The safety of natural medicines is exponentially higher than that of synthetic drugs, according to whichever statistic is examined" (Schnaubelt, Intelligence, p. 75).

Latrogenic causes (errors by medical professionals) are the third leading cause of death in the United States. And most of those deaths are due to side effects or mismanaged drugs. Clearly Schnaubelt is right when he draws this conclusion: "Compared to the hundreds of thousands of deaths caused by the wrongful application of conventional medicines and the hundreds of thousands more deaths caused by known side effects of conventional drugs, the journeys to explore essential oils are innocent and utterly harmless."

All the complex constituents in an essential oil are not random accidents of nature but rather a marvelous assortment of synergistic components that have evolved or been created to become amazingly beneficial to humanity at a time when the pharmaceutical community is clearly letting us down by providing a steady stream of unsafe drugs that often have to be recalled years after they have been introduced.

It is clear that not all pharmaceutical drugs are harmful and all essential oils are perfectly safe. That idea would be naïve. There are definite rules of safety that must be applied to both.

But the rules at the front of this book are much clearer and far safer than page after page of small type following every advertisement for a pharmaceutical drug.

So it's time to disregard all the overwrought warnings and disclaimers and learn together from decades of experiences how to safely ingest essential oils and enjoy their remarkable benefits. Clearly there are some oils that should not be taken internally, and they will be clearly noted in this book. But making a blanket order to "never ingest essential oils" out of fear, clearly keeps us from enjoying many of their most important benefits.

Dr. Pénoël says that to use essential oils without ingesting them is like having a fine pocket knife but never opening the blade. You can use it as a small blunt hammer to poke around at things, but that's all. Without ingesting them they cannot be fully used for the purpose they were created.

By far the most effective internal use of essential oils is taking them in capsules. In his clinic Dr. Pénoël creates and prescribes capsules with unique blends of essential oils diluted with carrier oil and other substances. While it is a little time-consuming to make up

capsules using empty veggie or gelatin caps, the results are remarkable.

You will see instructions online focused on putting a drop or two of an essential oil in a capsule, filling it with a carrier oil and swallowing it. There is a far easier way, and with a little ingenuity there will evolve many other convenient ways to fill capsules and enjoy their benefits.

"Naturopathic physicians are well positioned to understand and make effective use of essential oils. Side effects are rare and self-limiting, making essential oils a prime illustration of primum non nocere, 'first do no harm.' Essential oils work quickly, safely, and reliably, and they add the benefit of increasing the confidence of both doctor and patient" (Schnaubelt, Intelligence, p. 150).

How to fill essential oil capsules

Start by purchasing a package of 00-sized or 0-sized empty veggie or gelatin capsules. Put 30 to 50 of them on a plate.

Mix the essential oils you want to use in a dropper bottle. Most blends will be diluted about 40% essential oils with 60% carrier oil. If you are using exceptionally strong oils like oregano, thyme, cinnamon, or clove, you will want to have a ratio that is more like 25% essential oils and 75% carrier oil. But if you are mixing both mild and strong oils, your ratios can allow for higher ratios of essential oils.

Mix your essential oil recipe of choice with your favorite carrier oil use the dropper to fill and cap each capsule. Put the capsules in an opaque bottle and store them in a cool place out of direct sunlight.

It is a myth that essential oils will instantly erode the capsules and make a mess. They can last up to 6 months or more without harming the capsules. That doesn't mean that there won't be an occasional faulty capsule, but for the most part you can fill a whole bottle of capsules in less than 30 minutes and have them on hand for the next infection that comes around. Then you can safely take them according to the clear instructions Dr. Pénoël and those he has taught will give you in this volume.

Each one of us should make it our goal to take a single capsule of an essential oil blend for prevention once a day.

Essential oils in water, juice, teas, and recipes

A simple drop of essential oils in your drinking water, juice, tea, and various recipes can be a pleasurable and healthy addition to your life. Essential oils can be very strong tasting, so you'll want to experiment with quantities. Sometimes, as Dr. Pénoël says, "if a little is good, a little less may actually be better." One drop of spearmint oil may be far better tasting than two in a big, cold jug of drinking water. And a trace on a toothpick may be even better than a drop of basil oil in a cup of tea. Experiment until you find the right ratios to please your tastebuds.

For the greatest benefits and flavors from essential oils, add them to your recipes as you take them off the burner, just before you serve them. Less of the essential oils will evaporate, and you will consume more of the health-giving molecules. Olive oil,

I always use essential oils in my drinking water

I always carry water with me to keep myself hydrated. I love adding a drop or two of peppermint, lemon, or orange to my water. I even add a drop to the drinking water in restaurants. I've noticed that I drink more water because it tastes better. I seldom get sick when I keep up this habit. (Be sure to shake the mixture well before taking each drink to disperse the oil as much as possible.)

for example, is a lot healthier when it is not overheated, so it may be beneficial for you to mix up an olive oil blend with your favorite spice oils and add the flavorful blend to your recipes just as you serve them.

Essential oils in the mouth

Dentists have been putting essential oils in the mouth for decades. Clove oil was one of the earliest deadening agents used by dentists. The mouth is one of the most active places in the body where microbes, bacteria, viruses, and fungi thrive. It is thought to be between 4 and 4,000-times more permeable than skin (Prathipati Padmaja, "Buccal Drug Delivery System http://www.pharmatutor.org/articles/buccal-drug-delivery-system?page=0,0).

Capillaries are close to the surface in the lining of the mouth (the buccomucosal lining). Aerobic and anaerobic bacteria lodge on and in the layers of the cheeks, tongue, gums, and in microscopic cracks and crevices of the teeth and bones of the mouth. Keeping the mouth clean and the good and bad microbes in safe balance can be a major challenge. That's why bad breath and all kinds of infections lodge in the mouth and spread throughout the body through the bloodstream into places you would least expect. For example, an abscessed tooth can be a major contributor to bone and other serious infections throughout the body.

Keeping the mouth free from dangerous microbes is a major challenge and a great opportunity to leverage the power of essential oils.

Essential oils have been used for years in commercial mouthwash. Mint flavorings have essential oil origins. But using diluted and undiluted essential oils safely and effectively in the mouth offers many possibilities for not only cleaning up and keeping in balance this most critical area of the body, but also delivering aromatic molecules throughout the body through the bloodstream.

When you drink aromatic water, some microbes may make their way into the bloodstream. But a drop of a mild essential oil under the tongue like frankincense, lemon, or tea tree may deliver much more antimicrobial power to the body.

Dr. Pénoël suggests the "lick trick" for sore throats and other respiratory conditions. "Simply swipe a trace of an essential oil like a protecting blend or tea tree on the back of the hand and lick it off. Dilute the oil in your saliva and distribute the aromatic mixture around your mouth. Tea tree is not very flavorful in a whole drop. But a single trace, when you see what it actually does for a sore throat, will have you coming back for more. When you bite your tongue and it gets infected or you get an infection anywhere inside your mouth, essential oils are wonderfully helpful.

The lick trick for a sore throat

I was picking up my son at the airport the other day. We had an hour drive to get home. He complained of a sore throat coming on, so I gave him my little bottle of tea tree I always carry with me. I told him how to lick a trace off the back of his hand every few minutes. All the way home I would remind him every minute or two to take another lick. He had to be reminded to take only a trace because a full drop tasted awful. By the time we got home his sore throat was completely gone, and it didn't come back.

Be sure to dilute the strong oils like cinnamon, clove, lemongrass, oregano, and thyme at a ratio of at least 20:80 (essential oil to carrier oil) before putting them in your mouth. Mild oils like tea tree and chamomile can be used undiluted in the mouth, but all others should be blended at least by 50% with a carrier oil. Flavor will dictate how strong a blend you can tolerate in your mouth. Your saliva will further dilute the oils.

"This double-blind, placebo-controlled, randomized, 2-week cross-over study showed that rinsing with essential oils [mouthrinse] reduced the level of bloodstream bacteria in subjects with mild-to-moderate gingivitis" (Fine et al. 2010).

Use essential oils for "oil pulling"

"Oil pulling" is "swishing" olive or sesame oil around the mouth and between the teeth for 15 to 20 minutes, then spitting the mixture out. It is an increasingly popular Ayurvedic therapy recommended by health care professionals not only for bad breath and gingivitis, but also for many other health concerns—headaches, migraines, acne, diabetic symptoms, asthma, and even teeth whitening.

Add your favorite essential oil to the mixture, and you will experience still better results. A single drop or less in a tablespoon of oil may be too strong for you. Try using a drop and add olive or sesame oil until the taste is perfect for you. Then try the therapy for a few days or weeks and see if you are experiencing the benefits. Try using any of the citrus oils, peppermint, spearmint, basil, clove, cinnamon, etc.

Household Uses

There are diverse ways to use essential oils to improve the cleansing power of the household products you are using, purify the air, and make household chores into more healthy aromatic experiences.

Recommendations:

- For its antiseptic and air purifying action, add a drop or two of your favorite antiseptic oil to each application of dishwashing soap, 10 to 15 drops to your bucket of mop water, a drop or two to your spray bottle of window cleaner, and 10 to 20 drops to 8 oz. of surface cleaner.

- Spray down surfaces of saunas, hot tubs, and jacuzzis with an aromatic surface cleaner to minimize infections, especially if they are used often. Splash scented water on hot sauna stones.

- For an aromatic insect repellant, blend 20 drops of a repellant oil like peppermint, lemongrass, cypress, Eucalyptus globulus, or others with a half teaspoon of household detergent and add the mixture to an oz. spray bottle of water. Spray areas where insects could enter your home.

- Since essential oils can separate from water and the detergent in your product may not always disperse the oils effectively, be sure to shake or mix product well with each use.

- To make painting the house a more pleasurable and healthy aromatic experience, mix 50 drops of your favorite essential oil in a gallon of paint.

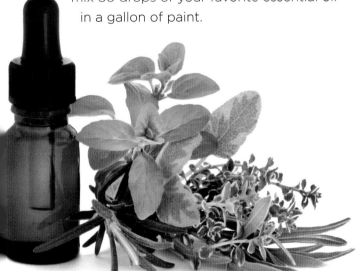

Working Day-to-Day with Essential Oils for Maximum Prevention

Essential oils only work when they are used. They're like healthy food. Only as they become a routine in your daily life will you experience the full promises of this book. As you become familiar with their amazing benefits, and comfortable with the simple safety rules, you will want to use them even more. Here are a few suggestions for inserting them easily into your daily activities. Compare the minimal cost of these few drops of aromatic health with the cost of recurring and chronic illness. They'll take no more time than brushing your teeth, but their rewards will be tremendous in health and emotional balance.

Keep your oils handy

- Many people carry small bottles of their most frequently used essential oils in carrying pouches on their key chains or belt or in their purse or pocket. Just make sure the lids are on tight.

- Create or purchase a no-spill wooden holder for your oils by drilling holes in a block of wood to match the size of your bottles. Then you can keep a dropper in the top for quick dipping, and they won't tip easily.

- Keep a supply of oils near the shower or bath where you can think about them and use them conveniently while your body is warm and damp.

- Keep oils in the kitchen where everyone can reach for a drop to put in their juice. Keep them with your spices so you can put a drop in a recipe just as it comes off the stove.

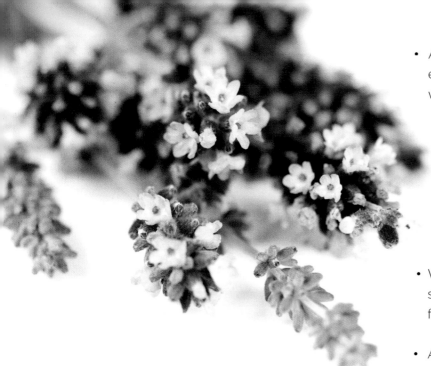

Make essential oils part of all your food and drink routines

- Enjoy a drop your favorite single or blend in your drinking water. Taste test one or two drops per quart of water.

- The best blends are created to taste delicious (or at least tolerable for most people) when diluted in water or herbal tea. Experiment until you have a recipe and routine that is perfect for you.

- Keep a pitcher of essential-oil-flavored water in the refrigerator for everyone to enjoy.

- Instead of taking trips to the drinking fountain, keep a supply of perfectly flavored water at your desk to enjoy throughout the day. You'll drink more water, and you'll be healthier.

- Keep toothpicks in the pouch or purse where you carry your oils. In restaurants, dip a toothpick in an oil and stir it into your glass of water or herbal tea. If you forget to carry toothpicks, ask for one at the restaurant.

- At the end of every meal while others are enjoying their coffee, ask for a cup of hot water or herbal tea and stir in a drop or trace of your favorite blend or single oil.

- Instead of your morning coffee, enjoy an herbal tea with a flavorful trace of essential oil. Or order hot water and add a drop of essential oil to get you going in the morning.

- When you order juice of any kind, be sure to stir in a drop or toothpick-trace of your favorite oil.

- As you take a dish off the stove, get in the habit of adding a drop of basil, lemon, peppermint, spearmint, orange, tangerine, lime, or one of the delicious blends. It will add a wonderful, memorable aroma your family will grow to love.

- Add a drop or trace of an essential oil to your salad dressings, vegetable dips, bean dips, sandwich spreads, salsas, and sauces.

- Before every meal, get your body relaxed and ready to enjoy the food by diffusing the aroma of basil, your digestion blend or another favorite oil. Your digestive system will work more efficiently under the influence of these wonderful aromas.

Start your day with essential oils

- Awaken to an aromatic alarm clock by putting your cold-air diffuser on a timer and add 20 drops of an energizing oil to brighten your mind and get you off to a great start.

- Use oils in your morning bath or shower. To fill the room with energy, add a drop of oil in each application of your shampoo or conditioner.

- Before exercising, put 4 to 5 drops of an energizing blend or single oil in a teaspoon of mixing oil. Quickly massage your muscles and joints. This will warm up, energize, and protect your muscles and joints for exercize. Your muscles and joints will recover more quickly as well.

- Make all your personal care aromatic by adding 10 to 20 drops of your favorite blend to 8 ounces of soft soap, shampoo, conditioner, shaving gel, or hair & skin mist. Be sure to use only fragrance-and-toxic-free personal care. You can also make your personal care more moisturizing by adding a few drops of an essential oil to a teaspoon of your favorite carrier oil and adding it to your lotions and creams.

- After your bath or shower while your skin is moist and warm, always apply a respiratory blend of oils to your throat, chest, and back on the points in this illustration.

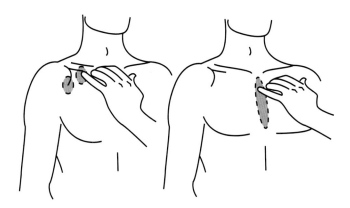

- Considering that your deodorant goes on your underarm area where a lot of your lymph nodes reside, you want an extra measure of immune protection there. Rub a drop of essential oil between your palms and apply to your underarm area before your deodorant. Dilute the essential oils with a little water or some carrier oil on this delicate part of the boy where the skin is extremely thin. It's also a good idea to use the least sensitizing oils like lavender, and Roman chamomile.

- Create an aromatic tooth powder by mixing 2 parts baking soda to 1 part fine-ground, natural salt. Thoroughly mix in drops of peppermint or clove oil to taste. Sprinkle some in your hand, wet your toothbrush, and enjoy brushing your teeth without the toxic chemicals.

- A trace of essential oil distributed around the mouth with your tongue is a much more effective mouthwash than the toxic commercial mouthwashes. Dip a toothpick in an essential oil or put a trace on your hand and lick it off.

- You can absorb a lot of essential oil molecules by simply fragrancing your lotion with oils. Mix 10 to 20 drops of your favorite blend in 8 ounces of lotion. Be sure to use a lotion base that's free from fragrance and toxic chemicals. A teaspoon of carrier oil will make your lotion even more moisturizing.

Enjoy essential oils at noon

- Using a toothpick, add a trace of your favorite essential oil to your restaurant water.

- Enjoy the aroma of basil to prepare your body for your meal.

- Prepare a diluted blend of your favorite savory spice oils with olive oil for sprinkling on salads, sandwiches, or in soup. Instead of spreading butter on your bread, dip it in this flavorful mixture.

Enjoy your evening with essential oils

- When you are ready to unwind at the end of the day, diffuse 10 drops of a calming essential oil to help erase the cares of the day. This five-minute ritual will give you more restful sleep and pleasant dreams.

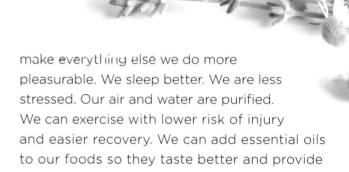

- If you exercise in the evening, warm up your muscles with an invigorating massage blend to protect your muscles and joints, but after your shower, cool down with a comforting blend.

- Make essential oils a part of your evening meal in your water and recipes.

- If you bathe or shower in the evening use calming oils to relax you and prepare you for sleep. If you are stressed, use a cup or two of Epsom Salts in a bath with one of these calming oils.

- During the cold and flu seasons use a respiratory blend in your aromatic bath.

- While your skin is still warm after your bath or shower, treat yourself to a foot massage using 4 to 5 drops of your favorite Comforting blend in a teaspoon of mixing oil.

- Use your aromatic tooth powder with peppermint or clove flavoring instead of toxic, chemical-laden toothpaste.

- A trace of an antiseptic oil or blend on the tongue distributed around the mouth is a much better mouthwash than the harsh commercial versions. Dip a toothpick in the oil or put a trace on your hand and lick it off.

Essential Oils and a Healthy Lifestyle

A holistic approach to health sees essential oils as an important element in an otherwise healthy lifestyle. We cannot hope to heal our physical and emotional problems by simply adding essential oils without also addressing the other lifestyle choices like clean air and water, exercise, sleep, a balanced diet, and wise stress management. Essential oils are a perfect complement to all these lifestyle choices. They

make everything else we do more pleasurable. We sleep better. We are less stressed. Our air and water are purified. We can exercise with lower risk of injury and easier recovery. We can add essential oils to our foods so they taste better and provide for better digestion.

However, for optimal health and deep healing, our basic choices, especially in diet and exercise need to be in place for essential oils to accomplish their most amazing work.

When patients finally show up at Dr. Daniel Pénoël's clinic they have often tried years of traditional allopathic cures with little success. His first interview involves a complete holistic assessment of their life—their stresses, their dietary habits, their sleep habits, everything. To leave anything out might be ignoring the most important element that becomes the key to breaking the cycle of disease.

In this assessment he often finds that a simple checklist of dietary and other guidelines uncovers some key issues that must be addressed before essential oils can even begin to start working at a deep level.

Without the benefit of personalized counseling that Dr. Pénoël and his wife give their patients, here are some basic guidelines for you to check to make sure you have the best chance for deep healing using essential oils.

Dr. Daniel Pénoël's 4 Basic Dietary Guidelines

#1: Do I eat foods close to the way nature created them?

Degenerative disease is a high price to pay for the convenience of over-processed foods. Nutritionally dead food, like synthetic essential oils, cannot give you the life your cells need. Do I choose to eat high-quality foods—organic where possible? Raw vegetables? Ripe fruit? Lightly steamed vegetables? Dried fruits? Frozen fruits and vegetables? Whole grains? Healthy fats—cold-pressed, heart healthy oils and nuts? Do I avoid processed meats and animal products that are full of hormones, antibiotics and preservatives? Do I avoid foods where the first few ingredients include refined sugars, processed flour (including whole-wheat flour rather than whole-grain flour), or animal fats? Don't fall for the deception that you can pop a few vitamin supplements to replace the complex nutrients found in whole foods.

#2. Do I eat light and stay satisfied?

Huge quantities of even the best foods will leave you feeling heavy and unhealthy. Adjust the quantity to your level of physical activity and the season. It is never healthy to be completely stuffed. Do you listen to your body and have a snack when you're hungry before you start feeling completely famished? Do you eat the amount of food that helps you remain satisfied, alert and able to work well, or do you eat too much and feel tired and groggy? It's healthy to have one light meal of fruit only, especially in the summertime. Add healthy snacks to your daily routine, and eat small amounts when you are a little hungry instead of becoming ravenous and bingeing just before bed or any time of day.

#3. Do I eat for variety?

To be healthy your body needs a complex assortment of glucids, lipids, protids, vitamins, minerals, trace elements, and enzymes in specific amounts. Nutrition, like essential oils, is extremely complex from a biochemical and analytical point of view. Nature is complex so we can live simply, but too much of some things can crowd out the nutrition your body needs. Most people these days eat much of one or all of these three—(1) excessive proteins and animal fats (especially meat and dairy products), (2) refined grains, and (3) industrial sugar. These three are at the root of most of civilization's degenerative diseases, and they keep us overfed and undernourished. Fill up on fresh fruits and vegetables in summertime and whole cereals, dried fruits, vegetables, and nuts during the cold seasons. Then you'll be entitled to a reasonable treat. But don't make the empty food the main event.

4. Do I eat slowly and mindfully?

As with all major human activities, the act of eating can be, in a sense, a healing ritual. If you feel tense and irritated and swallow your food at great speed, you are not likely to digest it properly, even if you are eating good food. Relax a few minutes prior to eating. Diffuse a calming, food-oriented spice oil. Precede your meal with a prayer of thanksgiving. Chew your foods mindfully and notice the tastes and aromas. Avoid arguments and conflicts while eating. Avoid eating in noisy places, especially in front of the TV.

How to retrain your taste buds using essential oils

Many people feel that if a food tastes good, it must be good for you. This might be true if we were living in nature one hundred percent of the time and if the only foods were the ones we would pick from the trees or collect from the earth! We are far from this.

Almost everything today is artificial. When infants are fed canned foods and sugary cereals, deserts, and drinks from a very early age, is it any wonder they cannot tolerate normal vegetables and fruits. Start with only healthy foods that are as close to nature as possible. Only then can you be guided by your tastes, knowing that you need time to reeducate your taste buds. Essential oils can help.

Take chocolate cravings, for example. Chocolate needs to become a treat again, not the main focus of your cravings. Give yourself a minute between the moment you start craving and when you eat it. Spend this minute inhaling an essential oil that you love. Check how you feel. You may find that your craving is slightly diminished. Make a fully conscious decision to treat yourself to only a small piece of chocolate. It's not a compulsive or uncontrolled act. You can fully enjoy a small piece instead of devouring twenty pieces like a "chocolate slave." If you will take this "mindful minute" over a period of 28 days, you are likely to master your addiction. And you will feel proud of your new freedom to enjoy one of the better things of life in a healthy and controlled way.

Use this "mindful minute" with an essential oil to reset whatever craving gets you in trouble. Is it the big fluffy white rolls at the restaurant that get you in trouble? Use a mindful moment with an oil and perhaps an herbal tea to reset your craving. Is it the gigantic dessert you've been looking forward to? Take a "mindful minute" before ordering. Order hot water for an aromatic tea first. Or maybe it's just a whiff from a bottle to reset your limbic brain. Then share that decadent dessert with others instead of devouring the whole thing yourself.

You come in from a long day of work late at night and head for the refrigerator or the pantry where the treats are hidden. Take a moment to turn on the diffuser. Take a few deep breaths and make a decision to make yourself a healthy sandwich instead of taking on that whole box of Oreos. Have a couple of Oreos to finish off your snack.

Troubleshooting Effectiveness of Essential Oils

It's aggravating to follow instructions in a book, and not get the results you're after. "What's wrong?" you ask. "Do I have a poor quality oil? Were the instructions wrong? Was I missing something?" You go to the Internet and find the same instructions in a dozen places. "I guess essential oils just don't work for me," you conclude.

It would be a tragedy for you to reach that conclusion, because they do work, and they work wonderfully.

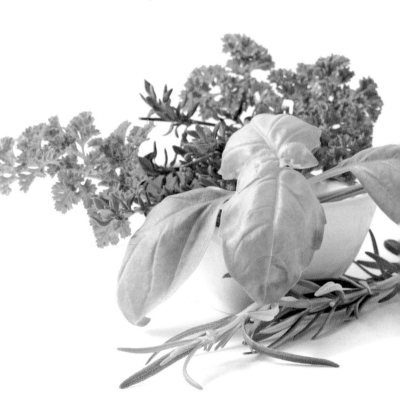

Instead, let's troubleshoot some of the reasons this one trial may have not worked for you so you don't give up on essential oils entirely.

What could have gone wrong?

Poor-quality oils

Please refer to the chapter on essential oil quality to help you recognize if the oils you've purchased are clinically reliable.

Poor-quality advice

There is a lot of information on the Internet that has been copied and pasted from the original books on essential oils by Tisserand, Worwood, Lawless, Davis, and others. Much of it is written for what Dr. Pénoël calls, "*timid, English-style aromatherapy*." Many of the dilutions recommended are just not strong enough to do the job. They may have some minor effect, but not what you would expect in a clinical setting.

Then there are the books and websites that give instructions and promise results that make no sense if you understand how essential oils actually work. You see instructions for curing cancer and other serious diseases that are way beyond the capacity of essential oils. This kind of advice hurts the industry and lowers the confidence of those who trust us to deliver results. The scientists come to disrespect us so they won't conduct trials of essential oils, and we have trouble convincing anyone to try our convincing and logical instructions.

The clinical use of essential oils has grown tremendously over the last 3 decades. As people try the instructions and therapies recommended by experts, they begin to focus on sharing those that work and ignore those that don't. The Internet is a tool we can use to keep each other honest and verify the value of what is recommended.

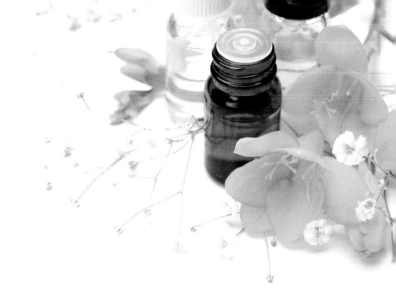

In this book we offer several valuable tools to help you identify those instructions that are the most likely to consistently work for you.

- We show ratings by Marcel Lavabre and by Dr. Pénoël on therapies and oils that they indicate are most effective and powerful. You'll see +++++P for Dr. Pénoël's ratings in L'Aromatherapie Exactement or +++++L for Lavabre's ratings in Aromatherapy Workbook.

- You'll also see a larger volume of research and more success stories centered around certain therapies and certain oils.

- You're always going to have more consistent and reliable success with the main essential oils—tea tree, peppermint, lavender, basil, geranium, lemon, oregano, etc.—simply because they've proven themselves over and over for multiple uses. That doesn't mean that other lesser-known oils aren't going to be just as effective or possibly even more effective. It just means that the more common oils have had more opportunity to prove themselves and their instructions.

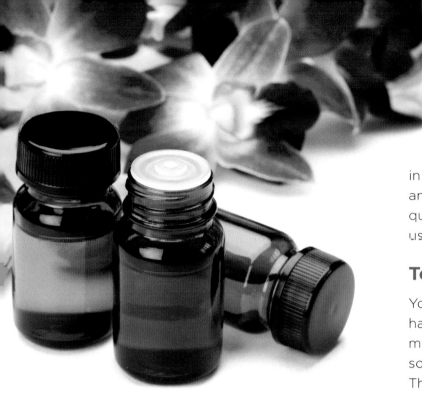

essential oils and finding them safe and effective for in-home use in 50:50 dilutions and in capsules as they are recommended in this book. They are verifying quality claims and endorsing the bolder clinical use of clinical quality essential oils. Competition is also helping us find the truth of the matter.

Too much oil

You wouldn't put a tablespoon of salt in a half-cup of water for an eye wash. It's too much. It would do harm. You need a saline solution that matches the salinity of tears. The same is true for essential oils. They are powerful and highly concentrated. So, when you're taking them in teas, water, and recipes, you'll need to use some care to regulate the amount of oil you're using.

There is a misconception we all share at one time or another that tells us if a little works well, then more must work better. In matters of flavoring and many safety issues exactly the opposite is often true.

Take peppermint, for example. It has a cooling action and can be highly effective in a spray for sunburn. But putting peppermint straight on a second-degree burn would be a big mistake. In its undiluted, highly concentrated state, it is no longer cooling but rather irritating. It's too much.

If your application of essential oil didn't work as well for you as you expected, you may want to check the instruction and adjust the quantity in your blend. This can make a big difference in some applications. For example, diffusing more than 20 drops of an essential oil is too much for your brain and your lungs to take at one time. Using undiluted, powerful essential oils like oregano, cinnamon, or thyme all over your

Too little oil

The "timid" English aromatherapists have cautiously written many volumes of frightening advice about the dangers of using too much essential oil in a blend. They use the word "poison" a lot and forbid many oils for children and pregnancy that have been clinically proven to be safe. In a way they have done the industry a disservice because many medical professionals in England have embraced their "timid" approach to aromatherapy. It's largely used for aromatic calming, and incidental help for various conditions, and for those purposes a tiny drop of essential oils can go a long way. In such timid dilutions the quality of the essential oils is not that critical, and the timid results are still real.

However, the medical, clinical, French approach to essential oils use has proven itself safe and highly effective all over the world. Dr. Pénoël and others have trained professionals like Jane Buckle, Ron Guba, and Kurt Schnaubelt who frankly feel that the timid approach doesn't take advantage of all that essential oils have to offer. Millions all over the world are trying face for acne would be dangerous and likely to do harm. You also wouldn't slather undiluted oregano all over your body to get rid of moles, or even diluted oregano. But these strong oils in careful dilution, applied judiciously, offer outstanding clinical benefits.

Expecting results too quickly

Beware of your mindset where essential oils are concerned. If you are too focused on the allopathic mindset because of using over-the-counter drugs, you may miss the outstanding benefits of essential oils. For example, the holistic model that Dr. Pénoël teaches recommends that when we have a respiratory infection, we don't want to stop the flow of mucous. We want to get it out of the way as quickly as possible so we can accomplish a deep and permanent healing. The over-the-counter, synthetic drugs will dry up and clog up the mucous—preventing deep healing and actually extending the disease and giving it a better chance of returning later on.

Our personal experience with Dr. Pénoël's healing of upper respiratory infections is this: If we act quickly, and apply all the therapies he recommends, the symptoms are very manageable, we can work full days with a full-time job throughout the whole illness, and a few days later come out more energetic than before.

Essential oils often work slower than the allopathic drugs, but they work more thoroughly and permanently to restore balance, energy, and vitality.

With this in mind, it's important to remember Dr. Pénoël's advice to continue with his therapies for several days after symptoms are gone. This prevents what he calls "morbid transfer," which is having the infection transfer to other organs for more serious manifestations. Or, it prevents the disease from returning again too soon. Be patient with essential oils. They are safe, they

are pleasurable to use, and they provide deep and lasting healing.

Here's another rule of thumb he uses for thorough healing. When you have suffered with a condition for many years, it may take you one month of serious therapy to clean up a year of damage to your body. For example. If you have suffered with chronic headaches for 5 years, it may take you 5 months of serious cleansing to rid yourself of them. A quick symptomatic headache remedy, like peppermint on the temples, may provide some relief, but if you want to be free of the headaches entirely, you will need to pay the price. There are many conditions of this nature that only a deep cleansing with multiple instructions can accomplish. You can't expect to permanently undo serious damage with a single, quick fix. Allopathic medicines are most often designed to control the symptoms, not permanently cure the ailment. They are not capable of accomplishing the kind of deep healing that many of these essential oils can. But we must be patient and obey instructions to get long-lasting and even permanent results.

Lifestyle habits getting in the way

Dr. Pénoël has many stories of patients who came to him for an ailment, and he had to turn them away because they were not willing to change some lifestyle habits that were doing more harm than essential oils could cure. His whole clinical orientation is toward holistic medicine. You heal the whole person with good nutrition, clean air, sensible exercise, and proper stress management. Then, the essential oils will do their work wonderfully. If you have tried a serious therapy using essential oils that didn't work for you, you may want to read Dr. Pénoël's 4 dietary guidelines and try again. Or you may want to add more clean air, exercise, and pure water to your life.

Expecting results that cannot be delivered

This is an error that many of the books and websites fall into. We have read the books, attended many lectures, and listened to many so-called experts who claim to cure things that simply cannot be cured with essential oils. Yet, because they want to sell more oils, they persist in holding out hope and selling large quantities of oils to people desperate to believe their stories.

Dr. Pénoël has a lot of experience with this in his clinic because he is often contacted as the medical professional of last resort when all allopathic treatment and drugs have failed. It's often a cancer that has spread too far or people who have lost their eyesight and their limbs to diabetes. So much could have been done using essential oils for prevention earlier in their lives, but the best use of essential oils for these people is calming them while they await the inevitable or make it through surgeries. The allopathic route or even some other alternative routes are the best route for them to take at these serious stages of degenerative disease.

As Jane Buckle says, essential oils will not grow a new valve in your heart, but they will certainly make a valuable contribution to your calming and healing after the surgery. And that alone could save your life.

If you were disappointed by a recommendation that you thought promised a cure, you may want to revisit the actual promise. The oil recommended for your heart condition may have merely been "palliative," for calming you and helping your body recover after surgery. Many books merely use medical terms that are hard to understand like "vulnerary," (wound healing capability), or "carminative" (eliminating gas). But they don't indicate how reliable the action or what you should actually expect. The effect may be relatively mild, and some other therapy may be far superior.

If there is virtually no evidence-based research behind the claims, then you're probably not going to experience the results you expect. At least start by trying therapies that have plenty of anecdotal evidence borne out in clinical practice, of which there are a great many in this book.

That's why we have inserted Dr. Pénoël's rankings of therapies and effectiveness of various treatments because they represent clinical and in vitro findings by actual medical chemists and licensed medical doctors.

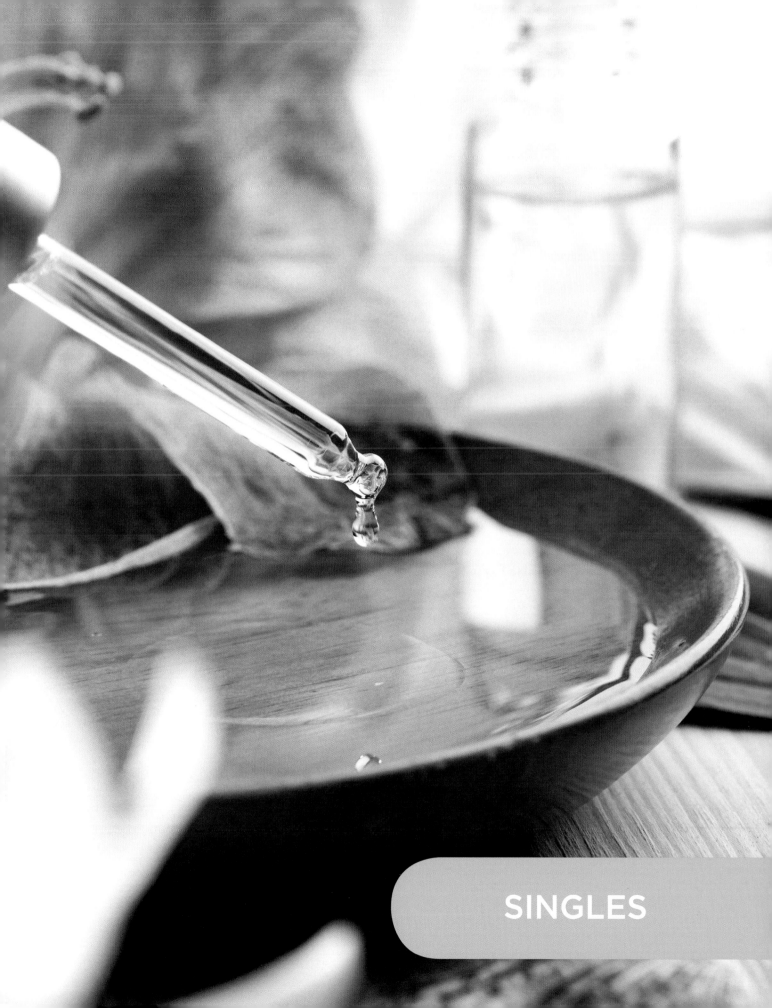

SINGLES

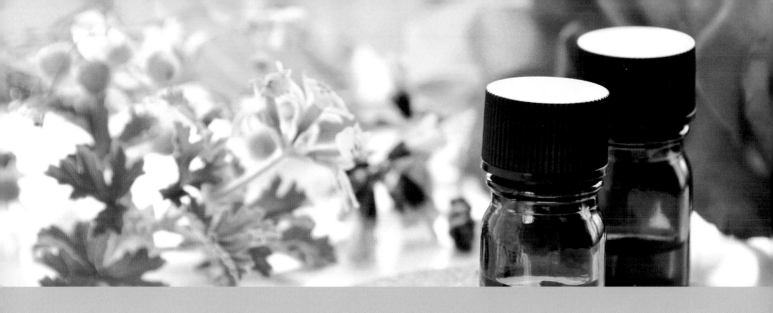

SINGLES

LEGEND

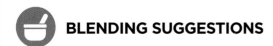
BLENDING SUGGESTIONS

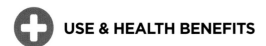
USE & HEALTH BENEFITS

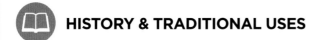
HISTORY & TRADITIONAL USES

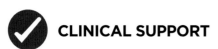
CLINICAL SUPPORT

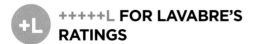
+++++P FOR DR. PÉNOËL'S RATINGS

+++++L FOR LAVABRE'S RATINGS

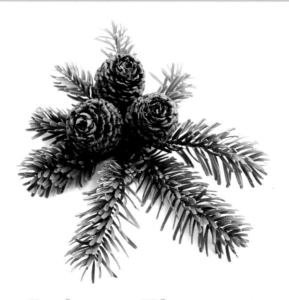

Balsam Fir

Abies balsamea

Family: Pinaceae
Origins: Eastern North America
Other names: Canadian Balsam, Balsam Tree, American Silver Fir, Balm of Gilead (oil),
Description: A tall evergreen tree
Extraction: Steam distillation from needles
Botanical Part Used: needles
Principal constituents: Mostly monoterpenes, pinene, phellandrene, and esters.

BLENDING SUGGESTIONS

- Relative strength: 3
- Among the middle notes that typically make up half or more of the blend
- Blends well with: pine, cedarwood, cypress, and sandalwood
- Description: fresh, woody, sweet, earthy, and balsam

HISTORY & TRADITIONAL USES

The resin has been used by American Indians for rituals and as therapy for burns, sores, cuts, and chest pain. It has also been used internally for coughs and topically for muscle pain. It is widely used as a fragrance in soaps, detergents, cosmetics, and perfumes.

USE & HEALTH BENEFIT

- For minor burns, cuts, and wounds; apply 50:50 dilution with carrier oil to affected area.

- For hemorrhoids apply 50:50 dilution with a carrier oil.

- To clear sinuses, mix a drop of balsam fir into a teaspoon of honey and lick it slowly. ++P ++++L

- To ease symptoms of asthma, bronchitis, excess mucous, or chronic cough; diffuse 10 to 15 drops. ++P ++++L

- For urinary tract infection, create a 50:50 blend with carrier oil and massage lower abdomen. +++L

- To calm depression, tension, stress, and anxiety, take an aromatic bath with 10 to 15 drops of oil with a cup of Epsom Salts. Also massage with a 50:50 blend of balsam fir with a carrier oil. Diffuse 20 drops of balsam fir. These therapies are all calming and will help to overcome insomnia.

- For stiff, painful muscles, rheumatism, and arthritis relief; massage larger areas with a 50:50 blend of balsam fir and carrier oil, apply undiluted to small areas (wrists, fingers, etc.), create a compress with a damp cloth, cover with a dry towel, and apply either heat or cold as needed. +P

- To stimulate endocrine system (thyroid), apply a compress over thyroid area or massage with a 50:50 blend of balsam fir and carrier oil and cover with a damp cloth, a dry cloth, and either apply heat or cool. ++++L

- To help ease symptoms of bronchitis, laryngitis, pneumonia, sinusitis, and other respiratory conditions; use 10 to 15 drops with a cup of Epsom Salts for a bath +++++L.

- As an aid in meditation, diffuse 20 drops +++++L.

- Layer with other oils in back and spinal Layer Therapy.

CAUTIONS: None when used in indicated quantities. In large doses it may be a purgative (Grieve, A Modern Herbal, p. 79)

CLINICAL SUPPORT

Balsam fir was found to be active against the S. aureus bacteria (Pichette, 2006).

Balsam fir oil was found to be active against all the solid tumor cell lines tested (Legault, 2003).

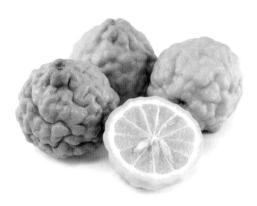

Bergamot

Citrus bergamia

Family: Rutaceae (citrus)
Origins: Southern Italy at the tip of "The Boot." Also grown in the Ivory Coast of western Africa.
Other names: Bergamot orange. Do not confuse with the herb by the same name: bergamot or bee balm (Monarda didyma).
Description: A small semi-tropical citrus tree, 4.5 meters high, that produces a small yellow fruit resembling a pear.
Extraction: Expressed
Botanical Part Used: The rind or peel of the nearly ripe citrus fruit
Principal constituents: about 300 compounds, mainly linalyl acetate (30-60%), linalool (11-22%), and other alcohols, sesquiterpenes, terpenes, alkanes, and furocoumarins (including bergapten, the phototoxic ingredient).

🌀 BLENDING SUGGESTIONS

- Relative strength: 2
- Among the top notes that typically make up less than 20% of the blend
- Blends well with: cypress, helichrysum, patchouli, frankincense, balsam fir, eucalyptus radiata, Roman chamomile, juniper, eucalyptus globulus, geranium, lavender, lemon, and ylang ylang
- Description: fruity, floral, citrusy, sweet, uplifting, lively, and fresh

📖 HISTORY & TRADITIONAL USES

Legend has it that Christopher Columbus brought the oil to Bergamo, Italy (in Lombardy in northern Italy) from the Canary Islands. It has been used extensively in traditional Italian medicine and throughout the Middle East, especially for oily skin conditions and fever. It gave its distinctive flavor to Earl Grey Tea and was an ingredient in the genuine eau de cologne. It is widely used in many food and beverage categories as a flavoring.

➕ USE & HEALTH BENEFIT

- To calm anxiety and nervous exhaustion, take a hot bath with 10 to 15 drops of bergamot in a cup of Epsom Salts ++P. Also works to stimulate digestion, settle the stomach, relieve gas, and improve appetite +++L.

- To calm inflammation of joints, muscles, organs, nerves, etc.; take an aromatic bath with 10 to 15 drops of bergamot mixed in a cup of Epsom Salts or massage afflicted area with a 50:50 blend of bergamot with carrier oil +++P.

- To help heal wounds apply undiluted to the wound or around it +++L.

- As a digestive stimulant, take a drop in your drinking water +++L.

- To help expel intestinal worms and parasites, take a 50:50 capsule of a bergamot/carrier oil blend daily with food.

- Apply a drop to each application of a mild stick or crystal deodorant.

- Lick a trace off the back of your hand as a mouthwash.

- To help lower a fever, take a warm (not hot) bath with 10 to 15 drops of bergamot in a cup of Epsom Salts.

- For treating depression and anxiety, diffuse 20 drops +++P ++++L.

- For stress, anxiety, agitation, and insomnia, diffuse 20 drops or put a few drops on a cotton ball inside your pillow case ++P ++++L.

- For inflammatory conditions of the organs, muscles and joints, especially for urinary tract infections, massage the afflicted area with a 50:50 blend of bergamot with a carrier oil. ++P

- For cold sores, use undiluted with eucalyptus radiata on the sore.

- Use a drop in drinking water or juice to enhance immunity or overcome colds, flu, fever, and other infections.

- To clear up acne and eczema, mix 20 drops 8 oz. of a mild cleanser or a couple of drops in each application. +++L

- To help with dandruff, use 20 drops in 8 oz. of shampoo and conditioner or a couple of drops in each application. Also mix with water and apply to scalp +++L.

- To help with a sore throat, mouth infections, or bad breath, lick a trace off your hand and distribute it around your mouth.

> CAUTIONS: None when used in quantities indicated. Phototoxic. Where it has been used topically, do not expose skin to direct sunlight for 12 to 24 hours.

✔ CLINICAL SUPPORT

Vogley, S. diffused bergamot essential oil in a psychiatric unit for the elderly noting enhanced communication, improved sleep (with a cotton ball with 2 drops of bergamot in the pillow case) and lowered agitation, depression, and anxiety (Vogley, 2002).

Bergamot has an anti-nociceptive effect on the central nervous system. This is a reduction in pain sensitivity. (Adorjan, B and Buchbauer, G. 2010).

"The antiseptic properties of Bergamot, allied to its really delicious fragrance, make it my first choice for treating acne, oily skins and all infected skin conditions" (Davis, p. 52). But do not expose the skin to direct sunlight for 24 hours after application because the bergapten, which increases the skin's sensitivity to sunlight and makes the skin more likely to burn.

Massage of the hands with the essential oils of bergamot, lavender, and frankincense had a helpful effect on pain and depression in hospice patients (Dobetsberger, C. and Buchbauer, G., 2011).

Bergamot essential oil released exocytotic and other chemicals in the hippocampus with evidence of neuroprotection in the case of pain. This supports the use of bergamot in treating symptoms of cancer pain, mood disorders, and stress-induced anxiety (Dobetsberger, C. and Buchbauer, G. 2011).

Singles

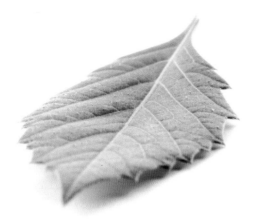

Birch

Betula lenta

Family: Betulaceae
Origins: Native to northern hemisphere of Europe and Asia
Other names: European white birch, silver birch
Description: A tall, decorative tree with white bark and light green oval leaves.
Extraction: Essential oil by steam distillation
Botanical Part Used: Wood
Principal constituents: Esters (99%), mainly methyl salicylate. Chemically almost identical to wintergreen, but from a completely different plant.
Odor type (doesn't blend well with anything, not listed)

🖌 BLENDING SUGGESTIONS

- Relative strength: 4
- Among the base notes that typically make up less than 30% of the blend
- Blends well with: Other woody and balsamic oils like juniper, cedar, pine, copaiba, balsam fir, and wintergreen as well as basil, bergamot, geranium, lavender, lemongrass, marjoram, and peppermint
- Description: Piercing, balsamic, sweet, sharp, and fresh

📖 HISTORY & TRADITIONAL USES

In Scandinavia and Russia birch twigs are bundled for use in saunas for promoting healthy skin. Preparations from the buds, leaves, and bark have been used for rheumatic and arthritic conditions. American Indians and early settlers enjoyed tea flavored with birch bark and wintergreen. This may have evolved into a preference for distinctively American "root beer" flavorings, chewing gum, and toothpaste.

➕ USE & HEALTH BENEFIT

- Relieve muscle and joint pain in rheumatoid and osteoarthritis using a 25:75 blend of birch and carrier oil for massage. Add a damp cloth covered by a dry towel and either heat or cool for a compress. Take a warm aromatic bath with 10 to 15 drops of birch in a cup of Epsom Salts. ++++L

- Patricia Davis suggests that birch is an ideal oil for muscle pain because it has powerful pain-relieving properties but at the same time is not very "hot" on the skin. "In rheumatism and arthritis it helps to drain the toxins which are the cause of pain" (Davis, p. 53). Apply undiluted on small, painful joints like fingers, wrists, and ankles but blend when applying to knees, elbows, shoulders, hips, etc.

- For tendonitis and tennis elbow, apply undiluted to affected area. +++P

- To relieve muscle cramps apply a 25:75 blend of birch and carrier oil. +++P

- To detoxify, release excess fluids, and increase urine flow (diuretic) and to help with urinary tract infections or kidney infections, use diluted 25:75 birch and carrier oil in massage or with a damp cloth compress with a dry towel and heat ++++L. An aromatic bath with 10 to 15 drops in a cup of Epsom Salts will help as well +++L.

- For mild skin conditions like acne, eczema, and skin ulcers, apply in 3 drops in a single application of a lotion, a liniment (water-based dilution), or 25:75 blend with carrier oil. Action similar to cortisone because of its methyl salicylate.

- For urinary tract infections, reducing a fever, lymphatic drainage, swollen legs and ankles (edema), gout, gallstones, kidney stones, ulcers, and bone pain; apply topically in a massage blend (25:75 birch to carrier oil) over area of concern. Also helps release accumulated toxins and increase circulation.

- Diffuse 20 drops to fill the room with its penetrating, elevating aroma.

> CAUTIONS: None when used in quantities indicated. Avoid during pregnancy. Avoid if you have epilepsy. Do not ingest. Do not use on children under 2 years of age. Do not use on the neck or chest of children under age 12. When topically applied it may increase blood-thinning effects. Do not overuse, especially on sensitive skin.

✅ CLINICAL SUPPORT

Patricia Davis says birch is her first choice for tendon inflammation "through overuse—usually due to repetitive tasks" (Davis, p. 54). She also has seen birch give dramatic results in treating cellulite when other treatments have failed (Davis, p. 53).

Bacterial infection with organisms resistant to antibiotics have increased during the last few decades worldwide. The authors tested essential oils from the stem, leaves and fruits of the four different birch species to microbial studies and found that they all had significant antimicrobial activity (Junor GO, et al., 2007)

Birch is safe when used according to instructions. Some books on essential oil safety recommend avoiding oils that contain methyl salicylate like wintergreen and birch. Methyl salicylate is closely related to acetylsalicylic acid or common aspirin.

Ron Guba notes that methyl salicylate is found in many common and popular over-the-counter creams for sprains that have a warming/cooling action. It is also abundantly used in candies and chewing gum. He suggests that 10 ml of wintergreen in a carrier oil massage at 2.4% dilution would give someone approximately 250 mg of methyl salicylate, roughly the equivalent of one aspirin tablet. Since only half that amount would be absorbed in a massage, it would be no more dangerous than rubbing half an aspirin on the body. Nevertheless, he warns against overuse or extended use of wintergreen for full-body massage if you are taking warfarin or any anticoagulant therapy (Guba R., "Toxicity Myths", p. 37-49).

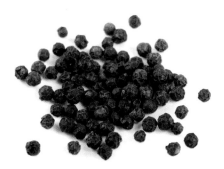

Black Pepper

Piper nigrum

Family: Piperaceae
Origins: Produced mainly in the tropics of Malaysia, China, Madagascar, Indonesia, India. Distilled in Europe and America.
Other names: Piper, pepper, Black peppercorn
Description: A woody vine with heart-shaped leaves and white flowers. It can climb 20 feet high. Berries turn from red to black peppercorns as they ripen.
Extraction: Essential oil by steam distillation

Botanical Part Used: Ripe peppercorns
Principal constituents: Mainly monoterpenes (70-80%): thujene, pinene, camphene, sabinene, carene, myrcene, limonene, phellandrene, & sesquiterpenes

BLENDING SUGGESTIONS

- Relative strength: 3
- Among the middle notes that typically make up more than 50% of the blend, but Black Pepper should be in small amounts in a blend.
- Blends well with: Frankincense, sandalwood, lavender, rosemary, marjoram, and other spice oils. Blends well with florals but only in tiny amounts.
- Description: spicy, peppery, musky, and warm.

HISTORY & TRADITIONAL USES

Used for both culinary and medicinal purposes in the East for over 4,000 years. Attila the Hun is reported to have asked for 3,000 pounds of black pepper as part of his ransom for the city of Rome (Davis, p. 246). Mendicant monks, who travel great distances each day on foot, maintain that their endurance is enhanced by taking 7 to 9 grains of pepper daily. The oil is used extensively in food preparation as well as in alcoholic beverages.

USE & HEALTH BENEFIT

- For stimulating the digestive glands, massage abdomen with a 50:50 blend of black pepper with a carrier oil +++P.

- To stimulate circulation, massage the afflicted area with a 50:50 blend of black pepper with a carrier oil.

- For toothache pain, apply to the gums around the afflicted tooth +++P.

- To break up and increase the flow of mucous allowing the lungs to clear, massage the chest and throat with a 50:50 blend with carrier oil.

- To stimulate the appetite and help overcome nausea, use a tiny amount of its warm spicy scent in a recipe.

- To improve circulation and give relief to aching muscles and joints, neuralgia, arthritis, stiffness, and sprains; use in a massage oil blended 50:50 with a carrier oil +++L.

- For chilblains (painful, itching inflammation of hands and feet brought on by cold temperatures or poor circulation), apply diluted 50:50 with carrier oil for massage.

> CAUTIONS: None when used in quantities indicated. Can redden sensitive skin when used in larger quantities, so use in moderation and in dilution.

CLINICAL SUPPORT

Piper nigrum, including its volatile oil, has demonstrated significant physiological benefits in preventing chronic ailments. It shows significant promise in improving cognitive brain functioning, boosting nutrient's absorption, and improving gastrointestinal functionality (Butt MS et al. 2013).

Essential oil of Piper nigrum shows strong antioxidant activity (Kapoor IP et al, 2009).

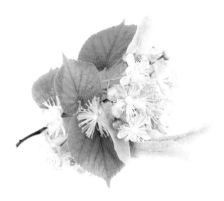

CAJEPUT

Melaleuca leucadendronL. Var cajuputi

Family: Myrtaceae
Origins: Grows wild throughout tropical Southeast Asia
Other names: White tea tree, white wood, swamp tea tree, punk tree, paperbark tree. Melaleuca leucadendron L. Var cajuputi and Melaleuca cajeputii are the same.
Description: A tall evergreen with spongy, flaky white bark, white flowers, and thick pointed leaves. It is in the same family as eucalyptus and tea tree.
Extraction: Essential oil by steam distillation
Botanical Part Used: fresh leaves, buds, and twigs
Blends well with: Juniper, peppermint, eucalyptus, and wintergreen.
Principal constituents: Cineol (65%), terpineol, terpinyl acetate, pinene, nerolidol, and others
Aromatic characteristics: Top note (5 – 20% of the blend). Scent medicinal, somewhat woody: Intensity: 3

BLENDING SUGGESTIONS

- Relative strength: 3
- Among the top notes that typically make up less than 20% of the blend.
- Blends well with: Juniper, peppermint, eucalyptus, and wintergreen.
- Description: medicinal, woody, camphoric, and penetrating.

HISTORY & TRADITIONAL USES

Used traditionally throughout East Asia for colds, headache, throat infections, toothache, aching muscles, fever, rheumatism, and various skin disorders. Also used in dentistry as an antiseptic. Used in throat lozenges and gargles. Its fragrance is used in soaps, detergents, cosmetics, and perfumes. It is occasionally used in flavoring foods and soft drinks.

USE & HEALTH BENEFIT

- For prevention and overcoming respiratory conditions of all types (asthma, bronchitis, excess mucous, coughs, sinusitis, and sore throat), diffuse 20 drops twice daily and apply a 50:50 cajeput/carrier oil blend topically on the chest and feet +++++L +++P.

- For respiratory, digestive, and antimicrobial benefits, create an aromatic bath using 10 to 15 drops of oil in a cup of Epsom Salts +++++L.

- For varicose veins and hemorrhoids, apply topically in 20:80 dilution cajeput/carrier oil ++P.

- To prevent or ease spasms of the muscles, digestive system, respiratory system (bronchial spasms), etc. (antispasmodic) apply a 50:50 blend of cajeput/carrier oil to the spasm area +++++L.

- Cajeput has some mild pain-relieving properties when topically applied in a 50:50 blend of cajeput/carrier oil.

- Massage to help cleanse and tone the urinary tract and digestive system, apply a 50:50 blend of cajeput/carrier oil to the lower abdomen.

Singles

- For radiation protection dilute 50:50 with carrier oil and apply topically ++P.

- For insect bites, oily skin conditions, and age spots; apply undiluted or 5 drops diluted in a teaspoon of water.

- For arthritis, muscle aches and pains, and rheumatism, apply in a 50:50 dilution with carrier oil +++L.

- For earache, apply three drops undiluted around the outer ear ++++L. Never put an essential oil into the ear canal.

- For urinary tract infections, apply topically in 50:50 dilution with carrier oil ++++L.

> CAUTIONS: None when used in quantities indicated. May be a skin irritant if you use too large a quantity undiluted on too large an area. Do not use if pregnant.

✔ CLINICAL SUPPORT

Cajeput is an effective antibiotic for topical application in modern medical practice (Jedlickova Z et al, 1992).

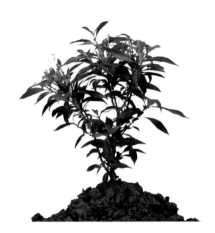

Camphor

Cinnamomum camphora

Family: Lauraceae
Origins: The camphor laurel is grown in Asia, particularly in Sumatra, Borneo, and Taiwan.
Other names: ravintsara, hon-sho, camphor laurel, gum camphor, Japanese camphor, Formosa camphor
Description: A tall evergreen similar in shape to a Linden. Clustered white flowers become red berries. The wood of trees over 50 years old produces the crude camphor, a white crystalline substance.
Extraction: Steam distillation
Botanical Part Used: Wood, root stumps, and branches
Principal constituents: Mainly cineol with pinene, terpineol, and others.

🌿 BLENDING SUGGESTIONS

- Relative strength: 4
- Among the middle notes that typically make up 50% of the blend or more, though camphor would only be a small part of any blend.
- Blends well with: peppermint, Eucalyptus radiata, Eucalyptus globulus, wintergreen, juniper, and rosemary.
- Description: camphoric, medicinal, woody, and penetrating.

📖 HISTORY & TRADITIONAL USES

Used traditionally to prevent infectious disease. A lump of the resin would be worn around the neck for protection. Used for nervous and respiratory diseases as well as heart failure. It is used as a solvent in the paint and lacquer industry. Used as masking agents in detergents, soaps, disinfectants, and other household products.

➕ USE & HEALTH BENEFIT

- For all types of infections—bacterial, fungal, and viral—apply undiluted to small areas (wrists, ears, etc.) and diluted 50:50 camphor/carrier oil to larger areas (shoulder, abdomen, etc.) +++P.

- For all types of respiratory conditions, create a 50:50 dilution and apply topically to the chest for its warming, stimulating, anti-inflammatory action.

- For physical exhaustion, bronchitis, chills, coughs, colds, fever, flu, and other infectious diseases, disperse 10 to 15 drops in a hot Epsom Salt bath ++P.

- For skin infections, skin inflammation, acne, age spots, and insect repellent, use topically in a 50:50 dilution camphor/carrier oil.

- For arthritis, muscle aches/pains, rheumatism, and sprains; apply topically in a 50:50 blend with carrier oil.

> CAUTIONS: None when used in quantities indicated. Some camphor chemotypes should not be used during pregnancy or on young children.

✔ CLINICAL SUPPORT

"Camphor exhibits a number of biological properties such as insecticidal, antimicrobial, antiviral, anticoccidial, anti-nociceptive, anticancer and antitussive activities, in addition to its use as a skin penetration enhancer" (Chen W. et al. 2013).

Julia Lawless recommends camphor for "acne, inflammation, oily conditions, spots; also for insect prevention (flies, moths, etc.)" (Lawless, p. 69).

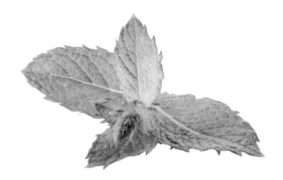

Chinese Spearmint

Menta spicata

Family: Lamiaceae (Labiatae)
Origins: Native to Mediterranean regions and throughout Europe, western Asia, and the Middle East. It is grown in the USA, Hungary, Spain, Yugoslavia, Russia, and China.
Other names: common spearmint, garden spearmint, lamb mint, pea mint, fish mint, spire mint, green mint
Description: A hardy perennial herb with green, lance-shaped toothed leaves. Spreads through underground runners. Lilac-colored or pink flowers in spikes.
Extraction: Essential oil by steam distillation
Botanical Part Used: Flowering tops
Principal constituents: Ll-carvone (50-70%), dihydrocarvone, phellandrene, limonene, and others.
Aromatic characteristics: Top note (5– 20% of the blend). Scent: minty, slightly fruity, lighter than peppermint: Intensity: 3

BLENDING SUGGESTIONS

- Relative strength: 3
- Among the top notes that typically make up less than 20% of the blend.
- Blends well with: lavender, lavandin, Eucalyptus radiata, Eucalyptus gobulus, basil, rosemary, and peppermint
- Description: minty, slightly fruity, lighter and more mild than peppermint

HISTORY & TRADITIONAL USES

Valued worldwide as a culinary herb. Used by the Greeks to scent their bath water. The infusion (tea) has been used for centuries to help with excess mucous, colic, nausea, indigestion, and gas. Applied topically, has been used to relieve headaches and as a cleansing agent for the skin of small children. It is used extensively in flavorings and fragrances.

USE & HEALTH BENEFIT

- To help with upset stomach, nausea, colic, fever, and food poisoning, create a mild spearmint tea with a little stevia or honey. Adjust the amount to create a pleasing flavor. Don't make it too strong, especially for children. Children respond better to mild flavoring. Their taste buds are more sensitive than an adult's, and if you use too much, they may come to dislike using essential oils entirely.

- As a fragrant antiseptic for household use, use 10 to 20 drops of essential oil in a few drops of mild household detergent. Mix with whatever amount of water you need for your project. See section under "Household Uses" in the "How to Use Essential Oils" chapter for more details.

- To prevent bronchial spasms, diffuse 20 drops and use a 50:50 spearmint/carrier oil blend for chest massage. Use on the abdomen to calm digestion and avoid spasms of the colon. Massage the blend on muscles to prevent muscle spasms +++L.

- To prevent and ease headaches and migraines, diffuse and massage the neck, temples, sinus, and jaw-joint areas of the face. +++L

- To lower a high fever and decongest and relax the respiratory system and digestive system, take an aromatic bath with 10 to 15 drops of spearmint in a cup of Epsom Salts ++L. This will also help symptoms of urinary tract infections.

- To decongest the sinuses +++L, ease coughing spasms, help with asthma symptoms, clear the bronchioles, and bring up excess mucous from the lungs +++L, diffuse and massage the sinus areas of the face, the neck, and the chest with a few undiluted drops of spearmint.

- To soothe your nerves +++L, relieve depression ++++L, and calm digestion ++++L, take a trace in an herbal tea or water using it in the same ways as peppermint.

- For acne, dermatitis, and congested skin conditions, mix 3 to 5 drops in a teaspoon of water and apply topically +++L.

- To calm the nerves and the digestive system, diffuse 20 drops +++L.

- To helps with scar formation, apply spearmint undiluted on a wound ++P.

- For calming respiratory conditions, digestive conditions, skin infections, and lowering fevers, make up capsules at 50:50 dilution with carrier oil and take for 3 times daily with food. This also helps in liver cleansing, especially when you include massage +++L.

- For all the digestive-calming functions listed here, use daily in drinking water, herbal teas, and recipes. +++L

- For respiratory relief from bronchitis, sinusitis, laryngitis, or simply a cold, put a few drops in a pan or bowl of hot water and breathe the aromatic steam. Reheat the water and add additional drops of oil as needed. You can increase the action by putting a towel over your head as you inhale the steam.

- For fatigue, headache, migraines, nervous strain, nervous exhaustion, and stress, apply topically on temples, back of neck, under nose, and on the outer ear +++L. Use as an antidepressant ++++L.

CAUTIONS: None when used in quantities indicated. Do not use on the necks and throats of babies and children under 12 years old.

 CLINICAL SUPPORT

Spearmint should be an ingredient in a blend targeting irritable bowel syndrome (Thompson A et al. 2013).

Spearmint and peppermint essential oils are effective and affordable alternatives for treatment of nausea associated with chemotherapy (Tayarani-Najaran Z, et al. 2013).

Spearmint essential oil significantly retards biofilm formation that can contribute to the development of treatments for preventing cavities (Rasooli I, et al. 2009).

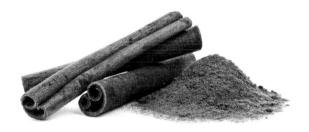

Cinnamon

Cinnamomum zeylanicum

Family: Lauraceae

Origins: Native to Sri Lanka, Madagascar, and Indochina. It is also grown in Jamaica, India, and Africa

Other names: Ceylon cinnamon, Seychelles cinnamon, Madagascar cinnamon, true cinnamon, cinnamon bark oil. Cinnamomum zeylanicum is the same as Connamomum verum. Zeylanicum merely refers to the fact that it is grown in Ceylon.

Description: a tropical evergreen with strong branches and thick bark. It has shiny leathery leaves and small white flowers that become blue-white berries. Leaves give off a spicy smell when crushed.

Extraction: Steam distilled essential oil

Botanical Part Used: Inner bark

Principal constituents: Aldehydes: trans-cinnamaldehyde (greater than 50%), hydroxycinnamaldehyde, benzaldehyde, cuminal; Phenols (up to 30%): eugenol (greater than 30%) and others.

 BLENDING SUGGESTIONS

- Relative strength: 5
- Among the base notes that typically make up less than 30% of the blend
- Blends well with: all citrus oils, cypress, frankincense, geranium, juniper, lavender, rosemary, and all spicy oils
- Description: spicy, warm, and sweet

📖 HISTORY & TRADITIONAL USES

The inner bark of new shoots is gathered every two years and sold as sticks for use as a culinary spice. It has been used for millennia for colds, flu, digestive and menstrual problems, rheumatism, and kidney complaints. Used in many food flavorings, especially in alcoholic and soft drink beverages, including Coca-Cola. Its fragrance and therapeutic actions are prized in toothpastes, nasal sprays, mouthwashes, cough syrups, and dental products.

➕ USE & HEALTH BENEFIT

- Because of its strong antimicrobial action and its familiar flavor, cinnamon will be a popular ingredient in many Protecting blends. It is typically too irritating to use undiluted on the skin, but in a blend or in a dilution with carrier oil, it becomes a powerful agent against infectious disease.

- To help overcome diarrhea, as a poison antidote, an anti-parasitic, an antiviral, an antibacterial, an antifungal, and to keep things from decaying, use cinnamon's a broad spectrum of antimicrobial action in foods, drinks, and capsules as well as topical massage blends +++P.

- To relieve a sore throat and get rid of bad breath take a trace of a blend containing cinnamon on the tongue and distribute it around the mouth ++++P.

- For urinary tract infection take a capsule containing cinnamon as a small percentage (less than 20%) 3 times daily with food ++P.

- To soothe inflammation of the small and large intestines, take a small amount in capsule (less than 20%) ++++P.

- To stimulate circulation, metabolism, and digestive action, massage the area of concern with a blend containing cinnamon (less than 10%).

- To energize and warm muscles for a workout or for warmth in healing, apply a blend with cinnamon as a minor ingredient (less than 20%).

- To disinfect the air and create a festive, spicy, holiday atmosphere, blend cinnamon (less than 20%) with various citrus oils and diffuse 20 drops of the blend.

- To warm and calm the digestive system, ease painful menstruation, improve circulation, and stimulate the appetite, take a trace of cinnamon in juice, herbal tea, or water.

CAUTIONS: None when used in quantities indicated. Do not apply to the skin of children under 5 years of age. It will be a skin irritant if it is applied undiluted or in too strong a concentration. Do not use as a single oil during pregnancy. Do not apply as a single oil, even diluted, directly to the mucous membranes. May have some minor blood thinning properties when taken with aspirin and blood pressure medications. May enhance the efficiency of antibiotics.

✅ CLINICAL SUPPORT

Cinnamon oil, lemongrass oil, cedarwood oil, clove oil and eucalyptus oil exhibit antibacterial property against S. mutans (Chaudhari, et al. 2012).

Aromatherapy with a blend of cinnamon, clove, rose, and lavender oil is effective in alleviating menstrual pain, its duration and excessive menstrual bleeding (Marzouk TM et al. 2013).

Cinnamon and clove, if taken together, can increase sleep times (Dobetsberger, C. and Buchbauer, G., 2011).

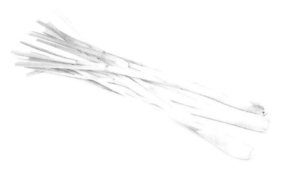

Citronella

Cymbopogon winterianus

Family: Poaceae (Gramineae)
Origins: Native to Java
Other names: Java citronella, Lenabatu citronella. Cymbopogon nardus and Cymbopogon winteriana
Description: Tall aromatic perennial grass
Extraction: Essential oil by steam distillation
Botanical Part Used: fresh and dried grass
Principal constituents: Mainly geraniol, citronellal with geranyl acetate, limonene, and camphene with monoterpene hydrocarbons.

BLENDING SUGGESTIONS

- Relative strength: 3
- Among the top notes that typically make up less than 20% of the blend.
- Blends well with: geranium, lemon, bergamot, orange pine and cedarwood
- Description: Citrus-like, slightly fruity, fresh, sweet

HISTORY & TRADITIONAL USES

Used for its aromatic and medicinal value in many cultures for fever, intestinal parasites, digestive and menstrual problems. It was used for rheumatic pain in Chinese medicine. It is used extensively as a fragrance in soaps, detergents, and industrial perfumes. It's a major ingredient in insect repellent and disinfectant products for home and garden.

It is used as a flavoring in most major food categories including alcoholic and soft drinks.

USE & HEALTH BENEFIT

- As an antiseptic and deodorant to cleanse the air, use 20 drops in a diffuser +++L ++P.

- For sanitizing and purifying, add 10 to 20 drops to household cleaning products ++++L ++P. See more instructions in the "How to Use Essential Oils" chapter.

- For a digestive stimulant and an antispasmodic to help with colitis, create a 50:50 citronella and carrier oil blend and massage the abdomen ++L.

- Use as an insect repellent both topically and in diffusion +++++L. Dilute 5 drops in a teaspoon of water and apply or blend 5 drops in a teaspoon of carrier oil and apply.

- To help with oily skin and excessive perspiration, add a drop or two to each application of skin care products, deodorants, and lotions. You can also add about 20 drops to an 8 oz. bottle of lotion.

- To strengthen immunity and prevent minor infections during cold and flu season, diffuse 20 drops at a time.

- To overcome headaches, migraines, and fatigue, diffuse 20 drops at a time.

- To ease neuralgia pain apply 5 drops of citronella in a teaspoon of carrier oil.

- To ease the inflammation of rheumatism apply 5 drops of citronella in a teaspoon of carrier oil+++P

CAUTIONS: None when used in quantities indicated. Avoid during pregnancy.

✔ CLINICAL SUPPORT

Locally delivered 2% lemongrass essential oil gel offers a new choice of safe and effective adjunct to scaling and root planing in periodontal therapy (Warad SB, et al., 2013).

Both Sweet Basil and Lemongrass are effective insect repellents against 3 types of mosquitos for approximately 2 hours of protection (Phasomkusolsil S, Soonwera M., 2010).

Citronella, clove, and geranium essential oils exhibited significant activity reducing the presence/quantity of important Candida albicans virulence factors (Budzyńska A, et al. 2014).

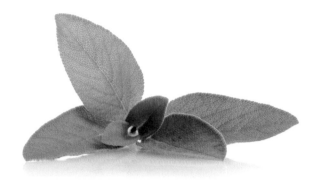

Clary Sage
Salvia sclarea

Family: Lamiaceae (Labiatae)
Origins: Southern Europe. Now cultivated worldwide, especially in the Mediterranean regions, Russia, the USA, England, Morocco, and central Europe.
Other names: clary, clary wort, muscatel sage, clear eye, see bright, common clary, clarry, and eyebright
Description: A sturdy biennial or perennial herb about 3 feet tall with hairy leaves and small blue flowers.
Extraction: Essential oil by steam distillation
Botanical Part Used: flowering tops and leaves
Principal constituents: Linalyl acetate (up to 75%), linalool, pinene, myrcene, and others.

🌀 BLENDING SUGGESTIONS

- Relative strength: 3
- Among the middle to base notes that typically make up more than 80% of the blend (middle notes 50% and base notes 30%).
- Blends well with: sandalwood, bergamot, cedarwood, cypress, juniper, and citrus oils.
- Description: herbal, spicy, sharp, warm, and camphoric.

HISTORY & TRADITIONAL USES

Used widely in the Middle Ages for digestive disorders, kidney disease, menstrual issues, and as a nerve tonic. An extract from the seeds was used for removing dust from the eyes. It cools inflammation and is used for respiratory infections. It is also used as a fragrance in soaps, detergents, cosmetics, and perfumes. It is used in food and beverage flavoring.

USE & HEALTH BENEFIT

- As a skin conditioner for wrinkles, aged skin, acne, boils, dandruff, hair loss, inflammations, oily skin & hair, apply a drop with each application of a hair care product or lotion. Add 3 drops to a teaspoon of water and apply to your skin +++L. Avoid putting an essential oil into the eyes. Apply 6 drops into a green clay masque.

- For high blood pressure, muscle aches and pains, create an aromatic bath with 10 to 15 drops of clary sage in a cup of Epsom Salts.

- For asthma, throat infections, or whooping cough, create an aromatic bath with 10 to 15 drops of clary sage in a cup of Epsom Salts.

- For colic, cramps, dyspepsia, and gas, take an aromatic bath with 10 to 15 drops of aromatic oils including clary sage mixed in a cup of Epsom Salts. Also apply a 50:50 blend of clary sage and a carrier oil over the abdomen.

- For painful menstruation or to help encourage regular menses, apply a 50:50 blend with a carrier oil to the lower abdomen. ++++L. Create an aromatic bath with 10 to 15 drops of clary sage in a cup of Epsom Salts.

- For depression ++++L, postnatal depression ++++L, migraines, nervous tension, and stress ++L; diffuse 20 drops of aromatic essential oils with clary sage as an ingredient.

- For circulatory issues: hemorrhoids, varicose veins, etc., apply a 50:50 blend of clary sage and a carrier oil.

> CAUTIONS: None when used in quantities indicated. Avoid during pregnancy. Do not use while drinking alcohol because it can promote a narcotic effect and amplify drunkenness.

CLINICAL SUPPORT

This small pilot study evaluated the effect of a topical application of the essential oils of lavender and clary sage on work-related stress of nurses in an ICU setting. Results demonstrated decreased perception of stress level in the intervention group during three 12-hour worked shifts (Pemberton E, Turpin PG., 2008).

The purpose of the study was to screen aromatic essential oils for antidepressant effects. The test studied chamomile, rosemary, lavender, and clary sage. Clary sage essential oil showed the strongest antidepressant action. It could be developed as a therapeutic agent for patients with depression (Seol GH, et al., 2010).

Singles

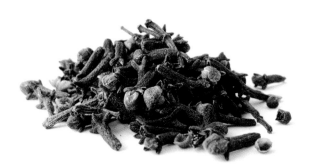

Clove

Syzgium aromaticum

Family: Myrtaceae
Origins: Native to Indonesia but cultivated worldwide especially in the Philippines and Madagascar.
Other names: Clove bud
Description: Slender evergreen with smooth grey trunk. Each rainy season long buds appear that become pink crowns at the tip. As they fade to deep red, they are taken from the tree and dried to become clove buds.
Extraction: Water distillation
Botanical Part Used: clove bud
Principal constituents: Eugenol (60 – 90%) eugenyl acetate, caryophyllene and other constituents.

🖐 BLENDING SUGGESTIONS

- Relative strength: 5
- Clove can be part of the middle notes, which make up about 50% of the blend or it can be part of the base notes, which make up less than 30% of the blend.
- Blends well with: vanilla, bergamot, lavender, lavandin, and ylang ylang
- Description: Citrus like, slightly fruity, fresh, sweet

📖 HISTORY & TRADITIONAL USES

Tradition has it that those who traded in spices like clove, cinnamon and other aromatics used in leather tanning, fragrancing, and other fragrant trades were more likely to be immune to the devastating plagues of the 15th century. Clove has been used as a pain killer in dental applications for many years. In addition to its popularity as a culinary spice, clove is a major flavoring agent in foods and drinks. It is also included as a fragrance in soaps, household products, and cosmetics.

➕ USE & HEALTH BENEFIT

- As a stimulant and antiseptic to help prevent respiratory conditions, use a small amount (less than 20% in a blend for diffusing +++++L.

- To reduce both muscle and joint pain through topical application, massage the area with a 25:75 blend of clove with a carrier oil +++++L.

- To energize and stimulate the digestive system, take a trace of clove in an herbal tea ++++L.

- To disinfect apply a diluted blend (25:75 clove/carrier oil) +++L.

- To enliven the senses and improve memory, diffuse a tiny amount of clove in a blend of other oils (20 drops at a time) ++++L.

- To help with acne, athlete's foot, or as an insect repellent, mix a drop of clove with a teaspoon of water or a water-based lotion.

- To help with bruises, cuts, infections, and wounds, use topically in a 25:75 blend with carrier oil.

- To help ease the pain of a toothache, apply a little clove oil undiluted to the gum of the tooth.

- To help with circulation, muscles and joint soreness, arthritis, rheumatism, and sprains, apply a 25:75 blend with carrier oil +++++L. This is a warming action. For a softer, cooling action use peppermint or a more calming oil like Roman chamomile or lavender.

- For asthma and bronchitis use a small amount of clove oil in an antimicrobial respiratory massage blend ++++L. For a single application, mix a drop or two in your hand with about a teaspoon of carrier oil.

- To help with nausea and painful digestion, take a capsule that includes a little clove as an ingredient (less than 20%) ++++L.

- To help build immunity to colds, flu, and minor infections, apply over lung areas in a 25:75 blend with carrier oil ++++L. Use this blend as a foot massage during cold and flu season.

> CAUTIONS: None when used in quantities indicated. Undiluted it can cause skin and mucous membrane irritation. Use in dilution for all topical applications. Avoid during pregnancy and lactation. Use caution when using with aspirin or blood-thinning medications because it thins the blood slightly. It may enhance the efficiency of antibiotics.

✔ CLINICAL SUPPORT

Clove oil, cinnamon oil, lemongrass oil, cedarwood oil, and eucalyptus oil exhibit antibacterial properties against S. mutans (Chaudhari, et al. 2012).

Clove, citronella, and geranium essential oils exhibited significant activity reducing the presence/quantity of important Candida albicans virulence factors (Budzyńska A, et al. 2014).

Cinnamon and clove, if taken together, can increase sleep times (Dobetsberger, C. and Buchbauer, G., 2011).

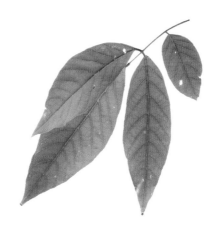

Copaiba
Copaifera officinalis

Family: Fabaceae (Leguminosae)
Origins: Northeast and central South America
Other names: Copaiba balsam, copahu balsam, copaiva, Jesuit's balsam, maracaibo balsam, para balsam. Copaifera langsdorffii and Copaifera officinalis are both copaiba.
Description: Wild, tropical tree with many branches and thick foliage.
Extraction: Essential oil by dry distillation
Botanical Part Used: Resinous balsam extracted from the trunk of the tree
Principal constituents: Mainly sesqueterpines and caryophyllene

🌿 BLENDING SUGGESTIONS

- Relative strength: 3
- Among the middle notes that typically make up more than 50% of the blend.
- Blends well with: lavandin, cedarwood, ylang ylang, and vanilla.
- Description: Soft, sweet, balsamic

📖 HISTORY & TRADITIONAL USES

Used in Europe for centuries to treat chronic urinary tract infections and bronchitis as well as chronic diarrhea and other intestinal problems

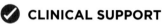

⊕ USE & HEALTH BENEFIT

- To release excess body fluids and flush toxins (diuretic), take in a 50:50 blend of copaiba and a carrier oil in capsules or gently massage swollen legs with the blend.

- To help bring up mucous from deep in the lungs (expectorant), diffuse 20 drops twice daily.

- To help dissolve and release mucous, put 5 drops in a bowl or pan of boiling water, cover head and inhale deeply. Reheat the water and add more drops of copaiba as needed.

- To help stimulate digestive, pancreatic, and liver functions, take a 50:50 capsule daily with food.

- To decrease inflammation in any area of the body (muscles, joints, bronchioles, skin, organs, etc.), take a copaiba capsule with a 50:50 blend of copaiba and carrier oil. Also massage the affected area of the body with the same blend +++P.

- For a bactericidal or antiseptic scalp treatment, add 20 drops of peppermint per 8 oz. of lotion, shampoos, or conditioners. Or, add one or two drops to each application.

- For a urinary tract infection take a copaiba capsule with a 50:50 blend of copaiba and carrier oil. Also massage the affected area of the body with the same blend +++P.

- To help clear up bronchial inflammation and decrease excessive respiratory mucous, massage sinus areas, under cheek bones, and neck with undiluted copaiba ++P.

- On small wounds and sores apply copaiba undiluted +P.

- To help clear up acne, mix with a mild skin cleanser

CAUTIONS: None when used in quantities indicated. Excessive doses may cause vomiting and diarrhea. If pregnant or under the care of a physician for a serious condition, consult your medical practitioner before use.

✔ CLINICAL SUPPORT

Copaiba oil is being considered as a viable alternative for treating a bacterial disease that destroys beehives—American foulbrood disease (Santos R.C. et al., 2012).

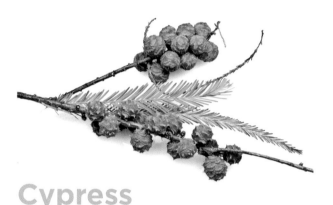

Cypress

Cupressus sempervirens

Family: Cupressaceae
Origins: Europe
Other names: Italian cypress, Mediterranean cypress
Description: Tall conical evergreen with small flowers and round brown-grey cones (nuts). Extraction: Essential oil by steam distillation
Botanical Part Used: needles and twigs
Principal constituents: Pinene, camphene, sylvestrene, cymene, carene and others

🌀 BLENDING SUGGESTIONS

- Relative strength: 3
- Among the middle notes that typically make up more than 50% of the blend.
- Blends well with: bergamot, clary sage, lavender, lemon, orange, and sandalwood.

- Description: fresh, herbaceous, slightly woody with evergreen undertones.

📖 HISTORY & TRADITIONAL USES

Ancient civilizations valued extracts from the cypress tree for medicine and for burning as incense. Chinese medicine uses the nuts of the cypress tree for liver and respiratory health and to stop excessive perspiration. It is also used as a fragrance in colognes, after shaves, & perfumes.

➕ USE & HEALTH BENEFIT

- To decrease colitis spasms, take a cypress capsule with a 50:50 blend of cypress and carrier oil. Also massage the affected area of the body with the same blend. ++P

- To help children stop bed wetting, apply a few drops of cypress in a carrier oil at the base of the spine two or three times a day for 20 days. If the child is at least 8 years old and can swallow a capsule, mix cypress 50:50 with a carrier oil, use a dropper to fill capsules, and have the child take a capsule 3 times a day ++P.

- Create a deodorizing foot massage oil to use daily by mixing cypress with carrier oil 50:50. ++++L

- To create an energizing and warming compress for any afflicted area, apply cypress undiluted to the area then cover with a warm damp cloth, cover that with a dry cloth and heat. ++++L

- To help with water retention (edema), massage legs with a 50:50 dilution of cypress with carrier oil. +++++L

- For oily skin mix 20 drops of cypress into 8 oz. of mild facial lotion or cream and apply 2 to 3 times daily.

- For a fragrant insect repellent, mix 5 drops of cypress with a teaspoon of water and apply to skin and clothing.

- To improve circulation in muscles and joints, decrease excessive perspiration, treat varicose veins, help with oily skin, decrease muscle cramps, control edema (swollen legs from fluid retention), and rheumatism, massage with a 50:50 blend of cypress with carrier oil.

- To relieve hemorrhoids, and help heal wounds a 50:50 blend of cypress with carrier oil.

- To help with respiratory conditions: asthma, bronchitis, and spasmodic coughing, diffuse 20 drops and massage the chest and throat with a 50:50 blend of cypress and carrier oil. +++L

- To ease painful menstruation and other menopausal problems, massage lower abdomen with a 50:50 cypress blend with a carrier oil.

- To calm nervous tension and stress, breathe the fragrant aroma of cypress in a tissue or handkerchief.

- To relieve varicose veins, apply cypress undiluted very gently—never massaging. It can also be blended with a cream or a 50:50 cypress and carrier oil blend, but be sure to apply it gently in the direction of the heart.

- To help control excessive perspiration, place a few drops of cypress in a few drops of water, rub palms together and apply to underarms. Men will also enjoy using cypress in this way as an aftershave for its woody, masculine aroma.

- Because of its antispasmodic action, it can be used diluted on the chest for treating asthma. You can also use a few drops on a tissue or handkerchief and inhale to help with an asthma attack. This may also be helpful for bronchitis, coughing spasms, and whooping cough.

- To control excessive foot perspiration, use cypress 50:50 with carrier oil for a foot massage or put 10 drops 1/2 cup Epsom Salts in a warm footbath.

- Patricia Davis suggests that cypress be applied topically to regulate excessive menstrual flow, especially in the early stages of menopause (Davis, p. 92).

> CAUTIONS: None when used in quantities indicated. Has some blood thinning properties. Use caution when taking aspirin or blood thinning medications.

 CLINICAL SUPPORT

Cypress oil possesses antioxidant and antiglycation properties that may be useful in the prevention of diabetic and cardiovascular complications (Asgary S. et al., 2013).

This study evaluated cypress essential oil and its ability to inhibit population growth of human cancer cells. Cypress oil exerted the highest cytotoxic activity against renal adenocarcinoma cells. The study also provided evidence on how cytotoxic activity of the oils is not always related to their major constituents (Loizzo MR. et al., 2008).

The essential oil of cypress leaves was studied for its antimicrobial activity against certain bacteria and fungi. Our results revealed that Cypress oil possesses significant antibacterial and antifungal properties (Manivannan R et al., 2005).

Cypress oil can be used to remedy the memory-lowering effect of using volatile solvents (Dobetsberger, C. and Buchbauer, G., 2011).

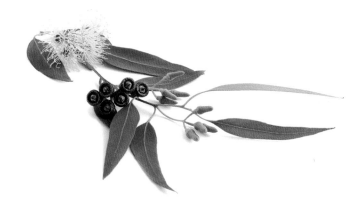

Eucalyptus Globulus
Eucalyptus globulus

Family: Myrtaceae
Origins: Native to Australia, cultivated in Spain, Portugal, Brazil, California, Russia & China
Other names: Blue gum eucalyptus, There are over 700 species of eucalyptus
Description: A tall evergreen with blue-green oval leaves. Creamy-white flowers and pale grey bark covered in a white power.
Extraction: essential oil by steam distillation
Botanical Part Used: fresh or partly-dried leaves and twigs
Blends well with: thyme, rosemary, eucalyptus radiate, lavender, marjoram, cedarwood, and lemon
Principal constituents: Cineol (70-85%), pinene, limonene, cymene, phellandrene, terpinene, aromadendrene, and others

 BLENDING SUGGESTIONS

- Relative strength: 5
- Among the top notes that typically make up no more than 20% of the blend.
- Blends well with: thyme, rosemary, Eucalyptus radiata, lavender, marjoram, cedarwood, and lemon
- Description: fresh, medicinal, slightly woody, earthy, evergreen

📖 HISTORY & TRADITIONAL USES

An Australian household remedy for respiratory illnesses like bronchitis and croup. The dried leaves of eucalyptus trees were smoked like tobacco for asthma. It has also been used for all kinds of fevers: malaria, typhoid, cholera, etc. It has been used for burns, boils, and wounds. Eucalyptus remedies have also been used for aching joints, bacterial dysentery, ringworms, and tuberculosis. It is used commercially in liniments, inhalants, cough syrups, ointments, toothpaste, veterinary, and dentistry products. It's also used in soaps, detergents, and toiletries. It is used as a flavor in many major food categories.

➕ USE & HEALTH BENEFIT

- To ease the pain of headaches, aching muscles, neuralgia, and rheumatism, mix 10 to 15 drops in a cup of Epsom Salts and soak in a hot aromatic bath.

- To decongest and help release mucous from deep in the lungs, and help with other respiratory issues (asthma, bronchitis +++P, excess phlegm (catarrh), coughs, sinusitis, and throat infections), massage lung area of chest and back with a 50:50 blend of E. globulus and carrier oil. Also apply to sinus areas of the face, under cheek bone, and around outer ears twice daily +++P +++++L.

- For a topical yeast infection, mix 2 to 5 drops of E. globulus in a teaspoon of water and apply to the affected area.

- To help relieve urinary tract infections, apply a 50:50 blend of E. globulus with a carrier oil to the lower abdomen++++L.

- To disinfect burns, blisters, cuts, scrapes, herpes infections (cold sores), insect bites, skin infections, and wounds, apply undiluted to the affected area ++++L.

- For an insect repellent, apply a 3 - 4 drops in a few drops of water and apply.

- To ease muscle aches and pains, increase circulation, relieve the pain of rheumatoid arthritis, and help to heal sprains; massage a 50:50 blend of E. globulus with a carrier oil on the affected area.

- For lymph node infections, massage a 50:50 blend of E. globulus with a carrier oil on the affected area. +P

- To help with a urinary tract infection and other infectious diseases: chicken pox, colds, epidemics, flu, and measles, massage a 50:50 blend of eucalyptus and carrier oil on the affected area twice daily ++++L.

- To relieve headaches massage the neck and shoulders with E globulus undiluted or diluted 50:50 with carrier oil.

- To relieve painful neuralgia, massage afflicted area with a 50:50 blend of E. globulus with a carrier oil.

> CAUTIONS: None when used in quantities indicated. Do not diffuse; use Eucalyptus radiata instead. Do not use if you have an epileptic condition.

✔️ CLINICAL SUPPORT

Eucalyptus oil, cinnamon oil, lemongrass oil, cedarwood oil, clove oil and exhibit antibacterial property against S. mutans (Chaudhari, et al. 2012).

Essential oils (EO) possess antimicrobial, anti-inflammatory, insect repellent, anti-cancer, and antioxidant properties. This study evaluated lemon, cypress, Eucalyptus globulus, and thyme. Thyme showed the best free-radical scavenging capacity. Thyme was also the most effective against lipid peroxidation along with lemon. Lemon demonstrated the best chelating power. Thyme showed the best anti-proliferative activity (Aazza S, et al. 2014).

Eucalyptus globulus, tea tree, and thyme have antiviral capacity against Herpes simplex virus. As whole oils they are more effective than their component parts and act in a dose-dependent manner. Tea tree shows promise in the treatment of influenza (Adorjan, B and Buchbauer, G., 2010).

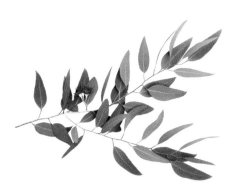

Eucalyptus Radiata

Eucalyptus radiata

Family: Myrtaceae
Origins: Australia
Other names: peppermint eucalyptus, fourth river peppermint eucalyptus, narrow-leaved peppermint eucalyptus. There are over 700 species of eucalyptus.
Description: A tall evergreen with blue-green narrow leaves and gray-brown bark that comes off in long strips. Summer flowers are creamy yellow.
Extraction: Essential oil by steam distillation
Botanical Part Used: leaves
Principal constituents: Oxides: 1,8 cineol (62-72%), caryoppyllene oxide; monoterpenes (up to 24%): alpha & beta pinenes , limonene, myrcene, p-cymene, alcohols and others

🍶 BLENDING SUGGESTIONS

- Relative strength: 3
- Among the middle notes that typically make up more than 50% of the blend.
- Blends well with: basil, geranium, lavender, lemon, rosemary, and sandalwood
- Description: slightly camphoric, sweet, and fruity, milder than E. globulus

📖 HISTORY & TRADITIONAL USES

Australian household remedy for respiratory illnesses and fevers like malaria, typhoid, cholera. Used for skin problems like burns, ringworms, skin infections, and wounds. Used commercially in liniments, inhalants, cough syrups, ointments, toothpaste, veterinary and dentistry. Used in soaps, detergents & toiletries. Used as a flavor in many major food categories.

➕ USE & HEALTH BENEFIT

- Safe to apply topically on children in a 50:50 ratio with a carrier oil.

- For cold sores (herpes simplex) and acne, apply topically with bergamot undiluted.

- For ear infections, apply undiluted around the outer ear +++P. Never put an essential oil down the ear canal.

- To reduce inflammation of the mucous membranes in the respiratory system, diffuse 20 drops twice daily. This also helps with hay fever.

- For calming nerves, diffuse 20 drops.

- To relieve pain of endometriosis and vaginitis, create a 50:50 blend of E. radiata with carrier oil and massage lower abdomen.

- For all respiratory conditions diffuse 20 drops of E. radiata. Avoid using eucalyptus globulus in a diffuser. It could actually promote coughing spasms. E. radiata is more mild and a more pleasant, aromatic oil for diffusing.

- To clear out excess hardened mucous in lungs, bronchioles, vocal chords, and sinuses, put 5 drops of E. radiata into a pan or bowl of boiling water. Cover head with a towel and inhale. Reheat the water and add more drops of oil as you desire. Blow into the water to release more aromatic steam. Re-heat the water and add more drops of oil as needed ++++P. Eucalyptus is exceptional for respiratory conditions because it reduces mucous and is anti-inflammatory, so it helps with bronchitis, sinusitis, and laryngitis. It also helps loosen and release mucous from deep in the lungs.

- To decongest and help release mucous from deep in the lungs, and help with other respiratory issues (asthma, bronchitis +++P, excess phlegm (catarrh), coughs +++P, sinusitis, and throat infections), massage lung area of chest and back with a 50:50 blend of E. globulus and carrier oil. Also apply to sinus areas of the face, under cheekbone, and around outer ears twice daily. +++P

- To ease the pain of headaches, aching muscles, neuralgia, and rheumatism, mix 10 to 15 drops in a cup of Epsom Salts and soak in a hot aromatic bath.

- For a topical yeast infection (candida), mix 2 to 5 drops of Eucalyptus radiata in a teaspoon of water and apply to the affected area.

- To help heal wounds apply undiluted to affected area.

- For an insect repellent, apply a 3 - 4 drops in a few drops of water and apply.

- To help with a urinary tract infection and other infectious diseases: chicken pox, colds, epidemics, flu, and measles, massage a 50:50 blend of eucalyptus and carrier oil on the affected area twice daily.

CAUTIONS: None when used in quantities indicated. Do not use if you have epilepsy. Use caution when ingesting if you are taking aspirin or blood pressure medications. It may have mild blood-thinning properties. Do not ingest.

✔ CLINICAL SUPPORT

Eucalyptus radiata and tea tree were found to be effective against Herpes simplex virus infections. (Schnitzler et al., pp. 343-7).

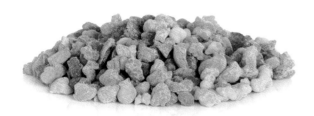

Frankincense

Boswellia carterii

Family: Burseraceae
Origins: A native to the Red Sea region of the Middle East. Grows throughout north east Africa—mainly Somalia and Ethiopia. It is also grown in China and distilled in Europe and India.
Description: A small shrub that yields a resin that is collected by making cuts in the bark. The milky liquid solidifies into a solid amber gum that is distilled for the essential oil or burned for incense.
Extraction: Essential oil by steam distillation
Botanical Part Used: Oleo gum resin
Principal constituents: Mainly monoterpene hydrocarbons, pinene, dipentene, limonene, thujene and others.

🌿 BLENDING SUGGESTIONS

- Relative strength: 3
- Among the bass notes that typically make up no more than 30% of the blend.
- Blends well with: sandalwood, vetiver, geranium, lavender, orange bergamot, sweet basil, black pepper, cinnamon, and other spices.
- Description: rich, deep, warm, balsamic, sweet, incense-like

📖 HISTORY & TRADITIONAL USES

Used from antiquity as an incense for burning in religious rituals and therapeutic treatments. In ancient Egypt it was an ingredient in cosmetics and perfumes. It has been used both in the east and the west for rheumatism, syphilis, respiratory conditions, urinary tract infections, digestive and nervous conditions. The gum is commonly used in soaps, cosmetics, and perfumes, especially in oriental spices and men's fragrances.

➕ USE & HEALTH BENEFIT

- To help control inflammation in the skin, organs, joints, and muscles, massage a 50:50 blend of frankincense and carrier oil on the areas of concern.

- To help speed up healing, apply frankincense undiluted to cuts, scrapes, and minor wounds +P.

- Helps ease painful menstruation and strengthen the uterus massage a 50:50 blend of frankincense and carrier oil on the lower abdomen.

- To help overcome insomnia apply 6 drops to a tissue, handkerchief, or cotton ball and inhale. You can put the cotton ball or handkerchief inside a pillowcase to help relaxation and restful sleep. Diffuse 20 drops of frankincense before bed.

- For skin conditions such as rashes, acne, psoriasis, or eczema, create a compress using green clay and a few drops of frankincense (possibly mixed with lavender) and hold it in place with a cling bandage. You can also use this for a facial masque.

- For blemished skin use a drop of frankincense in each application of a skin care lotion or cream. This also helps diminish wrinkles in dry, mature skin. Frankincense is safe enough to use undiluted within 1/2 inch of the eyes. It is both antiseptic and astringent ++++L.

- To reduce scarring use frankincense undiluted on wounds ++++L.

- To help calm an upset stomach, reduce gas, and overcome nausea, apply 6 drops to a tissue, handkerchief, or cotton ball and inhale. The aromatics can be kept in a plastic bag and used throughout the day.

- To clear out excess hardened mucous in lungs, bronchioles, vocal chords, and sinuses, put 5 drops of frankincense into a pan or bowl of boiling water. Cover head with a towel and inhale. Reheat the water and add more drops of oil as you desire. Blow into the water to release more aromatic steam. Re-heat the water and add more drops of oil as needed+++P. Frankincense also helps loosen and release mucous from deep in the lungs ++P.

- To decongest and help release mucous from deep in the lungs, and help with other respiratory issues (asthma ++P, bronchitis +++P, excess phlegm (catarrh), coughs +++P, sinusitis, and throat infections), massage lung area of chest and back with a 50:50 blend of frankincense and carrier oil. Also apply to sinus areas of the face, under cheek bone, and around outer ears twice daily ++P.

- For viral infections (colds and flu), take in a capsule in a 50:50 blend with carrier oil +++P.

- For a minor eye infection, create a weak compress with a tablespoon of warm salt water and 3 drops of Frankincense, soak a gauze pad in the mixture, squeeze out the excess water, and place it over the eye. The aromatic effect will help with the infection. Do not drop essential oils even in dilution directly in the eyes +++P.

- To stimulate and strengthen the immune system, take a capsule with a 50:50 blend of frankincense with carrier oil once a day with food +++P.

- Diffuse for depression ++P, anxiety, nervous tension, and stress +++++L. It has the remarkable ability to slow down the rate of breathing, which is useful for meditation and prayer.

- For painful menstruation and urinary tract infections, mix 50:50 with a carrier oil for a wonderful massage oil for the lower abdomen.

- Apply daily in a foot massage blend for all the therapeutic actions listed here and many more.

> CAUTIONS: None when used in quantities indicated. When taking both topically and orally, it may interfere with enzyme action in metabolizing medications.

 CLINICAL SUPPORT

Massage of the hands with the essential oils of bergamot, lavender, and frankincense had a helpful effect on pain and depression in hospice patients (Dobetsberger, C. and Buchbauer, G., 2011).

Frankincense as a night cream
Instead of using the expensive night cream I used to use, I now use a drop of frankincense in a couple of drops of carrier oil every night after I wash my face. It works so much better and keeps my face feeling healthy and moisturized.

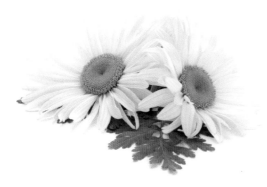

German Chamomile
MatAricaria recutita

Family: Asteraceae (Compositae)
Origins: A native to Europe and Northwest Asia. Also grown in North America and Australia. Most of the production today comes from Hungary and Eastern Europe.
Other species: German chamomile, pineapple weed, maroc chamomile
Description: An annual aromatic plant with small, delicate, daisy-like flowers.
Extraction: Essential oil by steam distillation. The oil is dark blue in color.
Botanical Part Used: Flowers
Principal constituents: Chamazulene, farnesene, bisabolol oxide, and others
Fruity, herbal, warm sweet

 BLENDING SUGGESTIONS

Relative strength: 3
Among the middle notes that typically make up more than 50% of the blend.
Blends well with: bergamot, neroli, and lavender
Description: fruity and herbal

 HISTORY & TRADITIONAL USES

Used historically for all kinds of nervous conditions and stress-related illnesses such as digestive upset, tension headaches, and sleep-inducing.

➕ **USE & HEALTH BENEFIT**

- As mild yet effective pain reliever for earache, toothache, and teething pain, apply undiluted around the outer ear and to the gum of the painful tooth. ++++L

- To ease allergic reactions, take a capsule with a 50:50 blend of German chamomile and a carrier oil once daily with food.

- To reduce inflammation of the skin, lungs, organs, muscles, and joints, apply undiluted or in a 50:50 dilution with a carrier oil over the afflicted area +++++L.

- For sensitive skin blend 20 drops into 8 ounces of a non-fragranced lotion or crème or a single drop per application. German chamomile is exceptionally mild yet wonderfully effective. ++++L

- To settle the digestive system (carminative) and reduce gas, take in a capsule 50:50 with a carrier oil 3 times a day with food. Or you can apply this blend topically over the stomach and abdomen. It will also be helpful to diffuse 20 drops of the oil ++++L.

- To reduce spasms of the digestive system, the muscles, the nerves, etc., take in a capsule 50:50 with a carrier oil 3 times a day with food. Or you can apply this blend topically over the afflicted area. It may also be helpful to diffuse 20 drops of the oil ++++L.

- For antibacterial and antifungal functions against infections like candida and strep throat, take German chamomile in a capsule 50:50 with a carrier oil 3 times a day with food. Lick a trace off your hand and distribute it to the affected area if it is in the mouth or throat. Apply an undiluted drop topically ++++L.

- To help the healing process, apply undiluted to the wound.

- To calm and cool a fever, take a warm (not hot) bath with 10 to 15 drops of German chamomile mixed in a cup of Epsom Salts.

- To help stimulate digestive and strengthen liver functions, take a 50:50 capsule of German chamomile with a carrier oil daily with food. This is also important in cleansing the liver and stimulating white blood cell production ++++L.

- To help stimulate the release of toxins through perspiration take a hot bath with 10 to 15 drops of German chamomile mixed in a cup of Epsom Salts. Helps cleanse the liver ++++L.

- For help in calming tantrums and anger, apply 6 drops on a cotton ball, tissue, or handkerchief and inhale. The cotton ball can also be put in a pillow case or pinned to the collar of pajamas ++++L. German chamomile is especially mild yet effective for use in therapy for children. It is calming without being depressing.

- To help eliminate intestinal worms, take a 50:50 capsule of German chamomile with a carrier oil daily with food.

- To calm painful menstruation, excessive menstrual flow, and symptoms of menopause; take a 50:50 blend with carrier oil in a capsule once a day with food. Or you can apply this blend topically over the stomach and abdomen twice daily ++++L.

- Use topically undiluted for skin care: acne, allergies, abscesses, boils ++++L, burns, cuts, chilblains, dermatitis, eczema +++L, scalp inflammation, insect bites, rashes, and sensitive skin.

- For arthritis, inflamed joints, muscle pain, neuralgia, rheumatism, and sprains, massage with lotion or carrier oil in a 50:50 dilution ++++L.

- To help with nausea and colic++++L, indigestion, and gas; massage a 50:50 blend of chamomile with a carrier oil on lower abdomen.

- To help with headache, insomnia, nervous tension, migraines, and stress, diffuse 20 drops and apply topically (undiluted) to the face, temples, and back of neck ++++L.

CAUTIONS: None when used in quantities indicated. May cause dermal sensitivity in some highly sensitive people. When taking both topically and orally, it may interfere with enzyme action in metabolizing medications. When taking diabetic medications, it may cause slight hypoglycemic effects when taken orally. When taken orally, it may have some blood-thinning effects.

✅ CLINICAL SUPPORT

German chamomile may be effective against pain and fluid retention (edema) in various inflammatory conditions. (Tomić M. et al. 2014).

German Chamomile was effective against Herpes simplex virus 2 and 1 by interrupting adsorption (Adorjan, B and Buchbauer, G., 2010).

Gastric diseases are increasing and becoming resistant to antibiotics. This study revealed that German chamomile and 3 other essential oils provided a safe antibacterial alternative to resistant strains of bacteria (Cwikla C. et al., 2010).

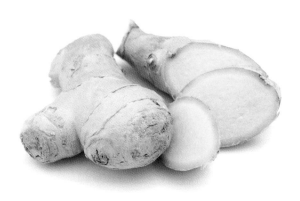

Ginger
Zingiber officinale

Family: Zingiberaceae
Origins: Native to southern Asia but cultivated in tropical areas of Nigeria, the West Indies, India, China, Jamaica, and Japan. The oil is distilled in the UK, China, and India.
Other names: Common ginger, Jamaica ginger
Description: A perennial herb with a tuberous rhizome root and a green, reed-like stalk with white or yellow flowers.
Extraction: Essential oil produced by steam distillation
Botanical Part Used: Root
Principal constituents: Gingerin, gingenol, gingerone, zingiberine, camphene, phellandrene and others.

🔄 BLENDING SUGGESTIONS

Relative strength: 4
Among the middle notes that typically make up more than 50% of the blend.
Blends well with sandalwood, vetiver, patchouli, frankincense, lime, neroli, orange, and other citrus oils.
Description: Sweet, spicy, woody, fresh, and sharp.

📖 HISTORY & TRADITIONAL USES

Has been used as a domestic spice and remedy for numerous conditions for thousands of years, especially in the East. In China it has been used for rheumatism, dysentery, toothache, malaria and many cold and moist conditions. It is best known as a digestive aid. It is currently used in cosmetics and perfumes, especially Oriental and male fragrances. It is extensively used in virtually all food categories including alcoholic and soft drinks.

➕ USE & HEALTH BENEFIT

- To increase circulation and ease the pain around muscles and joints with a warming action, apply a 50:50 blend with a carrier oil to the afflicted area. Or you can apply the oil undiluted if it is a small area like fingers and wrists. This will help with arthritis, muscle fatigue, muscle aches and pains, poor circulation, rheumatism sprains, and strains ++P.

- May have some minor aphrodisiac effects when applied topically in a 50:50 blend with a carrier oil. Apply to lower back. Do not apply to genitals +++P.

- For digestive relief from diarrhea, bloating, colic, cramps, flatulence, indigestion, loss of appetite, nausea, and travel sickness, apply 6 drops to a tissue, handkerchief, or cotton ball and inhale deeply. The oil can also be taken by mixing a drop in a teaspoon of honey +++P.

- To strengthen the system and relieve chills, fever, and other symptoms of colds, flu, or other infectious diseases, take capsule in a 50:50 blend with a carrier oil. Take a capsule as needed up to 3 times a day. You can also apply a 50:50 blend of the oil with a carrier oil to the chest, neck, sinus area, around ears, and to the abdomen.

- Take for nausea in pregnancy and for digestive relief from diarrhea, bloating, colic, cramps, flatulence, indigestion, loss of appetite, and travel sickness; apply 6 drops to a tissue, handkerchief, or cotton ball and inhale deeply. The oil can also be taken by a drop in honey +++P.

> CAUTIONS: None when used in quantities indicated. May be skin sensitive in some people and have some minor photosensitizing properties. After applying topically, avoid direct sunlight exposure for 12 hours. When taken orally with aspirin or blood thinners, it may have some blood-thinning effects.

 CLINICAL SUPPORT

In an animal study, ginger essential oil was able to consistently reduce the gastric ulcer in the stomach as seen from the ulcer index and histopathology of the stomach. Moreover, oxidative stress produced by ethanol was found to be significantly reduced by ginger essential oil. (Liju VB, Jeena K, Kuttan R., 2014).

Ginger possesses significant liver protective properties against fatty liver disease in an in vivo animal study (Liu et al., 2013).

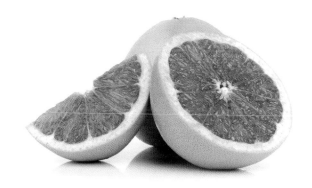

Grapefruit

Citrus paradisi

Family: Rutaceae
Origins: Native to tropical Asia and the West Indies. Now grown in California, Florida, Brazil, and Israel. The oil is mainly sourced in California from organic grapefruit.
Other name: shaddock (oil)
Description: A cultivated citrus tree with glossy leaves and large yellow fruit
Extraction: Cold expression
Botanical Part Used: Raw, fresh peel
Principal constituents: Limonene (90%), cadinene, paradisiol, neral, geraniol citronellal, sinensal, and others

 BLENDING SUGGESTIONS
Relative strength: 2
Among the top notes that typically make up less than 20% of the blend.
Blends well with lemon, bergamot, neroli, rosemary, frankincense, juniper, cedarwood, cypress, lavender, cinnamon, and clove
Description: Clean, fresh, citrusy, and a bit bitter.

 HISTORY & TRADITIONAL USES

Historically used for food, vitamin C, and protection against infectious diseases. Used as a fragrance in soaps, detergents, cosmetics, and perfumes. Used widely in desserts, alcoholic beverages, and soft drinks.

➕ USE & HEALTH BENEFIT

- To purify the air, diffuse 20 drops or mix 10 drops in 8 ounces of water, shake and spray to disinfect surfaces. ++P

- To detoxify, release swelling and water retention, stimulate stagnant lymph nodes, overcome cellulitis (swollen sore skin), and help with obesity, gently massage the areas of concern with a 50:50 blend of grapefruit and a carrier oil. +++++L

- To stimulate the digestive system to achieve more efficient metabolism and weight management, take a capsule containing a 50:50 blend of grapefruit and a carrier oil once daily with food.

- To stimulate healthy digestion, massage the abdomen with a 50:50 blend of grapefruit and a carrier oil. +++L You can also take an aromatic bath with 10 to 15 drops of grapefruit in a cup of Epsom Salts. Apply a few drops of grapefruit oil on cellulite or swollen areas while your skin is damp after a shower.

- To help with skin conditions such as acne, congested and oily skin, and hair growth, apply grapefruit (undiluted) topically or mixed with water for easier distribution.

- For exercise preparation, muscle fatigue, and stiffness, massage muscles and joints with a 50:50 blend of grapefruit and a carrier oil.

- To strengthen the immune system and prevent colds and flu, take a drop of grapefruit in 12 oz. of drinking water or herbal tea every day.

- For nervous system conditions: depression, stress headaches, nervous exhaustion, and performance stress, diffuse 20 drops of grapefruit twice a day.

CAUTIONS: *None when used in quantities indicated. When taken orally, it may interfere slightly with enzyme action in metabolizing medications. Somewhat photosensitizing: after applying topically, avoid direct sunlight exposure for 12 hours.*

✓ CLINICAL SUPPORT

Grapefruit oil inhibited the accumulation of triglycerides and efficiently inhibits adipogenesis (Haze et al., 2010).

Aromatherapy massage using grapefruit, cypress and other essential oils could be utilized as an effective intervention to reduce abdominal subcutaneous fat, waist circumference, and to improve body image in post-menopausal women (Kim HJ., 2007).

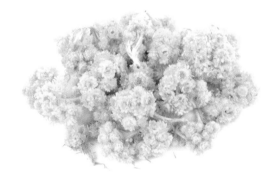

Helichrysum
Helichrysum angustifolium

Family: Asteraceae (Compositae)
Origins: Native to the Mediterranean area, especially eastern North Africa. Cultivated now in Italy, Yugoslavia, Spain, and France
Other names: Immortelle, everlasting, St. John's herb. Helichrysum italicum and Helichrysum angustifolium are the same.
Description: An aromatic herb with brightly colored daisy-like flowers that become dry as the plant matures, yet the dried flowers retain their bright color.

Extraction: Essential oil by steam distillation
Botanical Part Used: Fresh flowers and flowering tops
Principal constituents: Nerol and neryl acetate (30 – 50%), italiviones, geraniol, pinene, linalool, isovaleric aldehyde, sesquiterpenes, and others.

🥣 BLENDING SUGGESTIONS

Relative strength: 3
Among the middle notes that typically make up more than 50% of the blend.
Blends well with German and Roman chamomile, lavender, geranium, clove, and all citrus oils.
Description: Rich, sweet, honey-like, and fruity

📖 HISTORY & TRADITIONAL USES

Used in Europe for respiratory complaints like asthma, chronic bronchitis, headaches, migraine, liver diseases, skin conditions, burns, allergies, and psoriasis. Currently used as a fixative and fragrance component in soaps, cosmetics, and perfumes.

➕ USE & HEALTH BENEFIT

- To help in healing of tissue and especially nerves, apply undiluted to the wound or affected area. Nerves heal slowly so multiple applications over a period of time may prove useful.

- To help with tinnitus, apply undiluted to outer ear and areas around the ear, then pull on the ear in various directions to stimulate absorption. Multiple applications over time may result in significant improvement.

- For skin conditions of all kinds—acne, abscesses, allergic skin conditions, boils, burns, cuts, dermatitis, eczema, inflammation, spots, wounds, etc.—apply in a 50:50 blend with a carrier oil or undiluted directly on a small area. Also use in a facial masque with green clay ++++L.

- To help with conditions of the veins and capillaries such as phlebitis, pariphlebitis, rosacea, couperose, apply 3 drops of helichrysum diluted in a teaspoon of water or diluted 50:50 with a carrier oil to the afflicted area. If the area is small, an undiluted application is also fine. +++P If used on the face, a much higher 1:99 dilution should be used.

- To prevent or reduce a hematoma (a solid swelling of clotted blood), apply helichrysum (undiluted) ++++P. Helichrysum is the most powerful agent to use for a hematoma.

- For arthritis pain, muscle aches and pains, rheumatism, sprains, and strained muscles, massage with a 50:50 blend of helichrysum with a carrier oil +++P.

- For respiratory conditions: asthma, bronchitis, chronic cough, and whooping cough, massage respiratory areas of the body with a 50:50 blend of helichrysum and a carrier oil. ++P

- To help with liver and spleen congestion, take a capsule with a 50:50 blend of helichrysum and a carrier oil daily with food ++++L.

- To prevent bacterial infections: colds, flu, fevers, etc.; massage with a 50:50 blend of helichrysum and a carrier oil. Apply to the feet daily.

- To help depression, lethargy, nervous exhaustion, and other stress-related conditions, put 6 drops of helichrysum in a cotton ball, handkerchief, or tissue and inhale. You can also put a drop or

Singles

two in your palm, rub hands together,
place over nose and mouth and inhale
several times deeply.

- For the pain of neuralgia, massage area with 3
drops of helichrysum in a teaspoon of water or
a 50:50 blend of helichrysum and carrier oil.

CAUTIONS: None when used in quantities indicated.

 CLINICAL SUPPORT

Inhaling essential oils of peppermint, basil,
and helichrysum may reduce the perceived
level of mental fatigue/burnout (Varney
E, Buckle J., 2013).

"The essential oil of Helichrysum
italicum significantly reduces the multidrug
resistance of Enterobacter aerogenes,
Escherichia coli, Pseudomonas aeruginosa,
and Acinetobacter baumannii" (Lorenzi
et al., 2009).

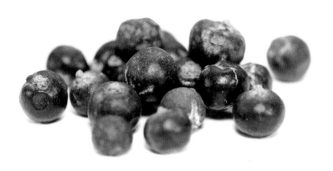

Juniper
Juniperus communis

Family: Cupressaceae
Origins: Grows throughout the northern
hemisphere in Asia, Europe, and North America.
The oil is produced mainly in Europe and Canada.
Other names: Common juniper
Description: An evergreen with narrow, stiff
blue-green needles. It has small flowers and
small, round berries.
Extraction: Essential oil created by steam
distillation
Botanical Part Used: Needles and berries
Principal constituents: Monoterpenes: pinene,
myrcene, sabinene with limonene, cymene,
terminene, thudene and others.

 BLENDING SUGGESTIONS

Relative strength: 3
Among the middle notes that typically make up
more than 50% of the blend.
Blends well with vetiver, sandalwood, cedarwood,
cypress, clary sage, pine, lavender, lavandin,
rosemary, and all citrus oils.
Description: sweet, woody, balsamic, fresh, and
turpentine-like.

 HISTORY & TRADITIONAL USES

Used traditionally for urinary tract infections,
respiratory infections, and digestive infections
and worms. Helps dispel uric acid in joints.
Also used for preventing ticks and fleas. Used
as a fragrance in soaps, detergents, cosmetics,

and perfumes, especially spicy ones. Used extensively in alcoholic and soft drinks as well as many food products.

⊕ USE & HEALTH BENEFIT

- To stimulate the liver and gallbladder, apply 3 to 5 drops in a teaspoon of carrier oil over the liver area (just below the rib cage) +++P. Also helps with infections of the liver and gallbladder ++P ++++L.

- To help relieve the pain and help prevent the formation of kidney stones, create an equal blend of cedarwood (25%), juniper (25%), and a carrier oil (50%). Massage to the kidney area of the back (just under the lowest ribs) 3 to 4 times a day +++P.

- To help with diabetes by stimulating the pancreas, mix 3 to 4 drops of juniper with a teaspoon of a carrier oil and apply it over the pancreas area of the abdomen ++P ++++L.

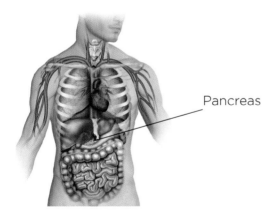

Pancreas

- For acne, eczema, and rashes apply 3 or 4 drops in a facial masque using green clay. You can also apply a 25:75 blend of juniper with a carrier oil to the affected areas and then cover with a damp cloth to help the oils penetrate. Just quickly mixing a few drops of juniper with water and applying topically is perhaps the simplest way to use the oil for skin conditions ++++L.

- To help relieve a urinary tract infection take an aromatic bath using 10 to 15 drops of juniper in a cup of Epsom Salts. You can also massage the lower abdomen with a 50:50 blend of juniper and a carrier oil. Add a hot, damp cloth to create a compress and then a dry towel and a hot water bottle or heating pad ++++L.

- To help relieve accumulation of uric acid creating gout and arthritic/rheumatic conditions, take an aromatic bath using 10 to 15 drops of juniper in a cup of Epsom Salts. You can also massage the painful area with a 25:75 blend of juniper and a carrier oil. Add a hot, damp cloth to create a compress and then a dry towel and a hot water bottle or heating pad +++++L.

- For hemorrhoids, mix a 25:75 blend of juniper with a carrier oil and apply to affected areas twice daily.

- For anxiety, nervous tension, and other stress-related conditions diffuse 20 drops of juniper twice daily. This will also help with colds, the flu, and other infections.

- For painful menstruation, prepare a compress by using a 50:50 blend of juniper with a carrier oil massaged on the abdomen. Then apply a damp, hot cloth. Cover it with a dry cloth and add a heating pad or hot water bottle.

> CAUTIONS: None when used in quantities indicated. If taking diuretics juniper may increase the activity.

✓ CLINICAL SUPPORT

This in vitro study of juniper essential oil demonstrated antibacterial and antifungal activity (Khoury M, 2014).

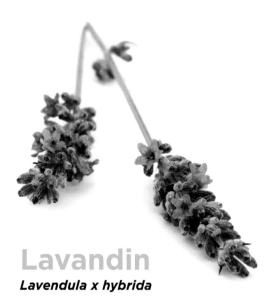

Lavandin

Lavendula x hybrida

Family: Lamiaceae (Labiatae)
Origins: Grows in the mountainous regions of southern France where parent plants grow wild. Now grown in Spain, Hungary, Yugoslavia, and Argentina.
Other names: bastard lavender
Description: A hybrid plant created by crossing true lavender (Lavendula angustifolia) with spike lavender (Lavendula latifolia). It is larger than true lavender with flowers that may be blue or grey.
Extraction: Essential oil by steam distillation
Botanical Part Used: Fresh flowering tops. It has a higher yield than true lavender.
Principal constituents: Linalyl acetate (30-32%), linalool, cineol, camphene, pinene and other constituents.

🜂 BLENDING SUGGESTIONS

Relative strength: 3
Among the top and middle notes that typically make up more than 70% of the blend (20% top notes and 50% middle notes).
Blends well with bergamot, clary sage, clove, cinnamon, citronella, cypress, thyme, patchouli, rosemary, and all citrus oils.
Description: Fresh, floral, sweet, and more herbal than lavender. Similar to true lavender but more penetrating and stimulating with a sharper scent.

📖 HISTORY & TRADITIONAL USES

This hybrid was created less than 60 years ago, so its history is only recent. It is used extensively in soaps, detergents, room sprays, hair preparations, and industrial perfumes. It is a flavor ingredient in many foods.

➕ USE & HEALTH BENEFIT

- To ease pain, help reduce infection (viral, bacterial, or fungal), and heal a minor wound, apply undiluted topically ++P.

- To calm, overcome shock, reduce stress, overcome depression, promote sleep, and overcome anxiety, emotional exhaustion, or restlessness, diffuse 20 drops of lavandin twice daily. Also apply undiluted topically to the solar plexus (just under the sternum on the chest) as well as the forehead, around the nose, and on the temples +++P.

- For an insect repellent disperse 20 drops of lavandin in a cup of water, shake, and spray areas you want to repel insects +++L.

- To calm convulsions and spasms of all kinds (muscle, digestion, respiratory, etc.), diffuse 20 drops of lavandin, massage with a 50:50 blend using lavandin and carrier oil, take an aromatic bath or foot soak with 10 to 15 drops of lavandin in a cup of Epsom Salts. ++P +++L

- Take advantage of its deodorant properties with a foot soak with 10 drops in 1/2 cup of Epsom Salts and a foot massage with a 50:50 blend with a carrier oil. You can also create a spray with 20 drops of lavandin in a cup of water for surface deodorizing or diffuse 20 drops to deodorize the air in a room. +++L

- For skin conditions: abscesses, acne, allergies, athlete's foot, boils, bruises, burns, dandruff, dermatitis, eczema, inflammations, insect bites and stings, insect repellent, lice, psoriasis, ringworm, scabies, sores, spots, sunburn, and minor wounds; apply undiluted to small areas or diluted 50:50 with a carrier oil to larger areas +++L.

- For an earache, apply lavandin undiluted on the outer ear.

- For lumbago, muscle aches and pains, rheumatism, and sprains, create a 50:50 massage blend of lavandin with a carrier oil, and apply to the afflicted area.

- For respiratory conditions: asthma, bronchitis +++P, excess mucous, bad breath, laryngitis, throat infections, and whooping cough; create a 50:50 massage blend of lavandin with a carrier oil, and apply to the afflicted area. You can also take a hot bath with 10 to 15 drops of lavender in a cup of Epsom Salts. Also diffuse 20 drops of lavandin twice daily +++L.

- For digestive issues: abdominal cramps, colic, gas, or nausea; take a 50:50 blend of lavandin and carrier oil in a capsule once a day with food. You can also massage a 50:50 dilution with a carrier oil onto the lower abdomen.

- To stimulate healthy menstruation or reduce menstrual pain, massage a 50:50 dilution with a carrier oil onto the lower abdomen.

- To decrease painful headaches, migraines, nervous tension, and stress related conditions, diffuse 20 drops of lavandin twice daily. Also use a 50:50 lavandin and carrier oil blend to massage face, forehead, back of neck, and back.

- To overcome shock or vertigo, diffuse 20 drops of lavandin twice daily. Also use a 50:50 lavandin and carrier oil blend to massage temples, forehead, and back of neck. Apply a cool, damp cloth over the lavandin to help it

penetrate. For use on the face dilute at a ratio of 5:95 lavandin with a carrier oil.

CAUTIONS: None when used in quantities indicated.

 CLINICAL SUPPORT

Preoperative anxiety is prevalent in surgical patients who may require anxiety medications, thus impacting preoperative teaching and patient satisfaction. This study demonstrated that lavandin is a simple, low-risk, cost-effective intervention with the potential to improve preoperative outcomes in decreasing anxiety and increasing patient satisfaction (Braden R, Reichow S, Halm MA., 2009).

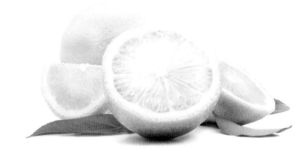

Lemon
Citrus limon

Family: Rutaceae
Origins: Native to Asia. Grows wild in the Mediterranean, especially in Spain and Portugal. Cultivated worldwide, especially in Italy, Sicily, Cyprus, Guinea, Israel, South and North America (California and Florida).
Other names: cedro oil
Description: Small evergreen tree with fragrant flowers and acidic yellow fruit.
Extraction: Cold expression

Botanical Part Used: outer part of the fresh peel of the fruit

Principal constituents: Limonene (about 70%) terpinene, pinenes, sabinene, myrcene, citral, linalool, geraniol, octanol, and others

🥣 BLENDING SUGGESTIONS

Relative strength: 3
Among the top notes that typically make up less than 20% of the blend.
Blends well with lavender, neroli, ylang ylang, sandalwood, Roman & German Chamomile, geranium, eucalyptus, juniper, lavandin, and all citrus oils.
Description: sweet, light, fresh, lemony, and fruity-floral

📖 HISTORY & TRADITIONAL USES

Juice and peel used in domestic food preparation. Fruit high in vitamins A, B, and C. Historically considered a "cure-all," especially for infectious diseases. Used for malaria and typhoid fevers. Important in curing scurvy. Juice is valuable for acidic disorders such as arthritis, rheumatism, dysentery, and liver congestion. Extensive use in flavorings many foods and drinks. An important fragrance in soaps, detergents, cosmetics, and perfumes.

➕ USE & HEALTH BENEFIT

- For skin conditions: acne, boils, chilblains, corns, cuts, oily skin, canker sores, insect bites, mouth ulcers, spots, varicose veins, and warts; apply undiluted to the small area +++P ++++L.

- For easing the symptoms of arthritis, cellulitis, obesity (fluid congestion), poor circulation, and rheumatism, create a 50:50 blend of lemon and a carrier oil and use for massage of the affected area +P ++++L.

- For high blood pressure, diffuse 20 drops of lemon twice daily +P ++++L.

- For a nosebleed, apply undiluted lemon oil followed by a cold, damp compress over the nose and another on the back of the neck.

- For respiratory conditions: asthma, throat infections, bronchitis, and excess mucous; take a blend of 50:50 lemon and carrier oil in a capsule 3 times a day with food. Put a drop of lemon oil in all your drinking water and herbal teas. Lick a trace of lemon oil off your hand and distribute it around your mouth to disinfect.

- For dyspepsia, nausea, and other digestive concerns, diffuse 20 drops of lemon, create an aromatic bath with 20 drops of lemon in a cup of Epsom Salts ++P ++++L.

- To strengthen the immune system to prevent colds, flu, fever, and infections, diffuse 20 drops of lemon oil twice daily +++++L.

- To help detoxify the liver, take a capsule of a lemon/carrier oil blend (50:50) twice a day with food.

- To help overcome nightmares and insomnia, diffuse 20 drops of lemon oil before bed and put 6 drops on a cotton ball or tissue inside your pillow case +P ++++L.

- To help overcome depression and anxiety, diffuse 20 drops of lemon oil. Take an aromatic bath with 10 to 15 drops of lemon in a cup of Epsom Salts. Massage the feet and hands with lemon oil (undiluted) ++++L.

- To disinfect the air in sick rooms, hospitals, and clinics, diffuse 20 drops of lemon 2 or 3 times daily. Also create a disinfectant spray with 10 drops of lemon in 8 ounces of water. Shake well and spray surfaces ++++L.

CLINICAL SUPPORT

Lemon oil could decrease both physical and psychological stress (Dobetsberger, C. and Buchbauer, 2011).

The results of this study suggest that lemon essential oil may suppress the growth of Acinetobacter species and could be a source of metabolites with antibacterial modifying activity (Guerra et al., 2012).

Numerous studies confirm that lemon oil exhibits a strong action against cancer cells including this study (Aazza. 2014).

Lemon capsules for a cold

My husband came down with a cold the other day and was concerned that it might progress into chronic bronchitis as it so often has in the past. He started making lemon capsules with 4 to 8 drops of lemon oil filled up with grapeseed carrier oil. He took four capsules before bed, and by morning the cold was gone without a trace. He kept taking a few capsules for a day or two just in case, and everything cleared right up. He also used lemon in his water for a few days after that just to be sure.

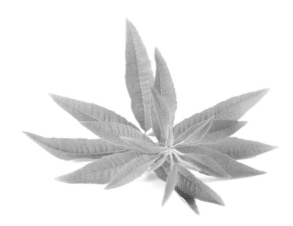

Lemon Verbena
Lippia citriodora

Family: Verbenaceae
Origins: Native of Chile and Argentina. Cultivated and found semi-wild in the Mediterranean regions of France, Tunisia, and Algeria—as well as Kenya and China. Oil mainly comes from South America and South Africa.
Other names: verbena, herb Louisa
Description: A perennial shrub that grows to 5 meters high. Small, pale green leaves and small light purple flowers. Often grown as an ornamental in gardens.
Extraction: Essential oil by steam distillation
Botanical Part Used: freshly harvested flowering stocks
Principal constituents: Mainly citral (30 – 45%) with limonene, myrcene, linalol, geraniol and others

 BLENDING SUGGESTIONS

Relative strength: 2
Among the top notes that typically make up less than 20% of the blend.
Blends well with neroli, lemon, and other citrus oils
Description: sweet, fresh, lemony, and fruity-floral

📖 HISTORY & TRADITIONAL USES

Used much like peppermint, spearmint, and neroli. Important for nervous conditions which manifest in poor digestion. Dried leaves are used for tea—refreshing, uplifting pick-me-up. Used for hangover. Used in perfumery and citrus fragrances. Eau de verveine is a popular related fragrance in Europe and America.

➕ USE & HEALTH BENEFIT

• Lemon verbena is a powerful sedative +++P. To help with insomnia, certain types of depression ++++P, nervous exhaustion, and the exhaustion associated with multiple sclerosis, massage feet and hands with a 50:50 blend of lemon verbena and a carrier oil. Also take an aromatic bath with 10 to 15 drops of lemon verbena in a cup of Epsom Salts. Diffusing 20 drops before bed will also help.

• To prevent or reduce a fever, take a warm (not hot) bath with 10 to 15 drops in a cup of Epsom Salts. Also apply lemon verbena undiluted to the fevered area of the body and apply a damp cool cloth over the oil.

• To stimulate the action of various organs (gallbladder, thyroid, pancreas, etc.), apply a 50:50 blend of lemon verbena with carrier oil over the area of concern.

• Lemon verbena is a powerful anti-inflammatory oil +++P. For inflammation of the small and large intestines ++P, Crohn's disease ++P, diabetes, intestinal parasites, and other conditions involving inflammation, apply a 50:50 blend of lemon verbena and a carrier oil over the affected areas. You may also wish to take a capsule of the blend with food once a day. This therapy is also helpful for cramps, indigestion, and liver cleansing.

CAUTIONS: None when used in quantities indicated.

✅ CLINICAL SUPPORT

"The essential oil of lemon verbena produced a significant reduction of the parasitemia, 85.4% with the peak at a dose of 250 mg/kg. It was also observed a reduction in the number of amastigotes and inflammatory infiltrates in the heart. The creatine kinase-MB plasma levels also decreased at dpi 28 as a result of such treatment.... The essential oil of ... lemon verbena has in vivo anti-Trypanosoma cruzi effect in mice" (Rojas J, Palacios O, Ronceros S., 2012).

Helicobacter pylori is an important bacteria responsible for peptic ulcers in humans. Although using antibiotics often improves these diseases, resistance to the antibiotics is emerging. The antimicrobial effect of essential oils and the development of resistance to the essential oils were evaluated in vitro and in vivo. Lemongrass and lemon verbena were bactericidal against H. pylori. Resistance to lemongrass did not develop even after 10 sequential passages, whereas resistance to clarithromycin (an antibiotic) developed under the same conditions. In in vivo studies, the density of H. pylori in the stomach of mice treated with lemongrass was significantly reduced compared with untreated mice. These results demonstrate that the essential oils are bactericidal against H. pylori without the development of acquired resistance, suggestingthat essential oils may have potential as new and safe agents for inclusion in anti-H. pylori regimens (Ohno T, et al., 2003).

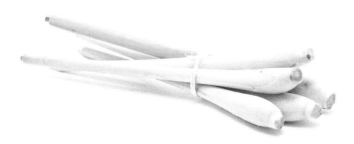

Lemongrass
Cymbopogon flexuosus

Family: Poaceae (Gramineae)
Origins: Native to Asia, probably Sri Lanka. Cultivated in the West Indies, Africa and tropical Asia. Main producers include Guatemala and India
Other names: East Indian lemongrass, Cochin lemongrass, native lemongrass, British India lemongrass, "vervaine Indienne" or France Indian verbena.
Description: A fast-growing, tall aromatic perennial grass that grows a meter and a half tall. Roots quickly exhaust the soil.
Extraction: Essential oil by steam distillation
Botanical Part Used: Fresh and partially dried grass
Principal constituents: Citral (up to 85%), geraniol, methyl eugenol, borneol, dipentene, and others.

BLENDING SUGGESTIONS

Relative strength: 4
Among the top notes that typically make up less than 20% of the blend.
Blends well with basil, clary sage, eucalyptus, geranium, lavender, tea tree, and rosemary
Description: Fresh, grassy, citrusy, pungent, earthy, and slightly bitter.

HISTORY & TRADITIONAL USES

- Used in Ayurvedic medicine for infectious diseases and fever. Acts as a sedative for the central nervous system. Insecticide and for food flavoring. Used as fragrance in soaps, detergents, cosmetics & perfumes. Flavor in many food categories, alcoholic beverages and soft drinks. Frequently used to adulterate and extend more expensive oils.

USE & HEALTH BENEFIT

- To use as an astringent and to open pores for release of toxins, take an aromatic bath with 5 to 10 drops of lemongrass in a cup of Epsom Salts +++L.

- To deodorize a room and prevent the spread of infections, diffuse 20 drops of lemongrass alone or in a blend with other aromatic essential oils +++L.

- To stimulate digestive functions and calm digestive problems like nausea, colitis, indigestion, gastric inflammation, irritable bowel syndrome, etc., massage the abdomen with a 5:95 blend of lemongrass with a carrier oil. Also take an aromatic bath with 5 to 10 drops of lemongrass in a cup of Epsom Salts. +++L ++P This therapy also helps with liver cleansing ++P.

- To help with various skin conditions: acne, athlete's foot, excessive perspiration, insect repellent (fleas, lice, ticks), opens pores, pediculosis, scabies, lice, etc.; apply a drop of lemongrass in a teaspoon of water, and apply to the skin or scalp. Or you can apply a 5:95 blend of lemongrass and carrier oil followed by extra carrier oil to make sure it doesn't sting the skin.

- To stimulate poor circulation, poor muscle tone, and slack tissue, massage the area with a 5:95 blend of lemongrass and carrier oil. This also helps with muscle pain.

- To increase circulation (vasodilation) +++P, and help with high blood pressure, headaches, etc., massage the affected area with a 25:75 blend

Singles

of lemongrass with a carrier oil. Also take an aromatic bath with 10 to 15 drops of lemongrass in a cup of Epsom Salts.

- For nervous exhaustion, insomnia, and multiple stress-related conditions +++P, massage the hands and feet with a 25:75 blend of lemongrass with a carrier oil. Also take an aromatic bath with 10 to 15 drops of lemongrass in a cup of Epsom Salts.

> *CAUTIONS: None when used in quantities indicated. Will sting the skin if it is not sufficiently diluted. Do not take in large doses if pregnant. Do not apply to mucous membranes (eyes, nose, mouth, vagina, or rectum). When taking both topically and orally, it may interfere with enzyme action in metabolizing medications. When taking diabetic medications, it may cause slight hypoglycemic effects when taken orally. When taken orally with aspirin or blood thinners, it may increase blood-thinning effects. May enhance the effects of antibiotics.*

✔ CLINICAL SUPPORT

Lemongrass essential oil exhibits antibacterial action against S. mutans (Chaudhari, et al. 2012). Also shows action of other oils against the same bacteria.

Lemongrass may inhibit cytokine production in vitro, thus the oil may have anti-inflammatory activity (Adorjan, B and Buchbauer, G., 2010).

Helicobacter pylori is an important bacteria responsible for peptic ulcers in humans. Although using antibiotics often improves these diseases, resistance to the antibiotics is emerging. The antimicrobial effect of essential oils and the development of resistance to the essential oils were evaluated in vitro and in vivo. Lemongrass and lemon verbena were bactericidal against H. pylori. Resistance to lemongrass did not develop even after 10 sequential passages, whereas resistance to clarithromycin (an antibiotic) developed under the same conditions. In in vivo studies, the density of H. pylori in the stomach of mice treated with lemongrass was significantly reduced compared with untreated mice. These results demonstrate that the essential oils are bactericidal against H. pylori without the development of acquired resistance, suggesting that essential oils may have potential as new and safe agents for inclusion in anti-H. pylori regimens (Ohno T, et al. 2003).

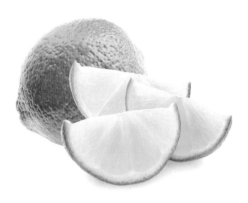

Lime
Citrus aurantifolia

Family: Rutaceae
Origins: Native to Asia but naturalized in many tropical and subtropical regions of the world. Cultivated mainly in south Florida, the West Indies, Central America, Mexico, and Italy.
Other names: Mexican lime, West Indian lime, sour lime
Description: small evergreen with smooth leaves and small white flowers. Fruit is green about half the size of a lemon.
Extraction: cold expression
Botanical Part Used: peel of the unripe fruit
Principal constituents: Limonene, pinenes, camphene, sabinene, citral, cymene, cineols & linalool and other

🥄 BLENDING SUGGESTIONS

Relative strength: 3
Among the top notes that typically make up less than 20% of the blend.
Blends well with: Neroli, citronella, lavender, lavandin, rosemary, clary sage, and all citrus oils
Description: Sharp, fruity, tart, citrusy, sweet, and lively

📖 HISTORY & TRADITIONAL USES

Historically used for medicinal uses similar to lemon including fevers, infections, sore throat, colds. Used as a remedy for dyspepsia. Used as fragrance components in soaps, cosmetics, detergents and perfumes. Used in the food industry, especially in soft drinks for the "lemon-and-lime" flavor.

➕ USE & HEALTH BENEFIT

- For skin conditions: acne, boils, chilblains, cuts, greasy skin, herpes infections, insect bites, mouth ulcers, and age spots; apply undiluted to small areas and dilute 50:50 with a carrier oil for larger skin areas.

- To improve circulation ++P for the treatment of arthritis, cellulitis, high blood pressure, nosebleeds, obesity (congestion), poor circulation, and rheumatism, massage the area of concern with a 50:50 blend of lime and carrier oil. You can also try taking a 50:50 blend of lime and carrier oil in a capsule once a day.

- For respiratory conditions: asthma, throat infections, bronchitis, and excess mucous; diffuse 20 drops of lime and enjoy an aromatic bath using 10 to 15 drops of lime mixed with Epsom Salts. Five drops of lime essential oil can also be used on the chest after a shower while the skin is still damp and while the pores are open. Create a cool compress on the chest using 5 drops

of lime to help with bronchitis by reducing inflammation. Put a cold, damp cloth over the oils and a dry towel over that. A cold ice pack may be used over that.

- To reduce spasms of muscles, coughs, asthmatic spasms, or digestive spasms (dyspepsia), take a 50:50 blend of lime and carrier oil in a capsule once a day. You can also massage the area of concern with a 50:50 blend of lime and carrier oil.

- To calm inflammation +++P of the muscles, skin, nerves, organs, cardiovascular system, etc., take a 50:50 blend of lime and carrier oil in a capsule once a day. You can also massage the area of concern with a 50:50 blend of lime and carrier oil.

- To use as a calming sedative ++P for anxiety, stress, or insomnia, take an aromatic bath with 10 to 15 drops of lime in a cup of Epsom Salts before bed. You can also massage hands and feet with a 50:50 blend of lime and carrier oil.

> *CAUTIONS: None when used in quantities indicated. Possible dermal sensitivity in some individuals. Can be phototoxic. After applying lime essential oil to exposed skin, stay out of the direct sunlight for 12 hours.*

CLINICAL SUPPORT

The need for developing more effective, safer, and cheaper weight-reducing drugs has become paramount in recent years. The effects of lime essential oils in reducing body weight, individually and in co-administration with ketotifen, an antihistaminic drug that causes weight gain, has been investigated using a mouse model. Groups treated with lime essential oil displayed a reduction in body weight and food consumption. Co-administration of the lime essential oil and ketotifen caused significant suppression in gaining weight, as well as decreased body weights of mice. The data obtained in this study suggested that lime essential oil plays an important role in weight loss and could be useful in the treatment of drug-induced obesity and related diseases (Asnaashari S et al., 2010).

Lime essential oil was studied for its potential spasmolytic effects on isolated rabbit jejunum, aorta, and uterus. The results indicated that the lime essential oil possesses important properties to relieve spasms in smooth muscle (Spadaro F et al., 2012).

The main compounds of lime essential oil have sedative effects. Therefore, the aims of this study were to determine the effect of lime essential oil massage on the physical and mental parameters of 40 volunteers. A single massage significantly decreased systolic blood pressure compared to controls, suggesting the stimulation of parasympathetic activity (Saiyudthong, S., 2009).

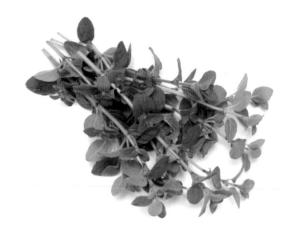

Marjoram
Origanum majorana

Family: Lamiaceae (Labiatae)
Origins: Native to the Mediterranean area. Major suppliers include France, Tusisia, Morocco, Egypt, Bulgaria, Hungary, and Germany.
Other names: knotted marjoram, sweet marjoram
Description: A tender, bushy perennial cultivated as an annual in colder climates. Dark green leaves and small grey-white flowers in clusters.
Extraction: Essential oil by steam distillation
Botanical Part Used: dried herb in flower
Principal constituents: Terpenes, terpineol, sabinenes, linalool, linalyl acetate, ocimene, cadinene, geranyl acetate, and others.

BLENDING SUGGESTIONS

Relative strength: 3
Among the middle notes that typically make up more than 50% of the blend.
Blends well with: Lavender, rosemary, bergamot, German and Roman chamomile, cypress, cedarwood, tea tree, Eucalyptus radiata, and Eucalyptus globulus.
Description: Herbal, green, warm, woody, camphoric, and spicy

📖 HISTORY & TRADITIONAL USES

A culinary herb and folk remedy. Used by ancient Greeks in fragrances, cosmetics, and medicines. A versatile herb with soothing, fortifying and warming effects. Aids digestive and menstrual concerns as well as nervous and respiratory complaints. Helps diseases of the chest, liver & spleen. Has been used for muscular and rheumatic pain, sprains, stiff joints, bruises, etc.

➕ USE & HEALTH BENEFIT

- For helping ease the pain of neuralgia, arthritis, and rheumatism +++P +++L, apply a 50:50 blend of marjoram and a carrier oil to the affected area. Also effective for painful joints, lower back pain, muscle stiffness, sprains, and strains.

- To calm respiratory spasms (cough, bronchitis, asthma, etc.), diffuse 20 drops of marjoram ++++L. Also diffuse 20 drops and take a hot aromatic bath using 10 to 15 drops of marjoram in a cup of Epsom Salts. These therapies are also helpful for digestive spasms.

- For a headache or migraine, create a compress using 3 drops of undiluted marjoram on the forehead and back of neck, or wherever the painful area manifests, with a cool damp cloth over it. Diffusing 20 drops of marjoram may also help.

- For canker sores, apply marjoram undiluted to the infected area. This can be effective for chilblains, bruises, and ticks as well.

- For help with insomnia, nervous tension, and stress related conditions, diffuse 20 drops of marjoram and massage feet and hands with a 50:50 blend of marjoram and carrier oil +++L.

- For symptoms of dystonia (manifest in muscle spasms and abnormal posture, typically due to a neurological disease or a side effect of drug therapy); apply a 50:50 blend of marjoram and carrier oil to the affected muscles, take an aromatic bath using 10 to 15 drops of marjoram in a cup of Epsom Salts, or diffuse 20 drops of marjoram +++P.

- To strengthen the immune system and prevent colds, flu, sinusitis, bronchitis, etc., take a capsule with a 50:50 blend of marjoram and carrier oil daily with food.

- To lower overactive sexual desire, take a hot bath using 10 to 15 drops of marjoram in a cup of Epsom Salts. Diffuse 20 drops of marjoram.

- For digestive conditions like colic, constipation, dyspepsia, diarrhea, inflammation of the colon and small intestines, colon infection, and gas, massage the abdomen with a 50:50 blend of marjoram and carrier oil.

- For symptoms of PMS, balancing the menstrual cycle, or painful menstruation, take an aromatic bath using 10 to 15 drops of marjoram in a cup of Epsom Salts.

CAUTIONS: None when used in quantities indicated.

✔️ CLINICAL SUPPORT

"The purpose of this study was to identify the effects of essential oil inhalation on blood pressure ... in 83 prehypertensive and hypertensive subjects. They used lavender, ylang ylang, marjoram, and neroli in a study [against similar synthetic fragrances]. The inhalation of an essential oil had immediate and continuous effects on ... stress reduction. Essential oils may have relaxation effects for controlling hypertension" (Kim IH, et al., 2012).

In vivo studies showed that marjoram has the potential for healing and protecting against the formation of gastric ulcers (Adorjan, B and Buchbauer, G., 2010).

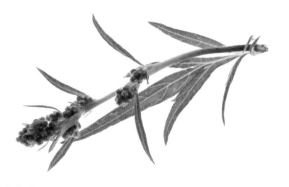

Mugwort
Artemisia vulgaris

Family: Asteraceae
Origins: A native of eastern Europe and western Asia. Now found in temperate zones worldwide. Oil is produced in southern France, Morocco, Germany, Hungary, India, China, and Japan.
Other names: Armoise, wild wormwood, felon herb, St. John's plant.
Description: A perennial herb that grows a meter and a half tall with purple stem and dark green leaves and small red-brown or yellow flowers.
Extraction: essential oil by steam distillation
Botanical Part Used: leaves and flowering tops
Blends well with: patchouli, rosemary, lavandin, sage, clary sage, and cedarwood.
Principal constituents: Thujone, cineol, pinenes, dihydromatricaria ester and others.
Powerful camphoric, bitter-sweet, herbal fragrance

🌀 BLENDING SUGGESTIONS

Relative strength: 5
Among the middle notes to base notes that typically make up more than 80% of the blend (50% middle notes, 30% base notes).
Blends well with: patchouli, rosemary, lavandin, pine, clary sage, and cedarwood.
Description: camphoric, bitter-sweet, musty, earthy, and herbal.

📖 HISTORY & TRADITIONAL USES

Historically associated with superstition and witchcraft. Seen as a protective charm against evil and danger. Legend has it that St. John the Baptist wore a girdle of the leaves while he lived in the wilderness. Traditionally used as a womb tonic for painful or delayed menstruation. A treatment for hysteria and epilepsy. Used to expel worms, control fever and cure dyspepsia. Also used to relieve gout and rheumatism. Used as fragrance in soaps, colognes, and perfumes. Limited use in flavoring due to high thujone content.

> *CAUTIONS This essential oil should not be used as a single oil. It can only be used as a minor ingredient in an aromatic blend. It is not used as a single oil due to its high thujone content. Do not use during pregnancy. A tiny amount in a blend is appropriate for aromatic use.*

CLINICAL SUPPORT

The in vitro tests here revealed that mugwort is a promising candidate for further research to develop novel anti-candida drugs (Obistioiu D, et al 2014). This study was done on the plant material, not the essential oil.

This study tested the inhibitory effect of Artemisia vulgaris (mugwort) on the yellow fever virus. The presence of mugwort produced a 100% reduction of virus yield in vitro. Mugwort showed antiviral activities against the yellow fever virus. The mode of action seems to be direct virus inactivation (Meneses R, et al., 2009). This study was done on the plant material, not the essential oil.

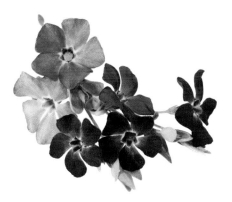

Myrtle

Myrtus communis

Family: Myrtaceae
Origins: Native to North Africa. It grows freely all over the Mediterranean region and is cultivated as a garden shrub all over Europe. The oil is mainly produced in Corsica, Span, Tunisia, Morocco, Italy, Yugoslavia, and France.
Other names: Corsican pepper
Description: A large bush with many branches. Brown-red bark and small leaves. White flowers followed with small black berries. Leaves and flowers are fragrant.
Extraction: Essential oil by steam distillation
Botanical Part Used: leaves, twigs, and sometimes flowers
Principal constituents: ,cineol, myrtenol, pinene, geraniol, linalool, camphene, and others

🜀 BLENDING SUGGESTIONS

Relative strength: 3
Among the top to middle notes that typically make up more than 70% of the blend (top notes 20% and middle notes 50%).
Blends well with bergamot, lavender, lemon, lemongrass, clary sage, lime, ginger, clove, cinnamon, lavandin, rosewood, rosemary, spearmint, thyme, and tea tree.
Description: Sweet and slightly camphoric with a hint of floral.

📖 HISTORY & TRADITIONAL USES

Leaves and berries have been used for drying and have been used for symptoms of diarrhea and dystentery, as well as mucous. Used for lung and bladder infections. The leaves and flowers were major ingredients in ancient skin-care preparations. Myrtle is used today in colognes and perfumes. It is used as a flavoring in meat sauces and seasonings with other herbs.

➕ USE & HEALTH BENEFIT

- As a treatment for acne, oily skin, and to open pores, use 5 drops of myrtle in a green clay masque.

- To help with hemorrhoids, apply a 50:50 blend of myrtle and a carrier oil to the affected area. The blend can also be used for varicose veins (apply with a delicate touch) and help with lymphatic drainage (massage).

- For diverse respiratory conditions: asthma, bronchitis, laryngitis, sinusitis, chronic coughs, and TB, diffuse 20 drops twice daily. Take aromatic baths using 10 to 15 drops of myrtle in a cup of Epsom Salts. Massage respiratory areas of the chest, neck, and face with a 50:50 blend of myrtle and a carrier oil. This is a mild oil for childhood coughs and chest colds +++++L +++P.

- To strengthen the immune system to prevent colds, flu, and other infectious diseases, diffuse 20 drops daily ++++L.

- For urinary tract or prostate infections or inflammation, apply a 50:50 blend of myrtle and carrier oil to the lower abdomen. You can apply a warm, damp cloth over the area with heat for a more penetrating effect. Also take an aromatic bath using 10 to 15 drops of myrtle in a cup of Epsom Salts ++++L.

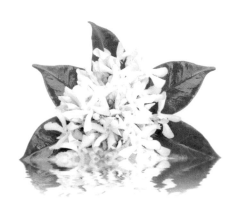

- As a liver cleanse and stimulant, use a 50:50 blend of myrtle and carrier oil for an abdominal massage and also to make capsules to take once a day.

- For insomnia take an aromatic bath using 10 to 15 drops of myrtle in a cup of Epsom Salts. Also apply a 50:50 blend of myrtle and a carrier oil to the hands and feet. Diffuse 20 drops of myrtle before bed time +++P.

- To treat an enlarged prostate (BPH), massage the lower abdomen with a 50:50 blend of myrtle and a carrier oil ++P.

- To stimulate thyroid activity (hypothyroid), massage the thyroid area of the neck and chest with a 50:50 blend of myrtle and a carrier oil.

> CAUTIONS: None when used in quantities indicated. Use only small doses orally. When taking diabetic medications, it may cause slight hypoglycemic effects when taken orally.

✓ CLINICAL SUPPORT

"The aim of this work was to evaluate ... the action of [myrtle essential oil] ... on the biofilm formation towards Candida albicans, Candida parapsilosis and Candida tropicalis. The effect of [myrtle oil] yielded encouraging results (Cannas S et al., 2014).

Topical application of myrtle oil exhibited a significant decrease in inflammation in this in vivo mice study (Maxia A, et al., 2011).

Neroli

Citrus aurantium bigaradia OR Citrus aurantium var amara

Family: Rutaceae
Origins: Tunesia and Morocco.
Other names: Orange blossom, orange flower, Citrus bigaradia
Description: An evergreen tree with glossy, dark green leaves and fragrant white flowers. Flowers are picked twice a year.
Extraction: Essential oil by steam distillation
Botanical Part Used: freshly picked flowers
Principal constituents: Linalol (about 34%), linalyl acetate (6 – 17%), limonene (about 15%), pinene, nerolidol, geraniol, nerol, methyl antrhranilate, indole, citral, and others.

⬤ BLENDING SUGGESTIONS

Relative strength: 3
Among the middle notes that typically make up more than 50% of the blend.
Blends well with virtually all oils—Roman and German chamomile, sandalwood,
clary sage, lavender, ylang ylang, lemon and all citrus oils.
Description: Fresh, light, floral, citrusy, delicate, slightly bitter with a terpine-like topnote.

HISTORY & TRADITIONAL USES

Named after a princess of Nerola in Italy who loved the perfume. Orange flowers were used in bridal bouquets and wreaths to calm nerves before retiring to the marriage bed. Dried flowers were used as a mild stimulant to the nervous system and as a blood cleanser. The floral water is used for cosmetic therapy.

 ## USE & HEALTH BENEFIT

To treat hemorrhoids and varicose veins, gently apply a drop of neroli with a half teaspoon of carrier oil to the affected area +P.

For many skin conditions: scars, stretch marks, thread veins, mature and sensitive skin, and wrinkles; apply in a drop with a few drops of carrier oil or even undiluted on small areas.

> CAUTIONS: None when used in quantities indicated. It is so expensive that it should typically only be used in a blend. A huge amount of flowers must be picked by hand to create a very small amount of this costly oil. Use it only drop by drop and properly diluted. It is mainly used for its psychological effect.

✔ CLINICAL SUPPORT

In this test neroli essential oil exhibited a marked antibacterial activity especially against Pseudomonas aeruginosa. Moreover, neroli oil exhibited a very strong antifungal activity compared with the standard antibiotic (Nystatin) (Ammar AH et al., 2012).

"The purpose of this study was to identify the effects of essential oil inhalation on blood pressure ... in 83 prehypertensive and hypertensive subjects. They used lavender, ylang-ylang, marjoram, and neroli in a study [against similar synthetic fragrances]. The inhalation of an essential oil had immediate and continuous effects on ... stress reduction. Essential oils may have relaxation effects for controlling hypertension (Kim IH, et al., 2012).

Neroli was as effective as Xanax (a benzodiazepine) in the treatment of induced anxiety in a gerbil study (Dobetsberger, C. and Buchbauer, G., 2011). Neroli essential oil has a protective effect on gastric mucosa; possibly due to stimulating an increase in mucous production (Adorjan, B and Buchbauer, G., 2010).

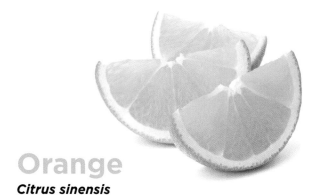

Orange
Citrus sinensis

Family: Rutaceae
Origins: Native to China, but extensively cultivated especially in California and Florida, around the Mediterranean. The oil comes mainly from Israel, Cyprus, Brazil and North America.
Other names: Sweet Orange, China orange, Portugal orange
Description: An evergreen tree, smaller than bitter orange and less hardy. Orange fruit.
Extraction: cold expressed
Botanical Part Used: ripe or almost ripe peel of fruit
Principal constituents: Over 90% monoterpenes, mainly limonene. Also contains bergapten for some phototoxicity.

 ## BLENDING SUGGESTIONS

Relative strength: 1
Among the top notes that typically make up less than 20% of the blend.
Blends well with cinnamon, frankincense, juniper, clove, neroli, lemon, clary sage, and rosewood.
Description: Sweet, fruity, citrusy, and fresh.

📖 HISTORY & TRADITIONAL USES

Fruit is highly nutritious with vitamins A, B, and C. In Chinese medicine the dried peel is used for coughs, colds, anorexia, and malignant breast sores. They are good for digestive disorders. Used extensively in soaps, detergents, cosmetics, and perfumes. Widely used as flavorings in food and drinks.

➕ USE & HEALTH BENEFIT

• For anxiety, nervous tension, stress-related conditions, and depression, take an aromatic bath using 10 to 15 drops of orange in a cup of Epsom Salts. Use a 50:50 blend of orange with a carrier oil to massage hands and feet ++P +++L.

• To assist in lymphatic drainage, use a 50:50 blend of orange and carrier oil and massage lymph areas of the neck and groin ++L. Take a hot bath using 10 to 15 drops of orange in a cup of Epsom Salts. This also helps with obesity and fluid retention +++L.

• To help with digestive problems, take a capsule of a 50:50 blend of orange and carrier oil daily. Diffuse 20 drops of orange daily. Take a hot bath using 10 to 15 drops of orange in a cup of Epsom Salts. Use a drop or trace of orange oil in your drinking water, juice, or herbal tea daily +++L.

• To prevent infection, diffuse 20 drops of orange daily ++P. Use a drop or trace of orange oil in your drinking water, juice, or herbal tea daily.

• To disinfect surfaces, blend 20 drops of orange oil in 8 oz of water in a spray bottle.

CAUTIONS: None when used in quantities indicated.

✅ CLINICAL SUPPORT

Sweet orange used in an aromatherapy massage found that the calming, sleep-inducing effects were probably due to the aroma rather than the massage (Dobetsberger, C. and Buchbauer, G., 2011).

Sweet orange oil had an anti-anxiety effect on rats (Dobetsberger, C. and Buchbauer, G., 2011).

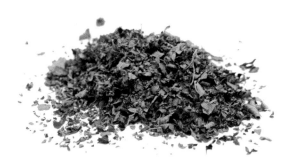

OREGANO
Origanum compactum

Family: Lamiaceae (Labiatae)
Origins: Mediterranean area, especially Morocco
Other names: oreganum (oil)
Description: A perennial herb, growing to about 32 inches tall dark green leaves and pink flowers.
Extraction: Essential oil by steam distillation
Botanical Part Used: dried flowering herb
Principal constituents: phenols (60-70%), monoterpenes, sesquiterpines, alcohols, monoterpenols, and others.

🥄 BLENDING SUGGESTIONS

Relative strength: 5
Among the middle notes that typically make up more than 50% of the blend, but oregano is so strong that it should be only a small percentage of a blend.

Blends well with: Basil, lemongrass, myrtle, thyme, and rosemary.

Description: herbal, sharp, warm, camphoric

📖 HISTORY & TRADITIONAL USES

Oregano has an ancient medicinal reputation for digestive upset, respiratory issues, colds, flu, and inflammation. In China it is used to treat vomiting, diarrhea, fever, jaundice, and itchy skin. The diluted oil is used for headaches, rheumatism, aches and pains, stings, and bites. Used as a fragrance component in soaps, colognes, and perfumes, especially men's. Some use as a flavoring agent in meat products and pizza.

➕ USE & HEALTH BENEFIT

- Oregano has a broad spectrum of action for virtually every system of the body: respiratory +++P ++++L, digestive, urogenital +++P, nervous, circulatory ++++L, and immune-strengthening. It is highly effective, but must be used with caution.

- To relieve menstrual pain and PMS symptoms, as well as help with urinary tract infections, apply a blend of 25:75 oregano to carrier oil to the lower abdomen. Add extra carrier oil to stop any sensitivity that may occur +++P +++L.

- To help expel worms and parasites, take a capsule containing a 25:75 blend of oregano with a carrier oil daily +++P.

- To relieve spasms (Antispasmodic) of the digestive system, the muscles, the nerves, the respiratory system, etc., massage the affected area with a 25:75 blend of oregano with a carrier oil +++L.

- Oregano has strong antimicrobial action at about the strength of penicillin but without its side effects. It is not only antibacterial +++P, but also antiviral +++P +++++L, and fungicidal +++P. You can apply oregano undiluted to a tiny area for strong antimicrobial action (acne, boils, infections, etc.), but have a carrier oil handy to use if it gets too hot. A few drops of oregano can be used undiluted for a back and spinal massage (Layer Therapy), but it must be layered with a carrier oil when it gets too hot. For a safer application, blend 25:75 with a carrier oil for infections of all types +++L. Avoid topical burning by adding extra carrier oil as needed. It can be warming but must not be burning.

- To settle the nerves and help with depression, add 2 drops of oregano to a tissue, cotton ball, or handkerchief and use throughout the day to inhale. You can keep this aromatic item in a plastic bag so it doesn't disperse into the air too quickly and lose its potency for aromatic inhalation.

- To help settle digestion and reduce gas, use as a minor ingredient in a 50:50 blend of milder oils with a carrier oil to be taken by capsule three times daily with food.

- To increase toxin release through perspiration and urine, massage topically as a minor ingredient in a 50:50 blend with other essential oils and a carrier oil. Also use a drop or two with other less strong oils in a hot bath. Mix the oils first with Epsom Salts so they disperse in the water and don't accumulate on the surface and sting sensitive skin.

- For infectious diseases of all kinds: respiratory, urinary tract, digestive, skin, etc.; take a capsule containing a 25:75 blend of oregano with a carrier oil 3 times daily with food +++L. A better choice might be an Protecting blend containing oregano. Taking a small amount of oregano regularly in this way increases energy and helps with nervous fatigue ++P.

- For skin infections, create a compress with a 25:75 blend of oregano and carrier oil or with a drop of oregano (with a 10 drops of other milder oils like tea tree) in a tablespoon of water. Soak a gauze pad in this solution and apply over the infection. Add heat to help the oils penetrate and disinfect.

- For a strong but safe antimicrobial action, massage the bottoms of the feet with a 50:50 blend of oregano and carrier oil. Use a hair drier to help the oils penetrate.

> CAUTIONS: None when used in quantities indicated. Can cause skin irritation. Always have carrier oil handy to dilute when it starts to feel too hot. Do not diffuse except as a minor ingredient in a blend. Do not use oregano on children under 12. Do not use when pregnant or lactating. Do not apply to mucous membranes (eyes, nose, mouth, vagina, or rectum). When taking diabetic medications, it may cause slight hypoglycemic effects when taken orally. When taken orally with aspirin or blood thinners, it may increase blood-thinning effects. May enhance the action of antibiotics.

✓ CLINICAL SUPPORT

Oregano is among the most effective essential oils in tests against 65 bacteria with varying resistance to antibiotics" (Mayaud L, et al., 2008).

Oregano exhibited the strongest antifungal activity of any of the 7 oils tested (Bouchra C, et al., 2003).

A combination of thyme and oregano can reduce the production of pro-inflammatory cytokines. (Adorjan, B and Buchbauer, G., 2010).

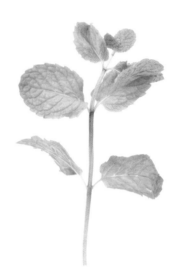

Patchouli
Pogostemon cablin

Family: Lamiaceae (Labiatae)
Origins: A native of tropical Asia, especially Indonesia and the Philippines. Also cultivated in India, China, Malaysia, and South America.
Other names: patchouli, puchaput
Description: A perennial bushy herb with fragrant, furry leaves and white flowers touched with purple.
Extraction: Essential oil by steam distillation
Botanical Part Used: Dried leaves
Principal constituents: Patchouli alcohol (approximately 40%), pogostol, bulnesol, and others.

BLENDING SUGGESTIONS

Relative strength: 4
Among the base notes that typically make up less than 30% of the blend.
Blends well with: vetiver, cedarwood, sandalwood, clove, lavender, bergamot, and clary sage.
Description: sweet, rich, and herbal

HISTORY & TRADITIONAL USES

The essence has been traditionally used to give fragrance to linens and clothes. It is believed to help prevent the spread of disease. In China, Japan and Malaysia the herb is used to treat headaches, colds, nausea, vomiting, diarrhea, abdominal pain, and bad breath. In Japan and Malaysia it is used to cure poisonous snake bites. It is used extensively in cosmetic preparations, soaps and oriental perfumes. It is used as a flavoring in many foods and drinks. It is used to mask many disagreeable tastes and smells.

➕ USE & HEALTH BENEFIT

- To help stimulate circulation +++P, massage the affected area with a 50:50 blend of patchouli and carrier oil.

- To help regenerate tissue +P ++++L especially for impetigo +++L, mix three drops of patchouli in a teaspoon of water—and apply to the infected skin. You can also dilute 3 or 4 drops in each application of a mild lotion. Try using a 50:50 blend of patchouli in a carrier oil as well to see which works better for you. Try these types of applications for acne ++P +++L, eczema ++++L, and other inflammatory skin conditions ++++L as well. Patchouli is an exceptional oil for all types of skin conditions.

- For fungal skin infections ++++L and dandruff ++++L, dilute three drops of patchouli in a teaspoon of water and apply to the scalp or the infected skin. You can also dilute 3 or 4 drops in each application of a mild lotion or if the infection is on the feet, apply undiluted (athlete's foot).

- As a calming antidepressant or to overcome anxiety or nervous exhaustion ++++L, massage hands and feet, or even the whole body with a 50:50 blend of patchouli and a carrier oil.

- To treat hemorrhoids and varicose veins, gently apply a 50:50 blend of patchouli with a carrier oil to the affected area. +++P

- Because of its pleasing aroma and benefits for the skin, patchouli can be added to many lotions, shampoos, conditioners, and creams at about 10 to 20 drops per 8 ounces of product.

- For quick healing of cuts, scrapes, and minor wounds; apply undiluted.

CAUTIONS: None when used in quantities indicated.

CLINICAL SUPPORT

Results of present study revealed that patchouli was capable of maintaining skin structural integrity caused by UV irradiation and it was useful in preventing photoaging. These protective effects were possibly due to its anti-oxidative property. Patchouli should be seen as a potential therapeutic agent for preventing photoaging (Lin RF, et al., 2014).

Patchouli oil exerts an anti-cancer activity by decreasing cell growth and increasing apoptosis in human colorectal cancer cells (Jeong JB, et al., 2013).

Patchouli is one of the few essential oils cited as a phlebotonic (a substance that helps stimulate poor circulation in the legs). (Price & Price, p. 262).

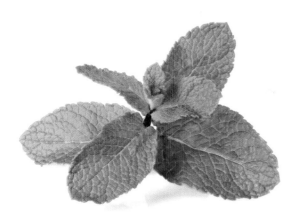

Peppermint
Mentha piperita

Family: Lamiaceae (Labiatae)
Origins: Naturalized throughout Europe and America but cultivated worldwide. The oil comes mainly from France, England, America, Russia, Bulgaria, Italy, Hungary, Morocco, and China.
Other names: brandy mint, balm mint
Description: a perennial herb with dark green serrated leaves that grows about 3 feet high.
Extraction: Essential oil by steam distillation
Botanical Part Used: the flowering herb
Principal constituents: Menthol (29-48%), menthone (20-30%), menthyl acetate, menthofuran, limonene, pulegone, cineol, and others.

🍶 BLENDING SUGGESTIONS

Relative strength: 5
Among the middle notes that typically make up more than 50% of the blend.
Blends well with: lavender, rosemary, marjoram, lemon, Eucalyptus radiata, Eucalyptus globulus, and spearmint
Description: minty, cool, sharp, and intense

📖 HISTORY & TRADITIONAL USES

Mints have been cultivated for their aromas and flavors since ancient times in the Far East. Peppermint has been used for many centuries for multiple complaints: indigestion, nausea, sore throat, diarrhea, headaches, toothaches, and cramps. It is a popular flavoring agent in many foods including chewing gum and candies as well as alcoholic and soft drinks. It is widely used in flavoring tobacco. It is used in soaps, toothpaste, detergents, cosmetics, colognes, and perfumes.

➕ USE & HEALTH BENEFIT

• To deaden pain from smashed fingers, a painful bump, a bruise, or a toothache, tap a trace or a drop undiluted on the painful area +++P.

• To relieve the itching of hives and eczema, apply a 50:50 blend of peppermint and oil (or water). ++P

• For temporary relief of headaches and migraines, apply topically (undiluted) to temples, forehead, back of neck, and in front of ears on jaw muscle +++P.

• To help decongest an enlarged prostate (BPH) use a 50:50 blend for a deep massage of lower abdomen. Avoid genitals. A more gentle massage is helpful for urinary and prostate infections.

• To help with pancreatic functioning +++P, prostate infections, shingles, yellow fever +++P, respiratory infections, candida, urinary tract infections, stomach flu, intestinal worms, or any bacterial, viral, or fungal infection, take a 50:50 capsule of peppermint and carrier oil 3 times daily with food.

• To calm the pain of shingles, neuralgia, and sciatica, apply a 50:50 blend of peppermint and carrier oil ++P.

• For a cooling, antiseptic scalp treatment, add 20 drops of peppermint per 8 oz. of lotion, shampoos, or conditioners. Or, add one or two drops to each application.

- Create a non-toxic peppermint tooth powder by mixing 2-parts baking soda to 1-part fine-ground, natural salt. Thoroughly mix in drops of peppermint oil to taste. Sprinkle some in your hand, wet your toothbrush, and enjoy brushing your teeth without the toxic chemicals of traditional toothpaste.

- To calm and cool a fever, take a warm (not hot) bath with 10 to 15 drops of peppermint mixed in a cup of Epsom Salts.

- For a refreshing, energizing, cooling pick-up, put a drop or trace of peppermint in drinking water, herbal tea, juice, and recipes. These cooling aromatic drinks also stimulate and calm the digestive organs and help with relaxation or calming the nerves. Be sure to shake to disperse it before you take each drink.

- For nausea, vomiting, and motion sickness, place 5 drops in a tissue, handkerchief, or cotton ball and inhale.

- To stay alert when drowsy, apply 6 drops to a tissue, handkerchief, or cotton ball and inhale. The aromatics can be kept in a plastic bag and used throughout the day.

- To stay alert while driving, apply 5 drops to a tissue, handkerchief, or cotton ball place in the vents of an automobile. If you feel yourself falling asleep while driving, do not use peppermint to try to stay awake. Instead, stop and take a nap. The effect of peppermint is of very short duration and should only be used to keep yourself fresh and alert.

- To heal a cold sore, apply a single drop or trace, undiluted, frequently.

- For painful menstruation, massage lower abdomen with a 50:50 blend of peppermint and carrier oil.

- To stay alert, overcome motion sickness, or ease a headache, put a drop in your palm, rub palms together, cup over nose and mouth, and inhale several times.

- Diffuse 20 drops of oil to help energize, improve concentration, help memorization, and overcome jet lag.

- To overcome charley horses and cramps, massage painful muscles with a blend of 5 drops in a teaspoon of carrier oil or use a 50:50 blend of peppermint and carrier oil.

- To ease sore throat pain or help with bad breath, lick a trace off the back of your hand and distribute around your mouth. Do this at the first tickle of a sore throat, and repeat every few minutes until pain subsides.

- To clear sinuses, mix a drop of peppermint into a teaspoon of honey and lick it slowly.

- To keep from fainting or to overcome shock, inhale 5 drops of peppermint from a tissue or handkerchief.

- To help stimulate digestive, pancreatic, and liver functions, take a 50:50 capsule daily with food.

- To reduce back or neck pain or organs influenced by the back, use peppermint as one of the layers in a back and spinal therapy (Layer Therapy).

- To help lower inflammation, stimulate circulation around surgical wounds, and promote healing, apply a blend of 5 drops in a teaspoon of carrier oil and gently massage the area.

CAUTIONS: None when used in quantities indicated. Do not give to babies under 30 months by ingestion. Do not apply topically to the neck and throat of *children under age 3. Avoid diffusing peppermint for children under 8. May increase jaundice in children. May enhance absorption of fluorouracil. Do not apply to mucous membranes (eyes, nose, mouth, vagina, or rectum). May enhance bioavailability of cyclosporine. May reduce the effectiveness of codeine. Do not apply peppermint over a large area of the body to reduce a fever or lower body temperature. Too much peppermint over a large area can create chills that can be dangerous and cannot be reversed.*

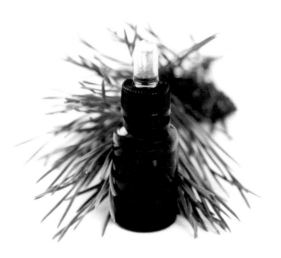

✓ CLINICAL SUPPORT

In this recent study peppermint was proven to help with the negative effects on the kidney from the use of a strong antibiotic (Ullah N. et al. "Mentha piperita in nephrotoxicity--a possible intervention to ameliorate renal derangements associated with gentamicin. *Indian J Pharmacol.*" 2014 Mar-Apr;46(2):166-70)

Inhaling essential oils may reduce the perceived level of mental fatigue/burnout (Varney E, Buckle J., 2013).

Peppermint and Motion Sickness

I used to get a lot of motion sickness. Now whenever I feel it coming on, I get out my peppermint and either put a drop in my drinking water if I have water handy, or I take a small trace on the back of my hand and lick it. It's strong, so I can't take too much, but I swish it around in my mouth. It seems to take away the motion sickness, and I feel better right away. I've noticed that I need to use it at the first hint of motion sickness, however, or it gets away from me. It doesn't work if I'm already green and ready to heave. Nothing works if I wait that long.

Pine
Pinus sylvestris

Family: Pinaceae
Origins: Native of Eurasia but cultivated throughout the eastern United States, Europe, and Russia.
Other names: Scotch pine, forest pine, scots pine, Norway pine, and pine needle (oil)
Description: A tall evergreen with a flat crown. It has long stiff needles that grow in pairs and cones.
Extraction: Essential oil by dry distillation
Botanical Part Used: needles
Principal constituents: 50 – 90% monoterpene hydrocarbons: pinenes, careen, dipentene, limonene, terpinenes, myrcene, and others.

BLENDING SUGGESTIONS

Relative strength: 4
Among the middle notes that typically make up more than 50% of the blend.
Blends well with: cedarwoood, rosemary, tea tree, sage, lavender, juniper, lemon, Eucalyptus radiata, Eucalyptus globulus, and marjoram
Description: strong, dry-balsamic, turpentine-like, woody, fresh

HISTORY & TRADITIONAL USES

The young shoots of the pine were mashed and added to bath water for nervous exhaustion, slow healing wounds, circulatory disorders, arthritis, and skin conditions. American Indians used pine needles to prevent scurvy. They also used pine needles in their mattresses to repel lice and fleas. Inhaling pine aroma helped relieve bronchial mucous, blocked sinuses, and asthma. The essential oil is used as an aromatic component in soaps, detergents, cosmetics, toiletries, and to a limited degree in perfumes. It is also used as a flavor ingredient in foods and beverages.

USE & HEALTH BENEFIT

- To relieve nerve pain, create a 50:50 blend of pine and a carrier oil and massage the painful area. If the area is small, you may apply the oil undiluted and add a carrier oil as needed.

- To help detoxify the lungs, the liver, the lymphatic areas, or the urinary tract, diffuse with 20 drops of pine or create a 50:50 blend of pine and a carrier oil and massage the affected area.

- For scrapes, cuts, and sores, apply pine undiluted to the area and add a carrier oil if needed.

- For treating lice, excessive perspiration, or scabies, you may want to mix 3 to 5 drops of pine in a teaspoon of water and apply. Or you can try diluting pine 50:50 with a carrier oil depending on what works best for you.

- For arthritis, gout, poor circulation, neuralgia, and muscle aches and pains, create a 50:50 blend of pine and carrier oil and massage the affected area.

- For urinary tract infections, create a 50:50 blend with a carrier oil and apply to the lower abdomen. Use a warm, damp compress and add heat to help the oil penetrate. Take capsules with a 50:50 blend of pine and a carrier oil. Take 3 capsules a day with food. +++L

- To overcome fatigue, nervous exhaustion, and other stress-related conditions, diffuse 20 drops of pine twice a day. +++P +++L

- To help with asthma, bronchitis, coughs, sinusitis, and sore throat, diffuse 20 drops of pine twice daily. Also create a hot bath using 10 to 15 drops of pine in a cup of Epsom Salts. Also use 3 to 5 drops of pine over your chest and neck after a shower while your skin is still damp. Heat a pan or bowl of boiling water, add 3 to 5 drops of pine, cover your head with a towel, and inhale. You can reheat and add more oil as needed. +++P ++++L

CAUTIONS: None when used in quantities indicated. When taken orally with aspirin or blood thinners, it may increase blood-thinning effects.

CLINICAL SUPPORT

Sick building syndrome is a term commonly used to describe the consequences of poor indoor air quality. Some species of fungi and their toxins cause difficulty in breathing, allergic rhinitis, watery eyes, headaches, and flu-like symptoms. Over recent years considerable interest has been developed for plant extracts that would be of great use for the improvement of air quality. The biological activity of pine essential oil was tested investigated to find out its fungicidal activity against airborne microorganisms. Minimum inhibitory concentrations of pine oil to 13 species (8 fungi, 2 yeast-like fungi, yeast and 2 bacteria) were determined. According to resistance to pine oil action, microorganisms grouped themselves as following: fungi, spore bacteria, yeast-like fungi, yeast, and bacteria (fungi being the most resistive and bacteria being the least resistive) (Motiejūnaite O, Peciulyte D., 2004).

The antimicrobial and antiradical activities of 15 essential oils were investigated. The results of the trials showed very high essential oils activity against all tested strains of microorganisms. The best antimicrobial activity against C. histolyticum was found at pine essential oil. The antioxidant properties were different in particular plant species. The highest% of inhibition after 30 min. of reaction was observed at Origanum vulgare (93%), and Lavandula augustifolia (90.22%) (Kačániová M, et al., 2014).

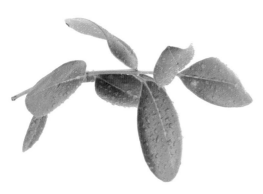

Ravintsara
Cinnamomum camphora

Family: Lauraceae
Origins: The **camphor laurel** is grown in Asia, particularly in Sumatra, Borneo, and Taiwan.
Other names: hon-sho, camphor laurel, gum camphor, Japanese camphor, Formosa camphor
Description: A tall evergreen similar in shape to a Linden. Clustered white flowers become red berries. The wood of trees over 50 years old produces the crude camphor, a white crystalline substance.
Extraction: Steam distillation
Botanical Part Used: Wood, root stumps, and branches
Principal constituents: Mainly cineol with pinene, terpineol, and others.

⊖ BLENDING SUGGESTIONS

Relative strength: 4
Among the middle notes that typically make up 50% of the blend or more, though camphor would only be a small part of any blend.
Blends well with: peppermint, Eucalyptus radiata, Eucalyptus globulus, wintergreen, juniper, and rosemary.
Description: camphoric, medicinal, woody, and penetrating.

📖 HISTORY & TRADITIONAL USES

Used traditionally to prevent infectious disease. A lump of the resin would be worn around the neck for protection. Used for nervous and respiratory diseases as well as heart failure. It is used as a solvent in the paint and lacquer industry. Used as masking agents in detergents, soaps disinfectants, and other household products.

⊕ USE & HEALTH BENEFIT

- As anti-infectious agent—antibacterial, antifungal, and antiviral +++P; apply a 50:50 blend of ravintsara with a carrier oil and massage the area of infection. Apply undiluted to small areas +++P.

- For its warming, stimulating, anti-inflammatory action for multiple respiratory conditions, create a 50:50 dilution with a carrier and apply topically to the chest, neck, and over sinus area of the face.

- For respiratory conditions like bronchitis, chills, coughs, colds, fever, flu, and other infectious diseases, diffuse 20 drops twice daily. Also disperse in an Epsom Salt bath, and massage in a 50:50 dilution.

- For physical exhaustion, disperse 10 to 15 drops of ravintsara in a cup of Epsom Salts for an aromatic hot bath ++P.

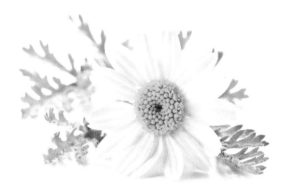

- For acne, skin inflammation, oily skin conditions, age spots, and as an insect repellent, use topically in a 50:50 dilution with a carrier oil.

- For arthritis, muscle aches/pains, rheumatism, and sprains, create a 50:50 blend with a carrier oil and massage on the painful area.

CAUTIONS: None when used in quantities indicated. Should not be used during pregnancy or on young children.

CLINICAL SUPPORT

"Cinnamomum camphora exhibits a number of biological properties such as insecticidal, antimicrobial, antiviral, anticoccidial, anti-nociceptive, anticancer and antitussive activities, in addition to its use as a skin penetration enhancer" (Chen W. et al., 2013).

Six essential oils including Eucalyptus citriodora, lemongrass, ravintsara, lemon, as well as two standard antibiotics, miconazole and clotrimazole, were tested in vitro for their anticandidial activity. All these essential oils exhibited higher activity than the two synthetic antibiotics (Dutta BK, et al., 2007).

Roman Chamomile
Anthemis nobilis

Family: Asteraceae (Compositae)
Origins: Originally from southwestern Europe. Now grown in North America, England, Belgium, Hungary, Italy, and France. Chamaemelum nobile and Anthemis nobilis are the same plant.
Other names: German chamomile, English chamomile, garden chamomile, sweet chamomile, true chamomile.
Description: Small perennial herb with daisy-like flowers that are larger than those of German chamomile. Smells like apples.
Extraction: Essential oil by steam distillation. The oil is pale blue.
Botanical Part Used: flowers
Blends well with: bergamot, neroli, geranium, and lavender
Principal constituents: esters, isobutyle, angelate, pinocarvone, and others.

BLENDING SUGGESTIONS

Relative strength: 4
Among the middle notes that typically make up more than 50% of the blend.
Blends well with: bergamot, neroli, geranium, and lavender
Description: Warm, sweet, herbal, fruity scent

HISTORY & TRADITIONAL USES

Used for over 2,000 years in herbal preparations throughout the world. It is said to promote the health of neighboring plants. Historic herbal volumes celebrate it for digestive disorders, anorexia, nausea during pregnancy, painful menstruation, and gas.

USE & HEALTH BENEFIT

• To help relieve pain, apply undiluted to small areas and 50:50 with a carrier oil for larger areas.

• For multiple skin conditions: acne, allergies, boils +++++L, burns, cuts, chilblains, dermatitis, eczema, inflammation ++P, insect bites, rashes ++P, sensitive skin, and infected wounds; apply undiluted to small areas and diluted 50:50 with a carrier oil to larger areas. For applications that would work better with a water and oil (like the scalp), mix 3 to 5 drops in a teaspoon of oil and apply. For infections, create a compress by applying a damp cloth over the oil, add a dry cloth and apply heat. This will help the oil to penetrate.

• For teething pain and toothache, apply undiluted to the gums.

• For an earache, apply undiluted on and around the outer ear. Do not insert essential oils into the ear canal.

• To help with spasms of all kinds: muscle, respiratory, nerves, digestive, etc.; create a 50:50 blend with a carrier oil and apply to the affected area. +++P

• To release intestinal parasites, take a capsule containing a 50:50 blend of Roman chamomile and carrier oil 3 times a day with food. +++P

• To treat emotional shock, place 6 drops on a tissue, a cotton ball, or a handkerchief, and inhale. You can also put 3 drops in your palm, rub palms together, put over nose and mouth, and inhale deeply several times. +++P

• To ease the pain of arthritis, inflamed joints, muscle pain, neuralgia, rheumatism, and sprains, massage the painful areas with a 50:50 blend with a carrier oil. Take an aromatic bath using 10 to 15 drops of Roman chamomile in a cup of Epsom Salts +++L.

• To help ease conditions of the digestive system: nausea, colic, indigestion, gas, etc.; take a capsule containing a 50:50 blend of Roman chamomile and carrier oil 3 times a day with food. You can also do an abdominal massage with a 50:50 blend of Roman chamomile and carrier oil. Diffuse 20 drops of Roman chamomile to ease nausea.

• To help stimulate digestion and strengthen liver function, take a 50:50 capsule of Roman chamomile with a carrier oil daily with food. This is also important in cleansing the liver and stimulating white blood cell production ++++L.

• To help with painful menstruation, menopausal symptoms, and excessive menstrual flow, do a low abdominal massage with a 50:50 blend of Roman chamomile and a carrier oil. You may want to apply a warm, damp cloth over the area with a heating pad to help the oil penetrate. Also try a capsule containing a 50:50 blend of Roman chamomile and carrier oil once a day with food ++++L.

• For help in calming tantrums and anger, apply 6 drops on a cotton ball, tissue, or handkerchief and inhale. The cotton ball can also be put in a pillow case or pinned to the collar of pajamas ++++L. Roman chamomile is especially mild yet effective for use in therapy for children. It is calming without being depressing.

- To help with headaches, migraines, insomnia, nervous tension, and stress, diffuse 20 drops of Roman chamomile twice a day. Take a capsule containing a 50:50 blend of Roman chamomile and carrier oil once a day with food. Massage your sinus areas, neck, shoulders, back, chest, abdomen, and feet with a 50:50 blend of Roman chamomile and carrier oil ++++L.

- To ease the pain of neuralgia or neuritis, gently apply Roman chamomile undiluted to the painful area +P.

- As a pre-anesthetic, inhale 2 drops of Roman chamomile in a tissue, cotton ball, or handkerchief +++P.

CAUTIONS: None when used in quantities indicated.

✔ CLINICAL SUPPORT

The use of complementary therapies, such as massage and aromatherapy massage, is rising in popularity among patients and healthcare professionals. This study assessed the effects of both massage and aromatherapy massage using Roman chamomile on cancer patients in a palliative care setting. There was a statistically significant reduction in anxiety after each massage. The aromatherapy group's scores improved on all subscales at the 1% level of significance or better, except for severely restricted activities. Massage with or without essential oils appears to reduce levels of anxiety. The addition of an essential oil seems to enhance the effect of massage and to improve physical and psychological symptoms, as well as overall quality of life (Wilkinson S, et al., 1999).

This study investigated the effects of a blend of lavender, Roman chamomile, and neroli on anxiety, sleep, and blood pressure of 56 patients in intensive care units. Patients received topical and inhaled treatments. Patients in the aromatherapy group showed significantly lower anxiety and improving sleep quality compared with conventional nursing intervention. Aromatherapy effectively reduced the anxiety levels and increased the sleep quality of patients admitted to the ICU (Mi-Yeon Cho, et al., 2013).

The purpose of this study was to investigate the effects of aromatherapy on the anxiety, sleep, and blood pressure (BP) of percutaneous coronary intervention (PCI) patients in an intensive care unit (ICU). Fifty-six patients with PCI in ICU were evenly allocated to either the aromatherapy or conventional nursing care. Aromatherapy essential oils were blended with lavender, roman chamomile, and neroli with a 6 : 2 : 0.5 ratio. Participants received 10 times treatment before PCI, and the same essential oils were inhaled another 10 times after PCI. Outcome measures patients' state anxiety, sleeping quality, and BP. An aromatherapy group showed significantly low anxiety (t = 5.99, P < .001) and improving sleep quality (t = −3.65, P = .001) compared with conventional nursing intervention. The systolic BP of both groups did not show a significant difference by time or in a group-by-time interaction; however, a significant difference was observed between groups (F = 4.63, P = .036). The diastolic BP did not show any significant difference by time or by a group-by-time interaction; however, a significant difference was observed between groups (F = 6.93, P = .011). In conclusion, the aromatherapy effectively reduced the anxiety levels and increased the sleep quality of PCI patients admitted to the ICU. Aromatherapy may be used as an independent nursing intervention for reducing the anxiety levels and improving the sleep quality of PCI patients.

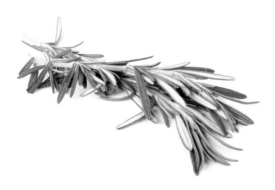

Rosemary

Roseamarinus officinalis

Family: (Labiatae)
Origins: Mediterranian area, but now cultivated worldwide. Oil producing countries are France, Spain, and Tunisia.
Other names: compass plant, incensier.
Description: A small evergreen bush with silver-green needle-like leaves and pale blue flowers.
Extraction: Essential oil by steam distillation
Botanical Part Used: fresh flowering tops
Principal constituents: Mainly pinenes, camphene, limonene, cineol, borneol, and others. There are possibly 3 chemotypes.

🅱 BLENDING SUGGESTIONS

Relative strength: 3
Among the middle notes that typically make up more than 50% of the blend.
Blends well with: lavender, lavandin, citronella, oregano, thyme, pine, basil, peppermint, cedarwood, cinnamon and other spices.
Description: strong, herbal, evergreen, minty, and fresh, with a woody-balsamic undertone

📖 HISTORY & TRADITIONAL USES

Rosemary has been used for thousands of years for food, medicine, and magic. It was regarded as sacred by many civilizations. It was burned to drive away evil spirits and protect people from the Plague during the Middle Ages. It has been traditionally used for respiratory and circulatory conditions, muscle and rheumatic pain, skin and hair conditions, liver disorders, digestive complaints, and nervous conditions.

➕ USE & HEALTH BENEFIT

- For varicose veins, create a 50:50 blend of rosemary and a carrier oil and gently massage the affected area.

- For skin conditions: acne ++++L, dermatitis ++++L, eczema ++++L, dry skin +++L, wrinkles, and scabies; apply undiluted and add a carrier oil as need to smaller areas, or create a 50:50 blend with a carrier oil and apply topically +++L.

- To stop a cut from bleeding, apply a drop of rosemary undiluted +++L. Use rosemary over the bridge of the nose with a cold, damp washcloth to stop a nosebleed. A cold aromatic cloth at the back of the neck will also help.

- As an insect repellent mix 3 drops of rosemary in a teaspoon of water and apply to skin and clothing. You can create a spray with 20 drops of rosemary in 8 ounces of water. Shake each time before spraying to disperse oil as much as possible into the water.

- To help stimulate hair growth or reverse hair loss and help with dandruff and greasy hair, mix 3 drops of rosemary in a teaspoon of water and apply to the scalp daily. Or mix 3 drops in a single application of a mild but not greasy hair care product and massage into the scalp ++++L. This will also help take care of a lice problem.

- To stimulate and strengthen the cardiovascular system to overcome exhaustion, poor circulation, symptoms of arteriosclerosis, headaches, and heart palpitations, have an invigorating massage with a 50:50 blend of rosemary and a carrier oil.

- To help with fluid retention, gout, muscular pain, and rheumatism, massage affected areas with a 50:50 blend of rosemary and a carrier oil.

- To help with respiratory conditions: asthma, bronchitis ++P, laryngitis, whooping cough, etc.; diffuse 20 drops of rosemary twice a day. Take hot aromatic baths using 10 to 15 drops of rosemary in a cup of Epsom Salts. Create a 50:50 blend of rosemary with a carrier oil and make capsules. Take a capsule 3 times a day with food. Use the same blend to massage the sinus areas, throat, and chest as well as the reflex areas on the feet. Use 3 or 4 drops of rosemary in a bowl or pan of steaming water. Put a cloth over your head and breathe the aromatic steam. Create a hot or cool compress over the affected areas—sinuses, throat, chest, etc.

- For digestive disorders: colitis, gas, diarrhea, liver disorders; create a 50:50 blend of rosemary with a carrier oil and create capsules. Take one 3 times a day with food +++P.

- Genito-urinary disorders: painful menstruation, hormonal regulation, infections, etc.; create a 50:50 blend of rosemary with a carrier oil and create capsules. Take one 3 times a day with food +++P.

- To strengthen the immune system to prevent colds, flu, and the spread of infections, diffuse 20 drops of rosemary twice a day.

- To help with mental fatigue, nervous exhaustion, and stress related conditions, diffuse 20 drops of rosemary and take an aromatic bath using 10 to 15 drops of rosemary and a cup of Epsom Salts. You can also inhale the aroma of rosemary by placing a few drops in your palm, rubbing your palms together, cupping your hands over your nose and mouth, and inhaling deeply several times. You can put 6 drops in a tissue, on a cotton ball, or on a handkerchief and inhale the aroma from time to time throughout the day. Keep in a plastic bag to keep the aroma from evaporating.

- For fatigue, depression, and cloudy or confused thinking (neurochatter), diffuse 20 drops of rosemary twice a day. Put 6 drops of rosemary in a tissue and inhale from it throughout the day to stay alert, energetic, and clear headed.

> CAUTIONS: None when used in quantities indicated. Avoid during pregnancy. Do not use on children under age 4. May increase risk of jaundice in children. Not to be used by epileptics. When taken orally it may increase blood-thinning effects. May enhance the effects of antibiotics. People with high blood pressure should avoid using rosemary long-term.

✓ CLINICAL SUPPORT

Self-administered abdominal massage with rosemary essential oil can increase attentiveness, alertness, liveliness, joyfulness, while increasingbreathing rate and blood pressure (Dobetsberger, C. and Buchbauer, G., 2011).

Rosemary essential oil has an anti-inflammatory and anti-nociceptive potential in an in vivo study (Adorjan, B and Buchbauer, G., 2010).

Rosemary has an anti-nociceptive effect on the central nervous system. This is a reduction in pain sensitivity. (Adorjan, B and Buchbauer, G., 2010).

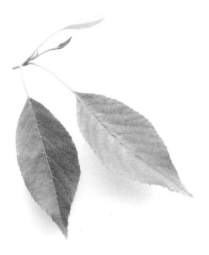

Rosewood

Aniba rosaeodora

Family: Lauraceae
Origins: Native of the South American rainforests of Brazil and Peru.
Other names: bois de rose, Brazilian rosewood
Description: Mid-sized tropical evergreen with red bark and yellow flowers. Endangered because it is being used for timber in clearing the rainforests of South America.
Extraction: Essential oil by steam distillation
Botanical Part Used: wood chips
Principal constituents: Linalol (80-90%), cineol, terpineol, geraniol, citronellal, limonene, pinene and others.

BLENDING SUGGESTIONS

Relative strength: 3
Among the middle notes that typically make up more than 50% of the blend.
Blends well with most oils, especially citrus, woody oils, and florals
Description: very sweet, woody-floral, with a spicy hint

HISTORY & TRADITIONAL USES

Wood is used for building, carving, and expensive cabinet making. Much rosewood is made into Japanese chopsticks. Used extensively in perfumery, soaps, toiletries, cosmetics. Used in major food categories and drinks.

USE & HEALTH BENEFIT

- To help with acne, dermatitis, scars, wounds, wrinkles, sensitive skin, dry or dull skin, create a masque with 7 drops of rosewood. Create a 50:50 blend and apply topically. Rosewood is mild and safe enough to apply undiluted on wrinkles and sensitive skin. Add carrier oils as needed. Rosewood helps to regenerate tissue.

- For depression, stress, headaches, nervous tension, or anxiety, create a 50:50 blend with a carrier oil and massage hands and feet. Have an aromatic bath using 10 to 15 drops of rosewood in a cup of Epsom Salts.

- To strengthen and stimulate the immune sysyem to help with colds, coughs, fevers, and infections +++P, create a 50:50 blend of rosewood and a carrier oil and massage the respiratory areas of the feet daily. Use 10 to 15 drops with a cup of Epsom Salts in an aromatic bath and about half that amount to soak your feet. Rosewood is safe for adults, children, and even babies to use for bronchial-pulmonary conditions.

- For a vaginal fungal infection, have an aromatic bath using 10 to 15 drops of rosewood mixed with a cup of Epsom Salts.

> CAUTIONS: None when used in quantities indicated. Exceptionally mild on the skin and the mucosal areas of the body. Rosewood is an endangered species in some areas of the world. Be sure to check to make sure it comes from a place where it is a renewable resource. This is a costly oil and should usually be used only in small quantities in blends.

✓ CLINICAL SUPPORT

Rosewood oil with its high linalool content, has sedative actions and can reduce neuronal excitability (Dobetsberger, C. and Buchbauer, G., 2011). Cinnamon bark, peppermint, chamomile, and rosewood are among the most common aromatherapy treatments that have been recommended for the relief of chemotherapy-induced nausea and vomiting (Mustian, KM, et al., 2011).

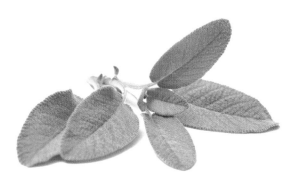

Sage
Salvia officinalis

Family: Lamiaceae (Labiatae)
Origins: Native to the Mediterranean area but cultivated worldwide, especially in Albania, Yugoslavia, Greece, Italy, Turkey, France, China, and the USA.
Other names: common sage, garden sage, true sage, Dalmatian sage
Description: A shrubby, perennial, evergreen herb that grows about 3 feet tall. Soft silver leaves and small blue-violet flowers.
Extraction: Essential oil by steam distillation
Botanical Part Used: dried leaves
Principal constituents: Thujone (about 42%), cineol, borneol, caryophyllene, and others.

 BLENDING SUGGESTIONS

Relative strength: 4
Among the middle notes that typically make up more than 50% of the blend.
Blends well with: bergamot, lavender lemon peppermint, rosemary, lemongrass, pine
Description: fresh, warm, spicy, herbal

 HISTORY & TRADITIONAL USES

Considered a sacred herb by the Romans. Used historically for respiratory conditions, menstrual issues, digestive concerns, inflammations of the mouth and throat, and improve memory. Highly valued as a culinary herb. It is used in pharmaceutical preparations like mouthwashes, gargles, and toothpastes. A fragrance in soaps, shampoos, detergents, antiperspirants, colognes, and perfumes, especially men's fragrances. Extensive use in meat flavorings and beverages.

USE & HEALTH BENEFIT

- For the flu, bronchitis, and sinusitis and a whole array of respiratory ear/nose/throat infections whether viral, bacterial or fungal, apply a 50:50 blend of sage and a carrier oil topically on the sinuses, throat and lungs. Take this 50:50 blend in a capsule, once a day with food. Create a cold compress for controlling bronchial coughing spasms using sage and a cold, damp washcloth over the upper chest. Diffuse 20 drops of sage twice daily. Take an aromatic bath using 10 to 15 drops of sage in a cup of Epsom Salts ++++P. To break up hardened mucous and bring up phlegm from deep in the lungs, put 6 drops of sage essential oil in a bowl or pan of boiling water, cover your head with a towel, and inhale the aromatic steam. Reheat the water and put in more oil as needed until your lungs and bronchioles start to loosen and clear.

- To encourage the breakdown of fat and reduce cellulite, create an aromatic compress or wrap by applying a 50:50 blend of sage and a carrier oil and then wrapping the area with a plastic wrap. Wrap up in a warm towel, blanket, or bathrobe and allow the oils to penetrate and break up the cellulite. Remove after 30 minutes or an hour.

- To heal canker sores and minor infected wounds, apply sage, undiluted several times a day. For more stubborn infections, create a compress by applying several drops of sage to the infection then putting a damp gauze over the wound, adding a cling bandage, then a dry towel, and finally adding a hot pad or a hot water bottle to help draw out the infection.

- To help reduce excessive perspiration, apply sage in the shower while the skin is still wet. Then pat yourself dry ++++L.

CAUTIONS: None when used in quantities indicated. Do not take topically or ingest in high doses. Do not use during pregnancy. If epileptic, do not use. Double the dilution instructions when using on children.

✔ CLINICAL SUPPORT

"[Sage,] in addition to treating minor common illnesses, might potentially provide novel natural treatments for the relief or cure of many serious and life-threatening diseases such as depression, dementia, obesity, diabetes, lupus, heart disease, and cancer. [Sage] essential oils have been used in the treatment of a wide range of diseases like those of the nervous system, heart and blood circulation, respiratory system, digestive system, and metabolic and endocrine diseases. In addition, sage essential oil has been shown to have carminative, antispasmodic, antiseptic, and astringent properties" (Hamidpour M, et al., 2014).

"[Sage] is used in traditional medicine as antiseptic, antiscabies, antisyphilitic, and anti-inflammatory, being frequently used against skin diseases. The oils revealed antifungal activity without affecting cell viability .... These findings demonstrated that bioactive concentrations of S. officinalis oils [make] them suitable to be incorporated in skin care formulations for cosmetic and pharmaceutical purposes (Abu-Darwish, MS, et al., 2013).

Salvia officinalis L. (Lamiaceae) is a Mediterranean species, naturalized in many countries. In Jordan, it is used in traditional medicine as antiseptic, antiscabies, antisyphilitic, and anti-inflammatory, being frequently used against skin diseases. This study aimed the assessment of the antifungal and anti-inflammatory potential of its essential oils, and their cytotoxicity on macrophages and keratinocytes. The oils were investigated by gas chromatography and gas chromatography-mass spectrometry and the antifungal activity was evaluated against yeasts, dermatophyte and Aspergillus strains. Assessment of cell viability was made by the 3-(4,5-dimethylthiazol-2-yl)-2,5-diphenyltetrazolium bromide assay and the in vitro anti-inflammatory potential was evaluated by measuring nitric oxide production using lipopolysaccharide-stimulated mouse macrophages. The main compounds of S. officinalis oils were 1,8-cineole (39.5–50.3%) and camphor (8.8–25.0%). The oils revealed antifungal activity against dermatophyte strains and significantly inhibited NO production stimulated by LPS in macrophages, without affecting cell viability, in concentrations up to 0.64 μL/mL. This is the first report addressing the in vitro anti-inflammatory potential of S. officinalis oil. These findings demonstrated that bioactive concentrations of S. officinalis oils do not affect mammalian macrophages and keratinocytes viability making them suitable to be incorporated in skin care formulations for cosmetic and pharmaceutical purposes.

For a long time, sage (Salvia) species have been used in traditional medicine for the relief of pain, protecting the body against oxidative stress, free radical damages, angiogenesis, inflammation, bacterial and virus infection, etc., Several studies suggest that sage species can be considered for drug development because of their reported pharmacology and therapeutic activities in many countries of Asia and Middle East, especially China and India. These studies suggest that Salvia species, in addition to treating minor common illnesses, might potentially provide novel natural treatments for the relief or cure of many serious and life-threatening diseases such as depression, dementia, obesity, diabetes, lupus, heart disease, and cancer. This article presents a comprehensive analysis of the botanical, chemical, and pharmacological aspects of sage (*Saliva*).

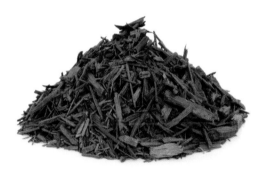

Sandalwood

Santalum album (India and almost not available any more) Santalum spicatum (Australia) check.

Family: Santalaceae
Origins: Native of tropical Asia, especially India, Sri Lanka, Malaysia, Indonesia, and Taiwan. India is the main producer. Some of the oil is distilled in Europe and the USA.
Other names: White sandalwood, East Indian sandalwood, sandalwood Mysore, sanders-wood, santal (oil)
Description: Small evergreen, parasitic tree with a brown-grey trunk and smooth branches. Leathery leaves and pink-purple flowers. The tree must be 30 years old before it can produce oil.
Extraction: Essential oil by steam distillation
Botanical Part Used: Dried and powdered roots and heartwood
Principal constituents: Santalols (90%), santene, teresantol, borneol, santalone, and others.

BLENDING SUGGESTIONS

Relative strength: 3
Among the base notes that typically make up less than 30% of the blend.
Blends well with: cypress, frankincense, lemon, myrrh, ylang ylang, patchouli, and spruce
Description: deep soft, woody-sweet, earthy, and balsamic, and long lasting.

HISTORY & TRADITIONAL USES

One of the oldest perfume sources. Used for incense, cosmetics, perfume, and embalming materials throughout Asia. A popular building material for temples. In Chinese medicine it treats stomach ache, vomiting, gonorrhea, and skin conditions. In India it is used for urinary and respiratory infections as well as diarrhea.

USE & HEALTH BENEFIT

- To decongest the lymphatic and cardiovascular system, create a 50:50 massage with sandalwood and a carrier oil, and massage affected areas of the body +++P.

- To help tone and strengthen the heart, create a 50:50 massage oil with sandalwood and a carrier oil and massage the heart area of the feet. Create an aromatic bath by using 10 to 15 drops of sandalwood in a cup of Epsom Salts ++P.

- For these skin conditions: acne, dry skin, cracked and chapped skin, or greasy skin; apply sandalwood undiluted on the area of concern, or if the area is large, apply a 50:50 blend of sandalwood. Can also be used as a moisturizer and aftershave on the sensitive tissues of the face +++L.

- To help ease the symptoms of bronchitis, excess mucous, coughs, laryngitis, or sore throat, diffuse 20 drops of sandalwood, take an aromatic bath using 10 to 15 drops of sandalwood with a carrier oil; or create a 50:50 blend of sandalwood and a carrier oil and respiratory areas of the body: chest and back, neck, and sinus areas of the face.

- For congestion of the organs in the pelvic region, create a massage oil using a 50:50 mixture of sandalwood and a carrier oil. Massage the lower abdomen and lower back. Also take hot baths using 10 to 15 drops of sandalwood and a cup of Epsom Salts ++P.

- To help with hemorrhoids and varicose veins, create a 50:50 mixture of sandalwood and a carrier oil and apply gently to the affected area.

- To help with neuralgia, sciatica (pressure on the sciatic nerve in the back leading to pain down the leg), and lower back pain, use sandalwood as one of the oils in the Layer Therapy with a hot compress.

- Create a 50:50 blend with sandalwood and a carrier oil to massage the affected areas. Take a hot aromatic bath using 10 to 15 drops of sandalwood in a cup of Epsom Salts.

- For a urinary tract infection and other associated urogenital conditions, create a 50:50 blend of sandalwood and carrier oil and apply to the lower abdomen. Use a warm, damp cloth over the area and apply a dry towel and heat to help penetration of the oils +++L.

- To elevate the mood and overcome depression, insomnia, nervous tension, and stress, diffuse 20 drops of sandalwood, take an aromatic bath using 10 to 15 drops of sandalwood with a carrier oil; or create a 50:50 blend of sandalwood and a carrier oil and massage hands, feet, and any area of

the body where you feel that your negative emotions seem to reside.

- To help with digestive disorders such as diarrhea and nausea, take an aromatic bath using 10 to 15 drops of sandalwood with a carrier oil; or create a 50:50 blend of sandalwood and a carrier oil and use the oil to massage the abdomen in a clockwise direction.

CAUTIONS: None when used in quantities indicated.

 CLINICAL SUPPORT

"... Isolates of herpes simplex virus type 1 (HSV-1) were analyzed in vitro for their susceptibilities to essential oils of ginger, thyme, hyssop, and sandalwood. All essential oils exhibited high levels of virucidal activity against [herpes simplex virus type 1] ... and reduced plaque formation significantly" (Schnitzler P, [Koch C.] Reichling J., (2007).

"We examined how aromatherapy massage influenced psychologic and immunologic parameters in 12 breast cancer patients. The results showed that anxiety was reduced in one 30 min aromatherapy massage .... Our results further suggested that aromatherapy massage ameliorated the immunologic state (Imanishi J, et al., 2009).

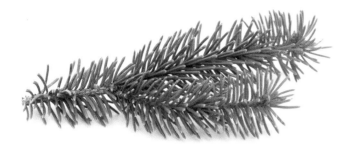

Spruce

Picea mariana

Family: Pinaceae
Origins: A native of northern North America, from Newfoundland to Alaska, and south to Pennsylvania and Minnesota.
Other names: black spruce
Description: A slow-growing, small upright evergreen coniferous tree having a straight trunk with a narrow, pointed crown. The needles are dark bluish green and the cones are the smallest of all of the spruces.
Extraction: Essential oil by steam distillation
Botanical Part Used: needles
Principal constituents: camphene, alpha pinene, limonene, bornyl acetate, borneol, and others.

BLENDING SUGGESTIONS

Relative strength: 3
Among the middle notes that typically make up more than 50% of the blend.
Blends well with: Eucalyptus globulus, Eucalyptus radiata, frankincense, helichrysum, birch, and wintergreen
Description: woody, fresh, earthy, sweet, and a little fruity

HISTORY & TRADITIONAL USES

Used by American Indians in their religious rituals.

USE & HEALTH BENEFIT

- For calming and uplifting your spirits, diffuse 20 drops of spruce daily. According to Dr. Kurt Schnabelt, spruce strengthens and supports the adrenal glands during times of stress and fatigue. This helps confirm that it is not only calming and sedating but also uplifting +++++L.

- To help overcome physical exhaustion, diffuse 20 drops of spruce regularly. Also massage your body (especially hands and feet) with a 50:50 blend of spruce and carrier oil ++++P.

- To help with hyperthyroidism (difficulty sleeping, nervousness, irritability, increased perspiration, heart racing, hand tremors, anxiety, difficulty sleeping, thinning of the skin, fine brittle hair, and muscular weakness), apply spruce undiluted to the base of the throat over the thyroid.

- For respiratory issues: asthma, bronchitis, sinusitis, laryngitis, etc.; diffuse 20 drops of spruce twice a day. Use in a cold compress for bronchial spasms by applying spruce undiluted over the upper chest then applying a cool, damp cloth to reduce inflammation in the bronchioles. Spruce can also be used, 2 to 3 drops per application in lotions and creams for respiratory benefits.

- To reduce prostate inflammation, create a 50:50 blend of spruce and a carrier oil and massage the lower abdomen once a day ++P.

- For calming spasms throughout the body—digestive, respiratory, nervous, muscular, etc.—create a 50:50 blend of spruce and a carrier oil and massage the affected area. A calming bath using 10 to 15 drops of spruce in a cup of Epsom Salts will also reduce spasms.

CLINICAL SUPPORT

Spruce "is a bronchial decongestant and an even more powerful adrenal stimulant than [pine]" (Rhind, 2012).

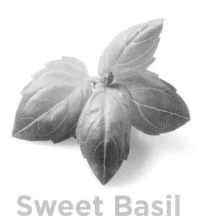

Sweet Basil

Ocimum basilicum

Family: Lamiaceae (Labiatae)
Origins: Produced mainly in India. Also grown in tropical Asia and Africa. Widely cultivated in the Mediterranean region, the Pacific Islands, and North and South America. The oil is distilled mainly in France, Italy, Egypt, Bulgaria, Hungary, and the USA.
Other names: Common basil, joy-of-the-mountain, "true" sweet basil, European basil, and French basil
Description: A tender annual herb with dark green leaves and green and pink flowers.
Extraction: Essential oil by steam distillation
Botanical Part Used: Flowering herb
Principal constituents: Linalol (40 – 45%), methyl chavicol (23%), small amounts of eugenol, limonene, citronellol, and others. Is it a pure tropical or sweet or in between.

 BLENDING SUGGESTIONS

Relative strength: 4
Among the top and middle notes that typically make up more than 70% of the blend (top notes 20%, middle notes 50%).
Blends well with: bergamot, cypress, helichrysum, lavender, fir, lemongrass, peppermint, spruce, marjoram, and wintergreen
Description: herbal, spicy, licorice, camphoric, lively

 HISTORY & TRADITIONAL USES

It is used for respiratory problems: bronchitis, coughs, colds, asthma, flu, and emphysema. Basil has been used traditionally as an antidote for poisonous insect and snake bites. It has been used to treat malaria and the plague. It improves circulation and digestion. In Chinese medicine it is used for stomach and kidney ailments. It is considered a "cooling" herb in Western traditions used for rheumatic pain, inflamed skin conditions, and to calm the nerves. It is a popular culinary herb in Mediterranean cuisine. It is used extensively in major food categories, especially in savory foods. It is also used as a fragrance in soaps, cosmetics, and perfumes.

USE & HEALTH BENEFIT

- To prevent spasms: muscles, respiratory, and digestive; mix with carrier oil in a 50:50 blend and massage over area of discomfort +++P.

- To ease itching of insect bites and as an insect repellent, apply undiluted or diluted with 5 drops in a teaspoon of water or 20 drops in an 8 oz. spray bottle. Be sure to shake the bottle to disperse the oil with each application.

- For anxiety, depression, fatigue, insomnia, migraine, and nervous tension, put 5 drops of basil in a tissue and inhale. You can also put 3 drops in your palm, rub palms together, cup hands over nose and mouth and inhale. Take an aromatic bath using 10 to 15 drops in a cup of Epsom Salts. Diffuse 20 drops. Create a 50:50 blend with a carrier oil and massage the areas of your body where negative emotions seem to congregate. It can also be used in these ways as a nerve tonic ++++L +++P.

- To clear confusion or "neurochatter", relieve mental exhaustion, stimulate the memory, and revive the mind, put 5 drops of basil in a tissue and inhale. You can also put 3 drops in your palm, rub palms together, cup hands over nose and mouth and inhale. Take an aromatic bath using 10 to 15 drops in a cup of Epsom Salts. Diffuse 20 drops. Create a 50:50 blend with a carrier oil and use as an abdominal, back, neck, head, and shoulder massage ++++L.

- To ease the pain of gout, muscle aches and pains, and rheumatism, create a 50:50 blend with a carrier oil and massage the affected area.

- To calm the digestive system, relieve gastric spasms, and reduce nausea and gas, take a drop or trace in drinking water, juice, or tea. Diffuse 20 drops daily. Create a 50:50 blend of basil and a carrier oil for an abdominal massage. +++L

- To calm cramps and spasms of the muscles, digestive system, respiratory system, and nerves, take an aromatic bath using 10 to 15 drops in a cup of Epsom Salts. Diffuse 20 drops. Create a 50:50 blend with a carrier oil and massage the affected area.

- To ease or prevent a migraine, create a compress using 10 drops of basil in 1/2 cup of cold water, soak a wash cloth, wring it out, and apply it to the forehead or back of the neck. Put a dry towel over it and keep it cool with a cold compress or ice pack ++++L.

CAUTIONS: None when used in quantities indicated. When ingested in high quantities it may have some blood thinning properties, promote show hypoglycemic effects, and may inhibit MAO enzymes with some minor effects on raising blood pressure, causing minor confusion, and diarrhea.

 CLINICAL SUPPORT

Basil lowers convulsions (Dobetsberger, C. and Buchbauer, G., 2011).

Basil was found to have the potential to improve the delivery of NSAIDs (Nonsteroidal Anti-inflammatory Drugs) like ibuprofen (Adorjan, B and Buchbauer, G., 2010).

Sweet basil for abdominal stress

I used to carry a lot of stress in my upper abdomen. I could feel it sitting there like a hard knot. When I started eating more fruits and vegetables, it eased up a bit. But I noticed that when I used a drop of sweet basil on a regular basis in my water or in capsules and applied it diluted right under my ribcage, the stress seemed to lighten up. I love putting a little basil in everything—water, recipes, herbal tea, tomato juice—anything. It seems to settle me down.

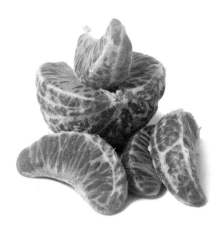

Tangerine
Citrus reticulata

Family: Rutaceae
Origins: Southern China. Originally called mandarin. Renamed tangerine when it was brought to Europe. The mandarin is cultivated mainly in Italy, Spain, Algeria, Cyprus, Greece, the Middle East, and Brazil. Tangerines are grown in Texas, Florida, and California.
Other names: mandarin, European mandarin, true mandarin, and Satsuma.
Description: A small evergreen with glossy leaves, fragrant flowers and a fleshy citrus fruit.
Extraction: Essence by cold expression
Botanical Part Used: outer peel of the fruit
Principal constituents: Limonene, methyl methylanthranilate, geraniol, citral, citronellal, and others

 BLENDING SUGGESTIONS

Relative strength: 3
Among the top notes that typically make up less than 20% of the blend.
Blends well with: basil, bergamot, Roman chamomile, German chamomile, clary sage, frankincense, grapefruit, lavender, lemon, orange, and spice oils like cinnamon and clove
Description: fresh, intensely sweet, citrusy, and floral

 HISTORY & TRADITIONAL USES

The origin of the name, "mandarin" comes from the fruit, which was regarded as a gift of the Mandarins of China. In Europe the oil has been valued as a safe children's remedy for digestive issues. Used as a fragrance in soaps, cosmetics, and perfumes ... especially in colognes. It is a flavoring used in candies and drinks.

✚ **USE & HEALTH BENEFIT**

• For skin care conditions: acne, congested and oily skin, scars, spots, and stretch marks; apply undiluted to small areas or create a 50:50 blend with a carrier oil. Add 3 drops to each application of lotions or creams.

• To prevent spasms: muscles, respiratory, and digestive; mix with carrier oil in a 50:50 blend and massage over area of discomfort +++P.

• To detoxify and release fluid retention as well as help with weight loss, create a 50:50 blend with a carrier oil and massage legs or other areas of fluid retention.

• For a digestive stimulant to help with hiccoughs, nausea, and gastric upset, put 3 drops in your palm, rub palms together, cup hands over nose and mouth, and inhale deeply several times. Create a 50:50 blend with a carrier oil for an abdominal massage. Take a drop or trace of tangerine in your drinking water, herbal tea, or juice. Diffuse 20 drops.

• For insomnia, nervous tension, restlessness, anxiety, and waves of stress, diffuse 20 drops of tangerine several times a day. Put 6 drops in a tissue, cotton ball, or handkerchief and inhale to help reduce negative emotions. This can be put inside a pillow case at night to help with restful sleep. Apply a 50:50 blend with a carrier oil to the hands using the "M" Technique. Use this blend for a foot massage ++++P.

CAUTIONS: *None when used in quantities indicated. May be photosensitizing. After applying to exposed skin, do not spend time in direct sunlight for 12 hours.*

✔ CLINICAL SUPPORT

"High pressure stress was found to induce immunosuppression accompanied with the enhancement of motor activity in mice. Citrus fragrance restored stress-induced immunosuppression and induced calm behavior in mice. The application of citrus fragrance to depressive patients made it possible to markedly reduce the doses of antidepressants needed for the treatment of patients" (Komori T, Fujiwara R, Tanida M, Nomura J. [Application of fragrances to treatments for depression]. *Nihon Shinkei Seishin Yakurigaku Zasshi*. 1995 Feb;15(1):39-42. [Article in Japanese]).

The anti-fungal and cytotoxicity activity of tangerine essential oil was analyzed. The results suggest that tangerine generates cytotoxicity in P. italicum and P. digitatum by disrupting cell membrane integrity and causing the leakage of cell components (Tao N, Jia L, Zhou H., 2014).

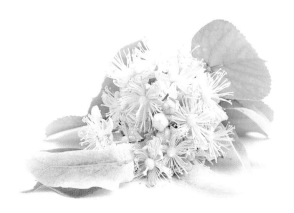

Tea Tree
Melaleuca alternifolia

Family: Myrtaceae
Origins: Australia.
Other names: narrow-leaved paperbark tea tree, ti-tree, ti-trol, and melasol.
Description: A small tree/shrub with needle-like leaves much like a cypress and yellow or purple flowers.
Extraction: Essential oil by steam or water distillation
Botanical Part Used: twigs and leaves
Principal constituents: Terpinene-4-ol (up to 40%), cineol, pinene, terpinenes, cymene, sesquiterpenes, sesquiterpene alcohols, and others.

BLENDING SUGGESTIONS

Relative strength: 3
Among the middle notes that typically make up more than 50% of the blend
Blends well with all citrus oils, cypress, clary sage, lavandin, pine, marjoram, clove, Eucalyptus radiata, lavender, rosemary, and thyme
Description: fresh, spicy, camphoric, warm, medicinal, woody, earthy, and herbal

Singles

📖 HISTORY & TRADITIONAL USES

The name comes from using the leaves in an herbal tea. Used by the aboriginal people of Australia for all types of infections. It is a very powerful stimulant to the immune system. It is used in soaps, toothpastes, deodorants, disinfectants, gargles, aftershaves, and spicy colognes.

➕ USE & HEALTH BENEFIT

- Tea tree is a major, broad-spectrum antimicrobial. It is safe but highly effective. It is antibacterial, antifungal, antiviral, and antiparasitic. It can safely be applied undiluted to small areas: abscesses, acne, blisters, cold sores ++++P, canker sores ++++P, minor burns, athlete's foot, insect bites, rashes, itches, warts, spots, and infected wounds.

- For larger areas of skin: acne, sunburns, dandruff, and insect repellent; it is best to mix 3 – 5 drops in a teaspoon of water and apply. In the case of a minor sunburn, you can mix 20 drops in a spray bottle, shake to disperse the oil, and spray it on the sunburn. For a diaper rash it is best to create a 50:50 blend with a carrier oil and apply. You may want to use a 20:80 dilution for diaper rash at first to see if it works just as well.

- To release toxins and excess fluids in swollen legs and arms, create a 50:50 blend with a carrier oil, and massage the appendages upwards towards the heart.

- To help with cardiac fatigue, slow blood flow to the brain, and sluggish circulation, create a 50:50 massage blend using tea tree and a carrier oil, and massage limbs, back, and abdomen.

- To help heal hemorrhoids and varicose veins, apply a 5:95 massage blend using tea tree and a carrier oil.

- Dr. Pénoël suggests that tea tree offers some protection from radiation exposure and helps with burns from radiation therapy when applied topically in a 50:50 blend with a carrier oil.

- For respiratory conditions: asthma, bronchitis, phlegm, cough, sinusitis, TB, whooping cough, etc.; diffuse 20 drops to help clear the air passages and the lungs. Use a diffuser with another 20 drops on a low setting throughout the night. Take an aromatic bath using 10 to 15 drops of tea tree in a cup of Epsom salts. Breathe the disinfecting aroma by putting 6 drops in a tissue, handkerchief, or cotton ball and inhaling through it throughout the day.

- For the first tickle of a sore throat, lick a trace of tea tree off your hand and use your tongue to distribute it to the infected area. If you do this every few minutes, you will feel the tickle or the pain begin to subside. Do not get too much oil each time, but do it frequently, every few minutes. Then, once the pain starts to diminish, do it throughout the day to keep the infection from returning. These same instructions can also be used for bad breath, oral fungus (candida/thrush), canker sores, cold sores, mouth abscesses, and gingivitis (inflammation of the gums) ++++P.

- For vagina, prostate, and various other genital and urinary tract infections, take an aromatic bath using 10 to 15 drops of tea tree in a cup of Epsom Salts. You can also take a capsule with a 50:50 blend of tea tree and a carrier oil 3 times daily with food. You can apply oils around the genitals with a 50:50 blend of carrier oil and tea tree, but do not apply essential oils, even in dilution directly on the delicate tissues of the genitals.

- For infections like colds, fever, flu, infectious illnesses (chicken pox), and shingles, diffuse 20 drops of tea tree a couple of times a day. Apply a 50:50 blend of tea tree and carrier oil topically on the area of infection. Take a tea tree capsule with this blend 3 times a day. Take aromatic baths using 10 to 15 drops of tea tree in a cup of Epsom Salts.

- To help with exhaustion, shock, and nervousness, take a few drops of tea tree in a tissue, handkerchief, or cotton ball and inhale. You can also add a few drops to your palm, rub palms together, cup your hands over your nose and mouth and inhale deeply several times. Diffusing 20 drops of tea tree will also help.

- For ear infections, apply tea tree undiluted around the outer ear. Do not put any essential oils inside the ear canal. Put a warm, damp cloth over the ear to help the oil penetrate. Use a hot water bottle or heating pad as well to help speed healing.

> *CAUTIONS: None when used in quantities indicated. Ingesting excessive amounts of 10ml or more have shown some toxic effects.*

 CLINICAL SUPPORT

Eucalyptus globulus, tea tree, and thyme have antiviral capacity against Herpes simplex virus. As whole oils they are more effective than their component parts and act in a dose-dependent manner. Tea tree shows promise in the treatment of influenza (Adorjan, B and Buchbauer, G., 2010).

Eucalyptus globulus, tea tree, and thyme have antiviral capacity against Herpes simplex virus. As whole oils they are more effective than their component parts and act in a dose-dependent manner. Tea tree shows promise in the treatment of influenza (Adorjan, B and Buchbauer, G., 2010).

Tea tree on cuts and scrapes

I have a large family so I'm no stranger to cuts and scrapes. I've used everything and nothing works better than tea tree on a cut. Whenever I see blood I reach for the tea tree because I know it will only be a matter of a day or two before there's hardly a memory of the cut. It also helps with the pain.

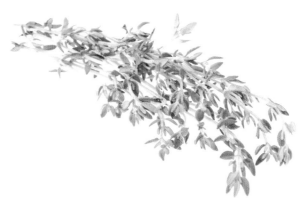

Thyme

Thymus vulgaris

Family: Lamiaceae (Labiatae)
Origins: Mediterranean region. Now found throughout Asia Minor, Russia, and central Europe. The oil is produced mainly in France, Israel, Greece, Morocco, Algeria, Germany, and the USA.
Other names: French thyme, garden thyme, red thyme (oil), white thyme (oil).
Description: A perennial shrub with small grey-green leaves and purple or white flowers.
Extraction: Essential oil by steam distillation.
Botanical Part Used: Fresh or partly-dried leaves and flowering tops
Principal constituents: Thymol and carvacrol (up to 60%), cymene, terpinene, camphene, and others. Check components given by Liebermuth. Have to dilute more if it is a strong thyme. I'm checking on this one too.

 BLENDING SUGGESTIONS

Relative strength: 4
Among the middle notes that typically make up more than 50% of the blend.
Blends well with: bergamot, cedarwood, juniper, melaleuca, oregano, and rosemary
Description: fresh, herbal, and medicinal

Singles

HISTORY & TRADITIONAL USES

Thyme was of the earliest known medicinal plants in the Mediterranean region. Used by Egyptians for embalming and by the Greeks for fumigating against infectious illness. Was used anciently in the preservation of meat. It's main historical applications were respiratory, digestive, and protection from infection. The oil is also used in mouthwashes, gargles, toothpaste, and cough drops. Thyme is used in surgical dressings. It is used as a fragrance element in soaps, aftershaves, and perfumes. It is extensively used in food and drink flavoring, especially in meat products.

USE & HEALTH BENEFIT

- Thyme is a powerful antimicrobial on the level of oregano and cinnamon. Use it with care and caution.

- For skin conditions: abscesses, acne +++P, bruises, cuts, scrapes, insect bites, gum infections, oily skin, wounds, and minor infections; apply thyme in 25:75 ratio with a carrier oil. A single drop in a teaspoon of oil for applying on an eczema infection may be the perfect ratio for you +++++L.

- As a circulation stimulating massage oil for the pain of gout, osteoarthritis ++++P, rheumatism, sprains, lower back pain, sciatica (back pain from a pressed nerve that radiates down the leg), sports injuries, and muscle aches and pains, create a 25:75 ratio with thyme and a carrier oil and massage the area around the muscles and joints ++++L.

- For stimulating circulation in cases of obesity, edema, and poor circulation, create a 25:75 ratio with a carrier oil and massage the limbs, back, shoulders, and abdomen, moving always toward the heart +++L.

- For respiratory conditions: asthma, bronchitis ++++P, coughs, laryngitis, sinusitis, sore throat,

and tuberculosis; diffuse a little thyme in a blend with other milder oils for a total of 20 drops. Thyme should be no more than 5 drops in the blend. Use thyme as one of the layers in a back and spinal massage: Layer Therapy. Have a carrier oil handy to dilute the oil if it gets too hot. Create a 20:80 massage oil for use on the back of neck, chest, and upper back. Do not use on the face. Massage the respiratory areas of the feet and hands. Create an aromatic bath using 10 to 15 drops of respiratory oils including no more than 5 drops of thyme. Blend the oils in a cup of Epsom Salts and disperse in bath water. All these therapies will also help with depression and nervous exhaustion +++L.

- For digestive disorders: diarrhea, gas, and nausea; create a 20:80 massage oil for use on the abdomen. Massage the digestive areas of the feet and hands. Create an aromatic bath using 10 to 15 drops of culinary spice oils like basil and marjoram including only 5 drops of thyme. Blend the oils in a cup of Epsom Salts and add them to your bath water.

- For genito-urinary infections +++P +++L, create a 20:80 massage oil for use on the lower abdomen. Use a warm, damp cloth a dry towel and heat over it to help the oils penetrate. Massage the lower abdominal areas the heels of the feet and hands. Create an aromatic bath using 10 to 15 drops of culinary spice oils like basil and marjoram including no more than 5 drops of thyme. Blend the oils in a cup of Epsom Salts and disperse in bath water.

- For viral infections: colds, chills, and flu +++++L; diffuse a little thyme in a blend with other milder oils for a total of 20 drops. Thyme should be no more than 5 drops in the blend. Use thyme as one of the layers in a back and spinal massage: Layer Therapy. Have a carrier oil handy to dilute the oil if it gets too hot. Create a 5:95 massage oil for the back of neck, chest and upper back. You can take this blend in a capsule 3 times a day. Massage the blend on your feet and hands. Create an aromatic bath using 10 to 15 drops of respiratory oils including no more than 5 drops of thyme. Blend the oils in a cup of Epsom Salts and disperse in bath water.

- For headaches, insomnia, general fatigue +++P, and stress, diffuse a blend of no more than 20 drops of oil with thyme as a minor ingredient (no more than 5 drops). Create a 20:80 blend with a carrier oil, and massage the shoulders, neck, and head. To avoid getting the hair greasy, blend 3 drops of thyme in a teaspoon of water to apply to the scalp and the back of the neck where the oil could come in contact with the hair.

- To stimulate various organs of the body ++++L: digestive, heart, liver, genito-urinary, endocrine glands, etc.; create a 20:80 blend of thyme with a carrier oil and massage the abdominal areas where those organs reside. Do not apply to genitals.

CAUTIONS: None when used in quantities indicated. Irritant to mucous membranes. Do not apply undiluted. Do not apply to mucous membranes (eyes, nose, mouth, vagina, or rectum). Do not take orally in large quantities over an extended period of time. When taking both topically and orally, it may interfere with enzyme action in metabolizing medications. When taking diabetic medications, it may cause slight hypoglycemic effects when taken orally. When taken orally with aspirin or blood thinners, it may increase blood-thinning effects. May enhance the effects of antibiotics.

✓ CLINICAL SUPPORT

Essential oils (EO) possess antimicrobial, anti-inflammatory, insect repellent, anti-cancer, and antioxidant properties. This study evaluated lemon, cypress, Eucalyptus globulus, and thyme. Thyme showed the best free radical-scavenging capacity. Thyme was also the most effective against lipid peroxidation along with lemon. Lemon demonstrated the best chelating power. Thyme showed the best anti-proliferative activity (Aazza S, et al., 2014).

Thyme has an anti-nociceptive effect on the central nervous system. This is a reduction in pain sensitivity. (Adorjan, B and Buchbauer, G., 2010).

A combination of thyme and oregano can reduce the production of pro-inflammatory cytokines. (Adorjan, B and Buchbauer, G., 2010).

Eucalyptus globulus, tea tree, and thyme have antiviral capacity against Herpes simplex virus. As whole oils they are more effective than their component parts and act in a dose-dependent manner. Tea tree shows promise in the treatment of influenza (Adorjan, B and Buchbauer, G., 2010).

A combination of thyme and oregano can reduce the production of pro-inflammatory cytokines. (Adorjan, B and Buchbauer, G., 2010).

Thyme has an anti-nociceptive effect on the central nervous system. This is reduction in pain sensitivity. (Adorjan, B and Buchbauer, G., 2010).

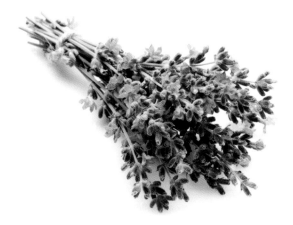

True Lavender
Lavandula officinalis

Family: Lamiaceae (Labiatae)
Origins: Mediterranean region. Now cultivated worldwide. Oil is mainly produced in France, Spain, Italy, England, Australia, Yugoslavia, Turkey, Russia, Bulgaria, and Greece.
Other names: garden lavender, common lavender. Lavandula angustifolia and Lavandula officinalis are the same. The word *officinalis* only refers to the fact that it is used for pharmaceutical purposes. It merely means "true lavender."
Description: A woody evergreen shrub about 3 feet tall with pale green, slender leaves and violet-blue flower on slender spikes. The whole plant is aromatic.
Extraction: Essential oil by steam distillation
Botanical Part Used: Fresh flowering tops
Principal constituents: Linalyl acetate (up to 40%), linalool, lavandulyl acetate, terpineol, limonene, ocimene and others. There are over 100 constituents.

BLENDING SUGGESTIONS

Relative strength: 2
Among the middle notes that typically make up more than 50% of the blend.
Blends well with most oils, especially the citrus oils, Roman chamomile, German chamomile, and clary sage
Description: floral, herbal, sweet, balsamic, and woody

HISTORY & TRADITIONAL USES

Lavender has been used traditionally as a folk remedy for digestive conditions, cosmetics, insect repellent, scenting linens, reviving, and soothing. It has been used to calm the nerves and ease palpitations, spasms, and colic. It relieves toothaches, painful neuralgia, sprains, and rheumatism. It is used extensively in pharmaceutical antiseptic ointments and as a fragrance in soaps, lotions, detergents, cosmetics, and perfumes. It is also used as a flavoring in foods and beverages.

USE & HEALTH BENEFIT

- Lavender has so many benefits, is so mild, and has such a pleasing aroma that it can almost be used for any health condition and considered the "universal oil" for almost anything.

- To ease pain, help reduce infection, and heal a minor wound, apply undiluted topically ++P +++L.

- To calm, overcome shock, reduce stress, overcome depression ++++L, promote sleep, and overcome anxiety or restlessness, diffuse 20 drops of lavender twice daily. Also apply undiluted topically to the solar plexus (just under the sternum on the chest) as well as the forehead, around the nose, and on the temples +++P.

- To calm a racing heart or pulse, apply topically in a 50:50 dilution with a carrier oil to the hands, feet, and on chest +P.

- To calm convulsions and spasms of all kinds (muscle, digestion, respiratory, etc.), diffuse 20 drops of lavender, massage with a 50:50 blend using lavender and carrier oil, take an aromatic bath or foot soak with 10 to 15 drops of lavender in a cup of Epsom Salts +++P ++++L.
- Take advantage of its deodorant properties with a foot soak with 10 drops in 1/2 cup of Epsom Salts and a foot massage with a 50:50 blend with a carrier oil.

- To eliminate intestinal parasites and worms, take a 50:50 blend of lavender and carrier oil in a capsule with food three times a day.

- For skin conditions: abscesses +++++L, acne, allergies, athlete's foot, boils, bruises +++++L, burns +++++L, dandruff, dermatitis, eczema, inflammations, insect bites and stings, insect repellent, lice, psoriasis, ringworm, scabies, sores, spots, sunburn, and minor wounds; apply undiluted to small areas or diluted 50:50 with a carrier oil to larger areas. Mix 3 drops in a teaspoon of water for a minor sunburn. You can also make a sunburn spray with lavender, helichrysum, and a little tea tree. Be sure to shake before each application to disperse the oils in the water +++L.

- For an earache, apply lavender undiluted on the outer ear.

- For lumbago, muscle aches and pains, rheumatism, and sprains, create a 50:50 massage blend of lavender with a carrier oil, and apply to the afflicted area.

- For respiratory conditions: asthma, bronchitis, excess mucous, sinusitis +++++L, bad breath, laryngitis, throat infections, and whooping cough; create a 50:50 massage blend of lavender with a carrier oil, and apply to the afflicted area. You can also take a hot bath with 20 drops of lavender in a cup of Epsom Salts. Also diffuse 20 drops of lavender twice daily ++++L.

- For digestive issues: abdominal cramps, colic, gas, or nausea; take a 50:50 blend of lavender and carrier oil in a capsule once a day with food. You can also massage a 50:50 dilution with a carrier oil onto the lower abdomen.

- To stimulate healthy menstruation or reduce menstrual pain, massage a 50:50 dilution with a carrier oil onto the lower abdomen +++L. Also effective for urinary tract infections +++++L.

- To decrease painful headaches, migraines, nervous tension and stress-related conditions, diffuse 20 drops of lavender twice daily. Also use a 50:50 lavender and carrier oil blend to massage face, forehead, back of neck, and back. ++++L

- To overcome shock or vertigo, diffuse 20 drops of lavender twice daily. Also use a 50:50 lavender and carrier oil blend to massage temples, forehead, and back of neck. Apply a cool, damp cloth over the lavender to help it penetrate.

CAUTIONS: None when used in quantities indicated.

 CLINICAL SUPPORT

"The purpose of this study was to identify the effects of essential oil inhalation on blood pressure ... in 83 prehypertensive and hypertensive subjects. They used lavender, ylang-ylang, marjoram, and neroli in a study [against similar synthetic fragrances]. The inhalation of an essential oil had immediate and continuous effects on ... stress reduction. Essential oils may have relaxation effects for controlling hypertension (Kim IH, et al., 2012).

Lavender, vanilla, and vetiver did not enhance arousal or wake-up, but did transiently reduce inhalation and enhanced exhalation for up to six breaths (Dobetsberger, C. and Buchbauer, G., 2011).

Massage the hands with the essential oils of bergamot, lavender, and frankincense had a helpful effect on pain and depression in hospice patients (Dobetsberger, C. and Buchbauer, G., 2011).

Lavender reduced reaction times and helped to sustain attention during longer tasks in a study of the effect of essential oils on learning (Dobetsberger, C. and Buchbauer, G., 2011).

The diffused aroma of lavender has an anti-stress effect, with stress levels significantly lowered (Dobetsberger, C. and Buchbauer, G., 2011).

Aromatherapy massage with Lavender can reduce pre-operative anxiety (Dobetsberger, C. and Buchbauer, G., 2011).

Lavender, administered via oxygen face mask, can reduce the application of pain relievers immediately after surgery (Dobetsberger, C. and Buchbauer, G., 2011).

Lavender baths for babies can significantly decrease stress in mothers and relax and induce sleep in babies (Dobetsberger, C. and Buchbauer, G., 2011).

Sunburn relief for a family of eight from a few drops of lavender

Last summer while we were visiting Disneyland my family of eight forgot the sunscreen and all got sunburns on our necks. All we had was one bottle with a few drops of lavender left in it. I knew it wouldn't work to put those few drops on all of us, so I decided to use a little of my drinking water in the palm of my hand and dilute the lavender in it. I was able to spread those few drops of lavender to everyone in the family, and the sunburn relief was instant for all of us. Lavender never ceases to amaze me!

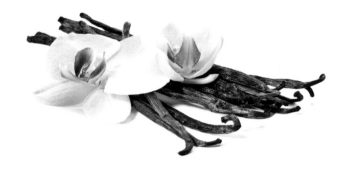

Vanilla
Vanilla planifolia

Family: Orchidaceae
Origins: Comes from Central America and Mexico. Also cultivated in Madagascar, Tahiti, the Comoro Islands, East Africa, and Indonesia. Oil is often processed in Europe and the USA.
Other names: common vanilla, Bourbon vanilla, Mexican vanilla, Reunion vanilla
Description: A perennial climbing vine with green stems and large, white, trumpet-shaped flowers. Vanilla bean pods mature for 8 to 9 months; after they are picked, they have to be fermented and dried for another 6 months.
Extraction: a resinoid or oleoresin obtained by solvent extraction
Botanical Part Used: fermented bean pods
Principal constituents: vanillin (1.3-2.9%) with over 150 other constituents including hydroxybenzaldehude, acetic acid, isobutyric acid, caproic acid, eugenol, furfural, and others.

🜶 BLENDING SUGGESTIONS

Relative strength: 5
Among the middle notes that typically make up more than 50% of the blend or the base notes that make up less than 30% of the entire blend. Vanilla can be overpowering, so do not use for more than 2 – 5% of the blend.
Blends well with: most oils, especially sandalwood, vetiver, balsam fir, and spice oils
Description: rich, sweet, balsamic, and vanilla-y

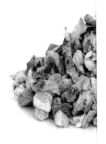

Virgin

Juniperus vir

Family: Cupr
Origins: Nativ
east of the Ro
Other names
southern red
Description:
reddish heart
Extraction: E
Botanical Par
and shavings:
Principal con:
cedrol (3 – 149

BLENDIN

Relative streng
Among the m
up more than
Blends well wi
vetiver, rosem
Description: m
smells like a sh

HISTORY

North America
for respiratory
up excess muc
of leaves, bark,
used to treat rh
venereal warts,

HISTORY & TRADITIONAL USES

Wherever vanilla is grown throughout the world, the flowers have to be hand-pollenated, except in Mexico where hummingbirds do the job. The flavoring is used in pharmaceutical products as a flavoring agent. It is a fragrance in perfumes, especially oriental blends. It is widely used in tobacco and food flavoring, especially ice cream and yogurt. Synthetic vanilla fragrance is widely used in candles, soaps, cosmetics, and toiletries.

USE & HEALTH BENEFIT

- Pleasant fragrance with all the familiar, comforting, emotional triggers associated with the familiar taste and aroma.

- Blend with other essential oils to create a more comforting, familiar emotional connection. Even though this oil may have limited therapeutic benefit, its value for turning less pleasurable blends into pleasant ones is a huge benefit. One tiny drop or even a trace of the powerful vanilla extract can make all the difference in how pleasant and acceptable a blend will be.

CAUTIONS: None when used in quantities indicated.

CLINICAL SUPPORT

While vanilla oil has no significant antimicrobial effect itself, it nevertheless serves as a highly effective masking agent for blending with other essential oils that have significant antimicrobial power—thyme, oregano, cinnamon, etc. (Gutierrez, L, et al., 2009).

Lavender, vanilla, and vetiver did not enhance arousal or wake-up, but did transiently reduce inhalation and enhanced exhalation for up to six breaths (Dobetsberger, C. and Buchbauer, G., 2011).

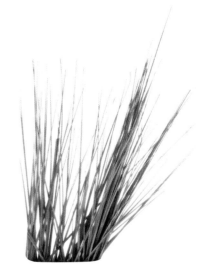

Vetiver

Vetiveria zizanoides

Family: Poaceae (Gramineae)
Origins: A native of southern India, Indonesia, and Sri Lanka, vetiver is also cultivated in Reunion, the Philippines, the Comoro Islands, Japan, West Africa, and South America. The oil is mainly produced in Java, Haiti, and Reunion. Some is distilled in the USA and Europe.
Other names: vetivert, khus khus
Description: A tall, tufted, scented grass with a straight stem, long narrow leaves and a complex network of roots and rootlets.
Extraction: Essential oil by steam distillation
Botanical Part Used: roots and rootlets
Principal constituents: vetiverol, vitivone, terpenes, and others

BLENDING SUGGESTIONS

Relative strength: 5
Among the base notes that typically make up less than 30% of the blend. A tiny amount is needed for most blends.
Blends well with: sandalwood, ylang ylang, patchouli, lavender, and clary sage
Description: heavy, earthy, balsamic, smoky, with sweet lemony undertones.

HISTOR

Through th
insomnia, p
rheumatisn
ingredient i
especially c
preservative

USE & I

- To calm s
  respirator
  and carrie

- To detoxif
  take a 50:
  a capsule

- For a war
  stimulate
  corpuscle
  vetiver an
  massage 1

- To help eli
  blend of v
  with food

- Apply top
  and woun

- To calm th
  insomnia

- For arthrit
  stiffness; b
  apply to jc

- Take advar
  aroma to r
  depressior
  a carrier oi
  For a relax
  of vetiver i

CAUTIONS: *None when used in quantities indicated. Avoid during pregnancy. Use only in dilution. May cause skin sensitivity in some individuals.*

✔ CLINICAL SUPPORT

Cinnamon oil, lemongrass oil, cedarwood oil, clove oil and eucalyptus oil exhibit antibacterial property against S. mutans (Chaudhari, et al., 2012).

The essential oil from a heartwood sample of Juniperus virginiana L. was evaluated for wound healing and anti-inflammatory activity by using in vivo experimental methods. Linear incision and circular excision wound models were used for assessment. The oil of Juniperus virginiana was found highly effective in anti-inflammatory activity (Tumen, I et al., 2013).

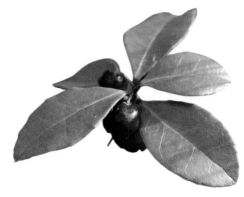

Wintergreen
Gaultheria procumbens

Family: Ericaceae
Origins: North America, China
Other names: Aromatic wintergreen, checkerberry, teaberry, gaultheria (oil)
Description: Small evergreen herb with scarlet berries.
Extraction: Essential oil by steam distillation
Botanical Part Used: leaves
Principal constituents: Almost exclusively methyl salicylate (98%). Similar to birch.

🌿 BLENDING SUGGESTIONS

Relative strength: 5
Among the middle notes and base notes that typically make up more than 80% of the blend (middle notes 50%, base notes 30%)
Blends well with: oregano, peppermint, spearmint, thyme, ylang ylang, and vanilla
Description: sharp, icy/hot, sweet, woody, somewhat minty

📖 HISTORY & TRADITIONAL USES

Strong, penetrating aroma similar to mint but more sharp. American Indians and early settlers made a tea flavored with birch or wintergreen leaves. Often associated with a synthetic flavoring used in toothpaste, mouthwash, mint candy, chewing gum, and soft drinks. Synthetic methyl salicylate is such a popular and common flavoring agent that true wintergreen actually made from plants is now a rare treat. It is challenging to locate a genuine non-synthetic version with the full complement of organic constituents you need for safe, therapeutic use.

✚ USE & HEALTH BENEFIT

- For a mild pain reliever (analgesic) for inflammation, swollen joints, sore muscles, tendonitis, muscular rheumatism, and cramps, apply 50:50 blend of wintergreen and carrier oil over the affected area.

- Anti-inflammatory +++P, apply a 50:50 blend of wintergreen and carrier oil over the area of inflammation.

- For cramps (antispasmodic) +++P, apply a 50:50 blend of wintergreen and carrier oil over the affected area.

- As a liver stimulant +++P for overall vitality, energy, and good health, apply a 50:50 blend of wintergreen and carrier oil over the liver area of the abdomen.

- As a vasodilator +P to calm high blood pressure and stimulate liver function, apply a 50:50 blend of wintergreen and carrier oil to the chest.

- To relieve a cough (antitussive), apply wintergreen to the trachea area (upper sternum), and add a little carrier oil to keep it from reddening your skin. Then place a cool, damp cloth over it and a dry one over that. Use an ice pack over that to cool and calm the cough. (Show an illustration of where this is on the body.)

- To settle digestion and gas (Carminative), massage the abdomen with a 50:50 blend of wintergreen with carrier oil. Also increases urine flow and releases toxins when massaged all over the body. Use 10 to 15 drops of wintergreen in a cup of Epsom Salts for a stimulating hot bath.

- To assist healthy menstruation (Emmenagogue), massage the abdomen with a 50:50 blend of wintergreen and carrier oil.

- To increase lactation (Galactagogue), create a mild compress with a 20:80 wintergreen to carrier oil ratio, and apply to breasts with a damp towel and a dry towel covering it. Add some heat if desired.

- Has a warming/cooling action for both cold and hot therapy

- To relieve the pain of arthritis, muscular rheumatism, and tendonitis +++P, gently rub 1-2 drops of wintergreen oil—diluted with 5-10 drops of carrier oil—into aching or swollen joints and bones. Use on muscles to relax aches and cramps and reduce inflammation. Rub into foot reflex points.

- To cool and calm hypertension (high blood pressure) and improve liver function +++P, use as a general, relaxing body massage.

- To decrease or eliminate dandruff, add a single drop to your daily handful of shampoo.

- To freshen the air and promote an alert mind and quick reflexes, diffuse 20 drops in a nebulizing diffuser.

- To prevent the formation and appearance of acne, add a drop to each application of mild facial cleanser or add 20 drops to 8 ounces of cleanser.

CAUTIONS: None when used in diluted quantities indicated. Do not ingest. Do not use on children under 2 years of age. Do not use on the neck or chest of children under age 12. Do not use if you are epileptic. Do not use if pregnant. When applied topically it may increase blood-thinning effects. Do not overuse, especially on sensitive skin.

Singles

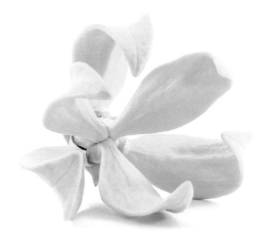

CLINICAL SUPPORT

Wintergreen is safe. Some books on essential oil safety recommend avoiding oils that contain methyl salicylate like wintergreen and birch. Methyl salicylate is closely related to acetylsalicylic acid or common aspirin. Ron Guba notes that methyl salicylate is found in many common and popular over-the-counter creams for sprains that have a warming/cooling action. It is also abundantly used in candies and chewing gum. He suggests that 10 ml of wintergreen in a carrier oil massage at 2.4% dilution would give someone approximately 250 mg of methyl salicylate, roughly the equivalent of one aspirin tablet. Since only half that amount would be absorbed in a massage, it would be no more dangerous than rubbing half an aspirin on the body. Nevertheless, he warns against overuse or extended use of wintergreen for full-body massage if you are taking warfarin or any anticoagulant therapy (Guba R., pp. 37-49).

Ylang Ylang
Cananga odorata

Family: Annonaceae
Origins: Tropical Asia, especially Indonesia and the Philippines. Major producers are Madagascar, Reunion, and the Comoro Islands.
Other names: flower of flowers
Description: A tall tropical tree with large, fragrant pink, mauve, or yellow flowers. Yellow flowers are considered the best for extracting the essential oil.
Extraction: Essential oil by water or steam distillation
Botanical Part Used: freshly picked flowers
Principal constituents: methyl benzoate e, methyl salicylate, methyl para-cresol, benzyl acetate, eugenol, geraniol, linalool and terpenes: pinene, cadinene, and others

 BLENDING SUGGESTIONS

Relative strength: 5
Blend among the middle-to-base notes that typically make up more than 80% of the blend (50% middle, 30% base). Ylang ylang is so potent that a very little goes a long way. It is a well-balanced oil with a top note, middle note, and base note. For this reason, it can be worn alone as a perfume, but experiment to get the correct dilution so it isn't overpowering.

Blends well with: rosewood, vetiver, lemon, grapefruit, marjoram, sandalwood, and bergamot
Description: intensely sweet, soft, floral-balsamic, slightly spicy

📖 HISTORY & TRADITIONAL USES

In Indonesia ylang ylang flowers are spread on the beds of newlyweds. Ylang ylang ointments with coconut oil are used for hair care, skin diseases, infectious diseases, and malaria. During the Victorian era ylang ylang was an ingredient in a popular treatment for hair growth. The oil was also used for insect bites. It was also used to regulate breathing and heart rhythm.

➕ USE & HEALTH BENEFIT

- To help control oily skin, use a drop in a single application of lotion or liniment. +++L

- Beneficial as an aromatic addition to other therapies in the treatment of diabetes +P. Diffuse 20 drops of various aromatic oils with ylang ylang as a small part of the blend (1 drop).

- As a scalp stimulant to help promote hair growth, apply a drop in each application of your hair care products +++L.

- To help control an irregular or racing heartbeat and high blood pressure, diffuse a drop with other aromatic oils ++++L.

- To reduce spasms: muscles, respiratory, or digestive; use in a Comforting blend containing ylang ylang diluted 50:50 with carrier oil. Massage the areas affected.

- For an alluring sexual tonic, use a small amount in a blend for diffusing 20 drops or creating a 50:50 blend with carrier oil for a massage +P ++++L.

- For a relaxing bath to help overcome depression or nervous exhaustion, use a small amount in a blend with other oils. Mix 10 to 15 drops of the blend with a cup of Epsom Salts.

- To help create a calming, euphoric emotional state, massage the feet with a blend of aromatic oils including ylang ylang +++L. An aromatic bath with Epsom Salts and a drop of ylang ylang mixed with other aromatic oils will help accomplish the same thing.

- To help overcome depressed or negative emotions of fear, anger, anxiety, or frustration, diffuse with other aromatic oils (a total of 20 drops).

CAUTIONS: None when used in quantities indicated.

✅ CLINICAL SUPPORT

"The purpose of this study was to identify the effects of essential oil inhalation on blood pressure ... in 83 prehypertensive and hypertensive subjects. They used lavender, ylang-ylang, marjoram, and neroli in a study [against similar synthetic fragrances]. The inhalation of an essential oil had immediate and continuous effects on ... stress reduction. Essential oils may have relaxation effects for controlling hypertension. (Kim IH, et al., 2012).

"This study provides ... evidence for the impact of the aromas ... on ... cognition and mood in healthy participants. One hundred and forty-four volunteers were randomly assigned to conditions of ylang-ylang aroma, peppermint aroma, or no aroma control. Peppermint was found to enhance memory whereas ylang-ylang impaired it, and lengthened processing speed. In terms of subjective mood peppermint increased alertness and ylang-ylang decreased it, but significantly increased calmness. These results provide support for the contention that the aromas of essential oils can produce significant ... effects on both subjective and objective assessments ... of human behavior" (Moss M, et al., 2008).

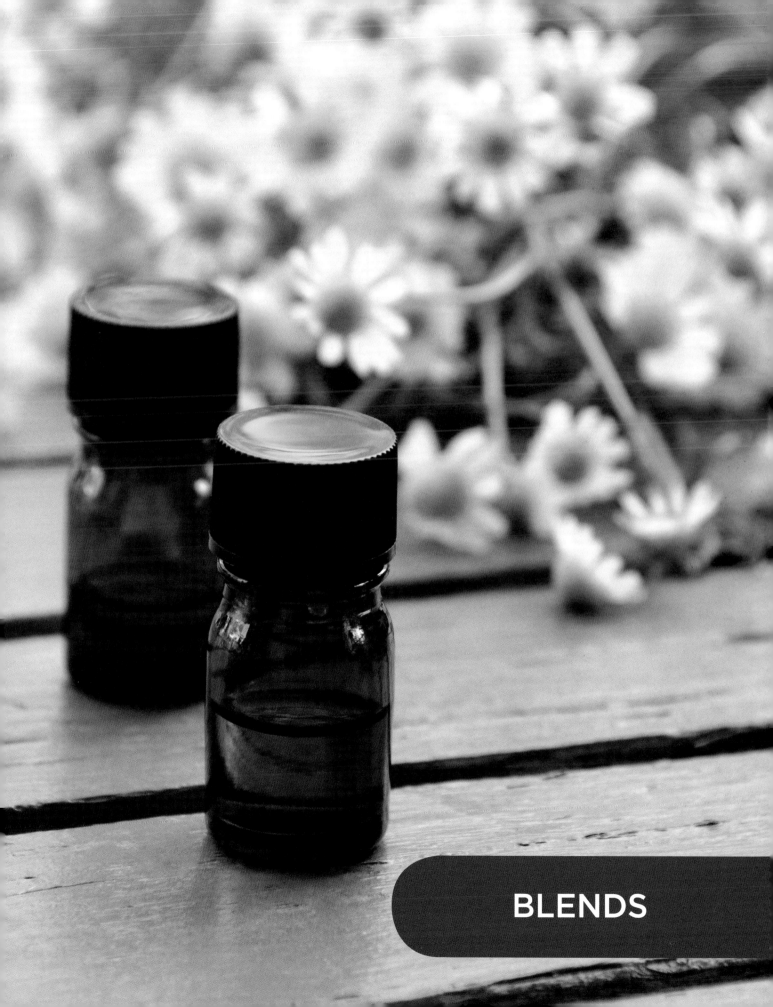

BLENDS

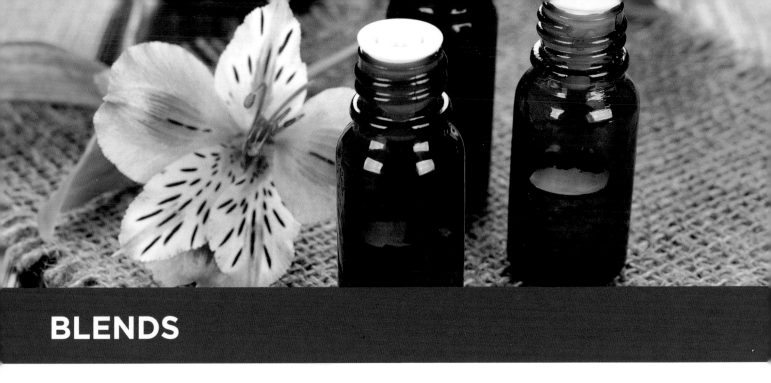

BLENDS

Nature has already blended some of the most amazing oils for you. They're called "singles." They each have multiple functions and capacities and as many as 300 or more chemical constituents capable of affecting multiple systems of the body as well as the emotions all at once. So with these versatile oils already at your fingertips, why would you want to blend them? We all like to see what we can do to organize nature in a way that makes things better—like organizing sounds to create tunes, organizing colors to create art, or organizing materials to create a building. It's a creative endeavor we humans can't resist. It's part art and part science. There are many reasons to use blends and even more reasons to create them.

Why use blends?

- **Convenience.** It's easy to grab a blend that we know consistently works well for headaches. We don't have to think about which oils or how much of each. It's all done for us with the best blending science and art. We don't have to learn anything—just grab and use.

- **Superior health benefits.** Master blenders know how to create a synergy where the combination is more powerful than the sum of the individual oils.

- **More pleasing aromas.** Eating your veggies is good for you. But veggies are easier to take in a delicious recipe. Blends are created not only for their effectiveness, but also for their pleasure. We're more likely to use them often if they smell nice. We don't want the embarrassment of someone turning up their nose and saying, "What's that smell?" Strong medicinal oils don't always smell great, so blends are created to balance those less agreeable aromas while retaining or improving their effectiveness.

- **More affordable.** Rather than purchasing a whole pharmacy of costly oils and learning by trial and error to blend them yourself, you can purchase a single blend and benefit from the power of synergy without the high price.

- **Low learning curve**. You don't have to learn all about blending or make mistakes through trial and error.

How to tell great blends from average blends

- **Pleasing aromas for each occasion.** Think of all the places you'll use a blend. Is it only for the bedroom and bathroom or will you want to use it in the kitchen, living room, at the office, or at the gym? Pick blends that will go where they are needed without embarrassment.

- **Flexible.** Since convenience is important, you want blends that are flexible enough to work for many practical uses.

- **Affordable.** They will be blended with your pocketbook in mind so you don't have to break the bank to enjoy the benefits of highly effective oils in small amounts.

- **Creativity & complexity.** The best blends will be like a sophisticated symphony of complex aromatic notes. You may not be able to identify individual aromas in the best blends, but like a fine gourmet recipe, they'll have that "je ne sais quoi," that special something that makes them great. Complex and surprising aromas will appear and disappear as you use them. They may smell different on the skin than when they're diffused. They will grow more delightful with consistent use. They will create wonderful aromatic memories both subtle and strong.

- **The right ingredients.** Oils will be selected from hundreds of possible choices. Master blenders are aware of precise chemotypes, subtle nuances, and all the medicinal potential and synergistic impact of multiple oils. From years of experience they know the rituals of blending for the exact effect you're after.

Why create your own blends?

With all this expertise from master blenders, why would you want to do your own blending? Here are several reasons.

- Maybe there isn't a blend available to match your specific need.

- You may want to try your hand at the creative art of blending. It can be remarkably satisfying to create your own "signature" blends. Just make sure you take good notes of precise recipes so you can recreate them when you run out.

- You read about a few oils that have what you need, but they're not found in one of the basic blends, so you need to create your own.

- Maybe you want to add more power to one of the basic blends or help them smell more pleasing.

How to create your own great blends

- In creating blends, it's helpful to recognize that essential oils are often divided into "top," "middle," and "low" notes. This is a musical pattern suggested by the 19th-century French perfumer Pliesse.

- The **top notes** have a fresh, light quality which is immediately recognized when the bottle is opened. But these notes have a quick evaporation rate, so they only last if they are mixed with lower notes. If you are using top-note oils alone, they will not linger, so you can put them on first thing in the morning, and they will have dispersed before you walk out the door for work. Top notes can be sharp and strong like peppermint, thyme, lemongrass, cinnamon, and clove. With these sharp high notes, you'll want to use very little in a blend because they can overpower other fragrances. Use, maybe 2 – 5% of the blend at the most.

- You can use softer top notes like the citrus oils (bergamot, orange, lime, tangerine, lemon, etc.). They can constitute from 10% to 40% of the blend, but they are typically no more than 20%. If you are creating a blend to use mainly in a diffuser, you can use more of the top notes.

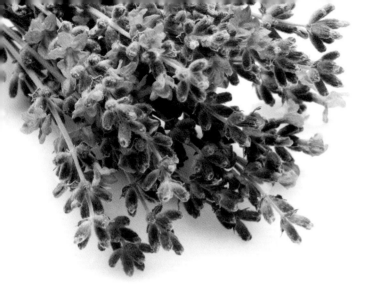

- The **middle notes** are the heart of the blend you are creating. They usually make up most of the blend—50% to 80%. This scent emerges sometime after the first impression. These notes give substance to the blend. They are typically warm, soft, and mellow. Sometimes they are called "enhancers." Typical enhancers are lavender, chamomile, marjoram, etc.

- The **base notes** are richer and heavier. They appear more slowly and linger longer than the middle notes. They can also act somewhat like a fixative to keep the lighter oils from dispersing too quickly. They increase the lasting effect of all the oils in the blend.

- Base notes will smell rather faint right out of the bottle, but when on your skin, they will begin to release their power. That's why you only truly experience the full fragrance when it has been on your skin for a minute or two. Base notes can linger for several hours.

- It is not necessary to use base notes in blends you're going to diffuse, though they do add depth and body to the aroma. They are, however, almost required for blends you'll apply to your skin (Lavabre, p. 107).

- Essential oils are often classified according to their dominant note. This is useful information

for those who are blending oils for perfumery, but it's also important to know how long the strong aroma you are using will be staying around. For example, because tea tree is a relatively high-middle note that doesn't last too long, you won't have to worry about a lingering aroma of tea tree throughout the day. The pleasant aroma of geranium, on the other hand, applied to the pad of a bandage is a middle note and could be with you all day.

- There are different opinions about which oils have predominant top, middle, or base notes. Some, like frankincense, patchouli, jasmine, and sandalwood are obviously bass notes. But perfumers and aromatherapists disagree on which are top and which are middle notes. In this book we will suggest a category, but depending on the growing conditions and climate, an oil that was once a top note may later become a middle note (Davis, p. 250). Some oils like ylang ylang and jasmine span several categories.

- **Fixatives** are often categorized as bass notes. They are typically heavier, and should be used sparingly. Patchouli, frankincense, and vetiver are fixatives. The base notes and fixatives are usually used in small quantities (between 5 – 20%).

- **Equalizers** are another useful category. These oils help get rid of hard, distinctive edges between sharper fragrances. Marjoram is a universal equalizer. Orange and tangerine are great equalizers with florals, spices, and other citrus oils. Balsam Fir is a great equalizer for other conifer oils (Lavabre, p. 108).

- **Personifiers** or **modifiers** are exceptionally powerful aromas. They are usually found among either the bass notes or the top notes. Examples include peppermint, oregano, thyme, clove, lemongrass, and cinnamon. Use them sparingly, one drop at a time, or they could overpower your blend.

- **Enhancers** are the most pleasant-smelling oils. They give a blend that pleasant, personal touch without overpowering it. They include bergamot, cedarwood, geranium, lavender, lemon, lime, sandalwood, spruce, and ylang ylang. Oils like rosemary, cajeput, and eucalyptus could also be considered enhancers, although they're less perfume-oriented and more appropriate for inhalation therapy—diffusers, saunas, steam rooms, etc. As a category, you may want up to 50% of your blend to be from enhancers.

- It's unusually challenging to describe a fragrance. We have a large vocabulary of words to describe sounds, colors, and textures. But aromas require a frame of reference. We use words like musky, fresh, fruity, green, floral, herbal, sharp, camphoric, sweet, clean, medicinal, citrusy, balsamic, spicy, woody, etc. Oils are usually a combination of these. For example, lavender is both herbal and floral.

- Before you create a blend, you want to decide its purpose and how you will use it. The more goals you try to achieve with a single blend, the more difficult it will be to create. Especially when you are starting out, create a specific blend for each of the functions of the body—the liver, circulation, mental focus, foot massage, etc. Decide if it is strictly a diffuser blend or if you want it to work in a bath, a massage, for ingestion, etc. A blend you use in a capsule doesn't have to be as fragrant as one you will use for emotional issues.

- Marcel Lavabre suggests that you create a blend like you would arrange for a meeting or social event. Some events are all business with medicinal goals and oils chosen strictly for ingestion in capsules. Blends for diffusing in your home are like public events where many people could be commenting on your choice of fragrance. You don't want fragrances fighting with one another. You don't want the subtle fragrances like bergamot being overpowered by the sharp oils of thyme or peppermint. Lavabre's advice for the beginner is "to use the stars only when you really need them and only one at a time, until you figure out who gets along with whom" (Lavabre, p. 113).

How to keep it simple and safe when creating your blends

- Use fewer rather than more ingredients. The safest would be 3 oils, for example, a top note at 30%, a middle note at 50% and a base note at 20%.

- Have your purpose clear before you start.

- Write down your recipe so if it turns out great, you can make more.

- Only go to the effort of creating a blend if you will be using it often.

- Check the "Singles" section of this book for suggestions on what blends well.

- Test your blend by using only a few drops of each oil rather than larger quantities. You can always make more.

- Let your blend rest for 24 hours before trying it.

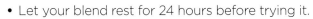
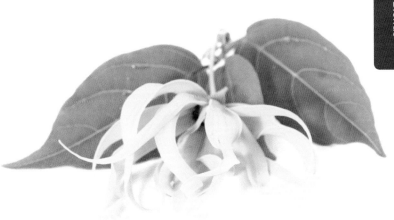

- Test it in various ways: (1) from the bottle, (2) on your skin, (3) diffused, (4) diluted, (5) in drinking water if appropriate, etc.

- Save yourself time and effort by sticking with one of your favorite time-tested blends and layer one or two other oils along with it to enhance its action.

- Use common sense like you would when creating a great recipe. Your sense of smell can become easily exhausted with overuse, and you may end up adding stronger and stronger aromas until you create something that could overpower other people. Use your favorite blends as a guide, and get input from friends who are new to the blends you are creating.

A Protecting blend

This is a blend you will be using often, so you want to choose it carefully.

EFFECTIVE for all kinds of antimicrobial uses (bacteria, viruses, parasites, fungi) and powerful enough to get the job done quickly before the microbes have time to multiply out of control and compromise your immune system.

TASTE. It must use only ingestible ingredients. It needs to taste good because you'll be putting it into drinks, water, and applesauce (for the children). If you're taking it in capsules and forget to take it with food, you don't want the aftertaste to be too disagreeable.

The aroma category	Examples	Blends well with	Doesn't work with
Floral	Lavender, ylang ylang, geranium, bergamot	Woody, fruity, sweet musky, and some green	Balsamic and some herbal
Citrusy	Orange, tangerine, lemon, grapefruit, lime, German chamomile	Versatile in large portions with most categories	Doesn't work well with balsamic and some herbal oils
Herbal	Basil, marjoram, rosemary, chamomile, ginger	Blends well with balsamic and woody	Not the best with florals
Spicy	Cinnamon, clove, black pepper, oregano, thyme	Use in small amounts—less than 5%	Too much can destroy any blend
Green	Spearmint, citronella, lemongrass, peppermint, Melissa, ginger	Blends well with most oils	Use the mints sparingly in any blend
Balsamic	Eucalyptus, cajeput, myrtle, tea tree, cypress, pine, rosemary, juniper	Best with woody and herbal. Makes blends seem medicinal	Not good with floral or fruity
Woody	Cedarwood, sandalwood, cypress, juniper, frankincense	Great bass notes in any blend. Use quantity under 20%	Small percentages primarily for bass notes
Minty	Peppermint, spearmint	Great with citrus, woody, herbal, and musky	Use sparingly
Medicinal	Tea tree, eucalyptus, cajeput	Blends with woody, herbals	Overpowering with floral
Musky/earthy	clary sage, frankincense, patchouli, vetiver, mugwort	Great bass notes	Use under 20% of the category: example, 20% of all the bass notes

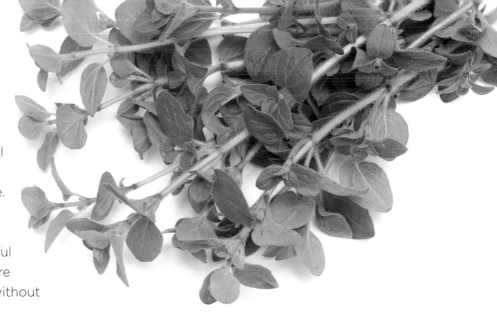

COMPLEXITY. It must have enough of the key antimicrobial ingredients so it could never become less effective by overuse. This complexity must cover the full range of microbes with the most powerful yet safe options available.

SAFETY. It must be safe enough that it can be used in many stressful situations. It can be taken anywhere and used for lots of applications without too much training.

PLEASING. Many antimicrobial oils can be strong smelling and offensive to some people. When you are in a stressful situation using your protecting blend in a crowd of people, you don't want someone adding to the stress by commenting, "What's that horrible smell?" That's why it may be a better choice to have the cinnamon and clove spices for your strong antimicrobials in the blend rather than too much oregano or thyme.

INSTRUCTIONS

The versatility of this blend makes it impossible to list all the potential uses. Here are a few of the countless ways you will be using it:

- Create your own capsules. Be sure to dilute 50:50 with a carrier oil. Use a weaker dilution for children: 30:70 or even 20:80, depending on the age. During a crisis, take a capsule 6 times a day with food. Take a capsule at breakfast, lunch, and dinner, with your food of course. But at 10 a.m. take another capsule with food, then again at 3 p.m. between lunch and dinner take a capsule with food. In the evening, take a capsule before bed with a little food.

- For regular prevention, take a single capsule daily with your vitamins at a meal.

- During cold and flu season use a drop or two in drinking water, herbal tea, juice, applesauce, and other recipes.

- When you have a sore throat or mouth infection of any kind, lick a trace off the back of your hand and apply it with your tongue to the afflicted area or merely distribute the molecules around your mouth for fighting the microbes that contribute to bad breath and other conditions.

- Use neat on cuts, scrapes, and scratches.

- Use for a compress, dry or with water. Use one drop or two on the pad of an adhesive bandage to disinfect a minor cut or scrape. Some latex adhesive bandages, though they are waterproof, won't adhere if you use too much oil. The gauze pad slips and makes a mess. Either use a bit less oil or an adhesive cloth bandage. You may want to dilute the oil for small children.

- Disperse in bath salts for an antimicrobial aromatic bath. Use in the shower.

- Wear on a face mask when you are exposed to a lot of infection. Carry a drop or two in a handkerchief or tissue and inhale from it frequently throughout the day.

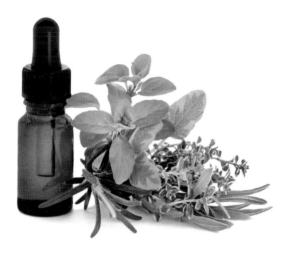

- Use it as one of the oils in back massage treatments for strong antimicrobial action.

- Use it for foot, hand, or ear reflexology treatments.

- Diffuse 20 drops a day during the cold and flu season or when there is an infection in your home.

A Respiratory Blend

This is a blend you will want to use daily for topical application and diffusing, so choose it carefully.

EFFECTIVE for all kinds of airborne as well as topical antimicrobial uses (bacteria, viruses, fungi).

AROMA. It must smell fresh and delightful—not too medicinal or you won't want to use it as often as you will need to. The fragrance should be temporary, not long-lasting.

TASTE. You may want to put it into drinks, water, applesauce (for the children) during cold and flu season, so you'll want it to taste fairly good. If you're taking it in capsules and forget to take it with food, you don't want a disagreeable aftertaste.

COMPLEXITY. It must have enough of the key antimicrobial ingredients so it could never become less effective by overuse. This complexity must cover the full range of microbes with the most powerful yet safe options available.

SAFETY. It must be safe enough that it can be diffused and used topically daily.

PLEASING. Many respiratory oils can be strong and strange to some people. You don't want those entering your home thinking, "What's that strong medicinal smell?" It needs to smell fresh and invigorating.

INSTRUCTIONS

The versatility of this blend makes it impossible to list all the ways to use this blend. Here are a few:

- Diffuse 20 drops daily, especially during cold and flu season.

- Create a 50:50 blend with a light carrier oil and use it in a spray bottle on your chest and back daily. See illustration for key locations.

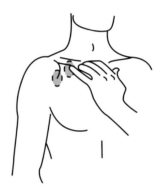

- Create a compress by applying the oil undiluted on the chest or around the neck and putting a hot, damp towel over it with a dry towel covering the damp one. If you are trying to stop a cough caused by bronchial inflammation, create a warm compress. If you feel you need a cold compress because of inflammation and tickling in the bronchioles that leads to coughing spasms, simply use a cool compress. Your body will tell you which will be better.

- Disperse in bath salts for a respiratory aromatic bath or foot soak. Use in the shower as instructed in the "How to Use Essential Oils" chapter.

- Wear on a face mask when you are exposed to a lot of infection. Carry a drop or two in a handkerchief or tissue and inhale from it frequently throughout the day.

- Use it as one of the oils in back massage treatments for respiratory conditions.

- Use it undiluted for foot, hand, or ear reflexology treatments focusing on the areas that correspond to the parts of your respiratory system.

- Use 3-4 drops in a bowl of hot water with a towel over your head. Inhale deeply. Reheat the water and add a few drops more as needed.

A Comforting Blend

This is a blend you will use often, both in public and in private, so you want to be one of your favorites.

EFFECTIVE for calming all kinds of emotional and physical stress (anxiety, insomnia, shock, fear, depression, etc.).

PLEASING AROMA. When you are in a stressful situation using this blend around other people, you don't want someone adding to your stress by commenting, "What's that strange smell?" You want it to be pleasing to all members of your family for frequent use.

TASTE. It may be used by ingestion in capsules or in drinks, so it should taste good with a single drop in drinking water.

COMPLEXITY. You'll want the blend to be sophisticated and interesting with no single fragrance shouting louder than the others. There can't be anything shrill, too sharp, or annoying in the blend.

SAFETY. It must be safe enough for frequent use in many stressful situations. While it will be used primarily for diffusing and topical use, it may also be ingested.

INSTRUCTIONS

- Diffuse 20 drops while preparing for a good night's sleep. Read something that helps calm you down while you inhale relaxing, aromatic molecules.

- Disperse in bath salts for a calming aromatic bath. Use in a shower before bed.

- During highly stressful times use a drop or two in drinking water, herbal tea, juice, applesauce and other recipes. You may even want to create your own capsules for calming, restful sleep. Be sure to dilute 50:50 with a carrier oil. Use a weaker dilution for children: 30:70 or even 20:80, depending on the age. During an emotional crisis take a capsule with food before bed.

- Place a few drops in a tissue, cotton ball, or handkerchief. Carry it with you and inhale as needed. Put the fragranced cotton ball inside your pillow case for a calming night's sleep.

- Use it for a calming, gentle, full-body massage.

- Use it both diluted and undiluted for foot, hand, or ear reflexology treatments.

- Wear it on a clay diffusing pendant around your neck.

- Use the "M" technique with a dilution of this calming oil

- Use the oil undiluted on those areas of your body where you seem to carry the most stress. After applying the oil, put a warm, damp cloth over the area, cover with a dry towel, and relax.

A Soothing Blend

This is a blend you will want to keep handy to stop a headache, calm a bruise, or apply to joints before the pain becomes unbearable. The quicker you get a handle on pain using essential oils, the lower the inflammation, and the more effective the therapy.

EFFECTIVE for all kinds of pain—headache, joints, muscles, backaches, bumps, bruises, etc. It must work both in cooling and warming situations.

AROMA. It must smell refreshing—not too sharp or medicinal so you'll want to use it often, whenever you need it. The fragrance should not be overpowering.

COMPLEXITY. It must have enough of a variety of pain-relieving ingredients to cover the full range issues that cause pain—inflammation, mental anxiety, antispasmodic, etc.

SAFETY. It must be safe enough that it can be used often without topical irritation. This is not a blend to ingest.

PLEASING. Many oils used to decrease pain can be strong and strange to some people. You don't want those entering your home thinking, "What's that strong, sharp, medicinal smell?" It needs to smell calming and soothing.

INSTRUCTIONS

Here are a few of many ways to use a Soothing blend:

- Use a few drops undiluted on a painful bruise or joint, especially small joints like hands, wrists, ankles, fingers, etc. For larger joints like knees, shoulders, back and hips, you may want to dilute the blend 50:50. Apply a cool or warm wet compress to increase penetration.

- Create a compress by using 3-4 drops of the Soothing blend in 3-4 teaspoons of water. Mix the oil and water as well as you can and soak a gauze pad in the solution. Apply it to the painful area and cover it with a cling bandage. This will penetrate even more quickly than the oil in water or the undiluted oil. A cold pack or even an ice pack over this compress can help bring relief to the inflamed area.

- You can create a green clay poultice using 5 to 10 drops of essential oils in a mixture of clay. Cover the poultice with a gauze and cling bandage. This with a cold compress can offer the most penetrating and constant relief to the area.

- For headaches you can apply a few drops undiluted at the temples and along the back of the neck.

- You can also apply cold compresses at the back of the neck and on the forehead.

- Use your hands, ears, and feet along with the Soothing blend to massage away pain in other areas of your body corresponding to the reflex points. Perhaps your shoulder is too tender to massage. Use your Soothing blend on the outside corner of your foot and your hand to unblock that area of your shoulder and provide healing energy there.

- Use a Soothing blend as one of the layers of oils in your Back and Spinal Therapy.

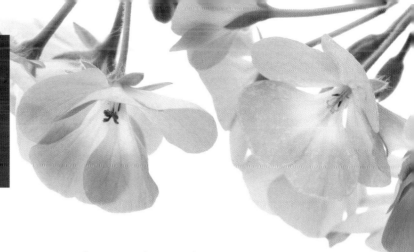

A Stress Control Blend

This is a blend you will want to use during the day to lower anxiety when you need it most. It is not designed to put you to sleep at the end of a stressful day, but to clear your mind and help you remain calm, but alert.

EFFECTIVE for all kinds of anxieties and phobias.

AROMA. It must smell refreshing—not too sharp or medicinal—so you'll want to use it often, especially in the work environment or around the house whenever anxiety or depression overtakes you. It should have a pleasing aroma, acceptable to anyone you work with.

COMPLEXITY. It must have enough of a variety of anti-anxiety ingredients to cover the full range of issues that cause the anxiety—lower nervous tension, decrease mental anxiety, improve mental awareness, provide focus, etc.

STAYING POWER. You don't want this blend to dissipate too quickly, that's why it's better as a topical than a diffusing blend.

SAFETY. It must be safe enough that it can be used often without topical irritation.

PLEASING. Many oils used to lower anxiety can be strong and strange to some people. You don't want those in your workplace thinking, "What's that strong, sharp, medicinal smell?" It needs to be relatively subtle and balancing—pleasing for everyone.

INSTRUCTIONS
Here are a few of many ways to use a Stress Control blend:

- It is for topical use only.

- Use undiluted on the temples, the back of the neck, and on areas of the head and neck targeted in craniosacral therapy (head, neck, jaw, ears, etc.). You can watch videos on YouTube to see the areas of the head massaged in these kinds of therapies.

- Apply a few drops to the palm of your hand. Rub your palms together, cup your hands over your nose and mouth and inhale deeply several times.

- Put a few drops in a tissue, cotton ball, or handkerchief. Keep in a small plastic bag and take it out to inhale when you feel the need. This method will keep the aroma from dissipating too quickly and filling the room.

- Massage a few drops undiluted on the reflexology areas of both the front and back of your hands.

- If you can take time out to massage your feet with this blend during the day, this can help unblock anxious emotions and bring quick relief. Focus on your toes, especially the Psi point on the inside of your big toe.

- Use the Stress Control blend as one of the layers in a Back and Spinal Therapy.

Blends

A Slimming Blend

This is a blend you can use to increase metabolism by creating an exothermic effect in your body. It can also assist in balancing and regulating blood sugars for slowing metabolism. It is primarily to be taken by ingestion. It can also help you control hunger. The oils in this blend, though spicy, will calm the digestive system and work to elevate your mood and enhance satiety.

EFFECTIVE for energizing and increasing fat-burning metabolism in your body.

TASTE can be sharp and spicy but it must be pleasant tasting or you will not use it often enough for it to be effective in the long run. It should be interesting and sophisticated enough in flavor that you can consistently use it several times a day for several months.

AROMA. It should have a spicy, yet pleasing aroma.

COMPLEXITY. It must contain a variety of thermogenic oils to increase the feeling of energy, help you feel satisfied, and also help burn the fat.

SAFETY. It must be safe for many types of ingestion—water, juice, herbal tea, recipes, etc. It should not be too hot on sensitive skin.

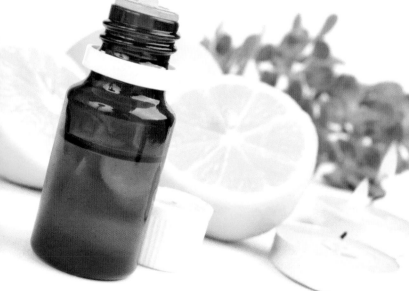

PLEASING. Some oils used for weight loss can be strong and strange to some people. You don't want people in your family or your workplace thinking, "What's that strong, sharp, smell?" It needs to be interesting yet somewhat familiar—pleasing for everyone.

INSTRUCTIONS

Here are a few ways to use a Weight Control Blend:

- Use 3 or 4 drops in 4 to 8 ounces of water 20 to 30 minutes before exercise and before each meal. You'll feel your body temperature go up within a few minutes.

- You can also drink it in a juice or an herbal tea. Use in citrus juices, apple juice, spicy cider, spicy teas, etc.

- You can dilute it 50:50 with a carrier oil and put it in capsules. Take one before exercise and 20 to 30 minutes before each meal.

- Add it to a recipe that is compatible with hot, interesting spices—marinated meat dishes, marinara sauce, salsa, etc.

- To help regulate appetite, apply a few drops in the palm of your hands. Rub your palms together, cup your hands over your nose and mouth and inhale deeply several times.

  - Put a few drops in a tissue, cotton ball, or handkerchief. Keep in a small plastic bag and take it out to inhale when you feel the need to avoid eating something you know you shouldn't.

  - As an added benefit, the citrus oils in the blend can be effective for helping to reduce cellulite. You can dilute the oil 25:75 with a carrier oil and create a body wrap. Apply the diluted massage oil to the cellulite area and wrap with plastic to increase penetration. The diuretic, fluid-releasing nature of the oils will help reduce the appearance of cellulite. Relax and enjoy the warm, penetrating oils. Add more carrier oil if the area becomes too hot or sensitive.

A Relaxing Massage Blend

This is a strong, spicy massage blend you'll want for warming your muscles, ligaments, and joints before and after exercise. It provides that extra degree of safety and comfort you need to maximize the effectiveness of your exercise. It will also help with your balance and form by sharpening your awareness and loosening the tension throughout your body. You won't feel as sore and stiff as you begin exercising, and you'll have quicker and easier recovery after exercise if you use this blend regularly. You can use it to increase circulation and release toxins.

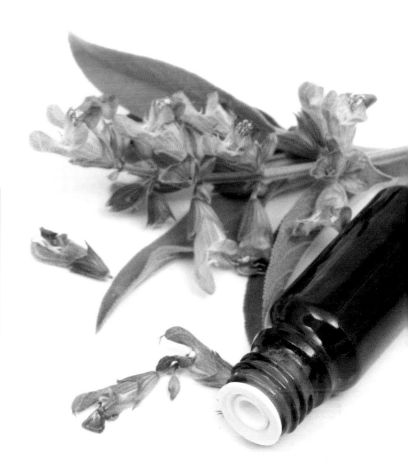

EFFECTIVE for energizing, stretching, and warming up ligaments and muscles.

AROMA. It should have a spicy, yet pleasing aroma that will be compatible with normal aromas in the home as well as the locker room.

COMPLEXITY. It must contain a variety of warming and relaxing oils to increase circulation, flexibility, balance, and energy.

SAFETY. It must be safe for all types of massage and topical application—liniments, massage oils, baths (always dilute with salt), and showers.

PLEASING. Some oils used for pre-exercise massage can be too strong and strange for some people. You don't want people in your family or your gym thinking, "What's that strange smell?" It needs to be interesting yet somewhat familiar— pleasing for everyone.

INSTRUCTIONS

Here are a few ways to use a Massage blend:

- Dilute at least 50:50 with a carrier oil, water, lotion, or witch hazel for a massage of the joints and muscles you will be using.

- After exercise cool down with another massage of your joints and muscles using your diluted Massage blend.

- Use the blend as one of your layers in a Back and Spinal Massage.

- For sore or tired muscles, apply the diluted blend and apply either a cold or warm, wet cloth with a dry towel over it Add a hot water bottle, heating pad, or ice pack over it to increase the penetration and healing. You can add plastic wrap to increase penetration and keep the aromatic molecules from evaporating.

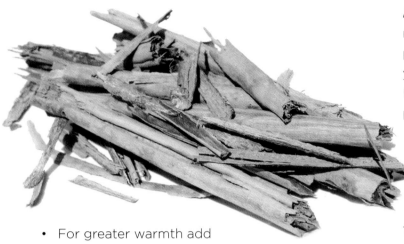

- For greater warmth add a little extra cinnamon or clove

- To calm the blend a little, add lemon, orange, grapefruit, lavender

A Purifying Blend

This is a blend you'll need for diffusing and disinfecting the air in your home or office. It will freshen, deodorize, and neutralize cigarette smoke and other disagreeable odors. Its disinfecting action can also cleanse cuts and scrapes. It can be an excellent blend for repelling insects and treating bites of spiders, hornets, mosquitos, wasps, and bees.

EFFECTIVE for purifying, disinfecting, and deodorizing the air, cleansing wounds, and repelling insects.

AROMA. It should have a clean, crisp, pleasing aroma that will be compatible with normal aromas in the home, car, or office.

COMPLEXITY. It must contain a wide enough variety of oils that it can perform all its functions powerfully, safely, and synergistically.

SAFETY. It must be safe for both diffusion and topical application.

PLEASING. Some oils used for pre-exercise massage can be too strong and strange for some people. You don't want people in your family or your gym thinking, "What's that strange smell?" It needs to be interesting yet somewhat familiar—pleasing for everyone.

INSTRUCTIONS

Here are a few ways to use a purifying blend:

- Diffuse 20 drops two or three times a day in the most active areas of your home.

- Put 4 to 8 drops on a tissue or cotton ball and put it in the vent of your car.

- Apply a few drops in the palm of your hands. Rub your palms together, cup your hands over your nose and mouth and inhale deeply several times.

- To disinfect and freshen items in the clothes dryer, put a couple of drops on a cloth and add it to the dryer.

- For small cuts, bruises, or bumps, apply the blend undiluted. For larger areas, dilute the blend 50:50 with a carrier oil.

- For minor cuts and scrapes, add the blend to the pad of an adhesive bandage and place it over the area.

A Balancing Blend

This is the first blend you'll want to use when layering oils for back massage. It should help relax the tiny myofascial and deep fascial connective tissues in the muscles and nerves along the spine, allowing the spine to naturally align and and allow other oils to penetrate and provide their healing energy. It can also be used for many other calming topical applications. Because this blend is more "yin," relaxing, and calming, it can be used as the opposite of your Massage blend to provide balance and relaxing energy after exercise. This blend is mainly for topical application, not ingestion.

EFFECTIVE for relaxing tension throughout the body and allowing for more natural alignment of the spine and deeper penetration of other oils.

AROMA. It should have a pleasing and emotionally calming aroma that will be universally acceptable and serve to lessen tension, stress, fear, and anxiety.

COMPLEXITY. It must contain a sophisticated blend of oils that will work together safely and synergistically.

SAFETY. It must be safe for all types of topical application.

PLEASING. This is the blend that will be used to set the stage for your entire massage session using a variety of oils and massage techniques. Therefore, it must make a wonderful trusting and calming first impression. It's the first bottle you will open to help your friends and family become comfortable with whatever type of massage you are planning.

INSTRUCTIONS

Here are a few ways to use an balancing blend:

- Apply either undiluted or diluted to the hands or feet to relax and calm before any massage session.

- Apply 6 to 8 drops along the spine as the first step in the layering of various oils for a Back and Spinal Massage. See the chapter on How to Use Essential Oils for step-by-step

- Use as a calming massage oil for relaxing the muscles and joints after exercise or before bed.

- Apply a few drops in the palm of your hands. Rub your palms together, cup your hands over your nose and mouth and inhale deeply several times.

- Because this blend is so universally pleasing for both men and women, it can be used to anchor emotional states you want to reinforce. When you are feeling happy and relaxed, use this oil often for hand or foot massage, or merely to inhale. Then in moments of stress or crisis, you can instantly return to those happy emotions by getting the bottle out and inhaling the aroma.

A Focusing Blend

You'll want this blend to be wonderfully fragrant for multiple emotional uses. It should strike a balance between relaxing and energizing so it creates a mood of trust and acceptance. Like the balancing blend, it should break down barriers of doubt and help you feel confident in sharing your aromatic treasures with others. It should be the most versatile of all your most pleasing emotional blends and single oils.

EFFECTIVE for opening a conversation of trust and acceptance. It should build confidence for an open and relaxed communication. This is a relationship-strengthening blend with the goal to help people come together with others and create something greater than any of them could do alone. It should be neither too masculine nor too feminine.

AROMA. It should have a pleasing and emotionally friendly aroma that will be universally acceptable and serve to break down emotional barriers.

COMPLEXITY. It must contain a sophisticated blend of oils that will not draw attention to themselves, but rather set a mood of faith, trust, and unity.

SAFETY. It must be safe for all types of topical application and diffusing.

PLEASING. This can be a great signature blend you can wear anywhere with confidence, so you will attract positive attention and open, friendly conversation.

INSTRUCTIONS

Here are a few ways to use a Focusing blend:

- Wear this blend as a fragrance to set people at ease and help open conversation. Apply it undiluted to temples, wrists, back of neck, chest, ears, and hands.

- Apply 3 to 5 drops to a tissue, cotton ball, or handkerchief and put it in vents of your car.

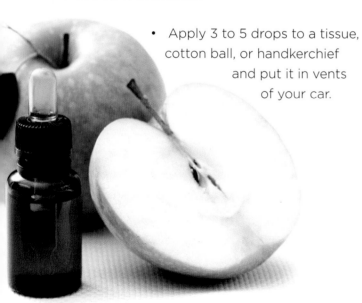

- Wear a clay pendant with several drops of the Focusing blend.

- Use liberally in a bath or shower. Add it to your shampoo or conditioner. Mix it into your lotions and other cosmetics.

- Apply a few drops in the palm of your hands. Rub your palms together, cup your hands over your nose and mouth, and inhale deeply several times.

- Because this blend is so universally pleasing for both men and women, it can be used to anchor emotional states you want to reinforce. When you are feeling extra cheerful and relaxed, use this oil often for hand or foot massage, or merely to wear or inhale. Then in moments of stress or crisis, you can instantly return to those cheerful emotions by applying the aroma.

Antioxidant Blend

You'll want this blend to deliver antioxidants to help protect your cells from the powerful dose of free radicals that attack your body every day from toxins, from outside your body as well as within.

Dr. Pénoël says that one of the most damaging effects of an overactive immune system is the low-grade infections in the body you may not even be aware of. This natural immune response produces large quantities of free radicals that contribute to premature aging and many degenerative diseases. We can deal with this daily toxic overload in two ways. (1) By providing a large quantity of antioxidants such as those found in this blend. (2) By lowering the need for the body's natural immune response by ingesting other systemic antimicrobial essential oils daily. He recommends doing some of both.

EFFECTIVE for fighting the extensive free radical damage in the body that we are all subject to daily. This helps prevent premature aging and the development of degenerative diseases related to free radicals. These antioxidant oils can also have many other functions such as clearing the excess mucous in the respiratory system and anti-inflammatory support. It will also support improved cognitive function.

PLEASING AROMA & TASTE. This should have a spicy yet calming aroma that will be flavorful when ingested in small quantities in water, juice, or recipes. Be sure to adjust the quantity you're using when flavoring anything.

COMPLEXITY. It will contain a robust yet sophisticated blend of oils that boost your antioxidant power. It will be important for you to find a blend that maximizes the most powerful antioxidant essential oils and blends them synergistically.

SAFETY. It must be safe for ingestion.

INSTRUCTIONS

- Mix the blend with an equivalent amount of carrier oil. Fill single 0 capsules using a dropper. Take one a day with food. This will probably be the most efficient way to get sufficient antioxidants into your system daily to make a significant difference.

- Use a toothpick to adjust the quantity of this oil for adding to your drinking water and various other juices and recipes. Enjoy it in every way that tastes good.

- Use 15 drops liberally in a bath with a cup of Epsom Salts. Or you can use about 10 drops after your shower while your body is still damp. Drive the molecules into your body with a hair dryer to maximize the penetration.

- You can also diffuse 10 to 15 drops of this oil in a nebulizing diffuser and breathe deeply to help the oils penetrate the lungs and pass into the blood stream where they will fight free radicals effectively.

"Essential oils are so complex in their make-up and interactions that the formulator may not be able to predict with certainty exactly how the final blend will perform. Neither will he or she know for certain, before the blend is mixed, exactly what its aroma will be" (Pénoël, Life Helping Life, p. 127).

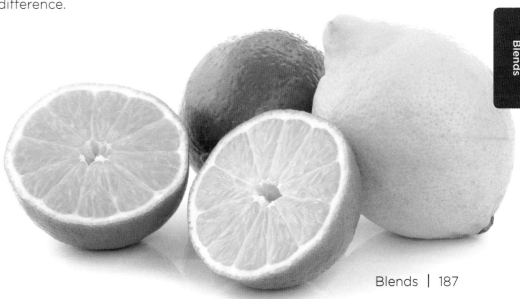

Suggested Blend Recipes

Circulation Blend

Our body is a complex network of tubes, and the more freely they flow, the healthier we are. Our lymph and circulation are a major component of the free-flow of fluids throughout our body. Massage designed to enhance circulation, especially of the legs, the abdomen and the back, bring wonderful benefits to the whole body.

Whereas the Massage blend is ideal for warming up muscles and joints before exercise, this Circulatory Blend is for enhancing free circulation to spread nutrition and energy throughout the body and eliminate toxins.

The purpose of the blend is to eliminate stagnation and toxins from the body by increasing healthy circulation through aromatic massage.

Suggested Recipe for a Circulation Blend

Lemon 30%, myrtle 25%, rosemary 20%, cypress 20%, cinnamon 3%, oregano 2%

This blend is less spicy than a massage blend. It can be used in place of a massage blend if your skin becomes sensitive to the spicier oils.

This massage blend is more herbal and medicinal than the Massage blend. You may want to use it when you can either go to bed or shower afterwards.

INSTRUCTIONS

Here are a few reasons and ways to use the Circulation Blend:

- A primary reason for this blend is to improve circulation in the legs and feet because we sit too much and move too little. This leads to many leg and joint problems that a little leg and foot massage with the Circulation Blend would help to solve. Dilute the blend in either water or carrier oil at 5 – 10% and apply in upward massage starting at the feet. Concentrate on the ankles and calves and move upwards onto the thighs if desired.

- Use the same dilution to massage the liver and the kidney area right under the ribcage in the front and the corresponding area in the back.

- Massage the lung area by stroking the soft tissue between the ribs as well as above and below the clavicle.

- Many people complain of cold hands and feet, which means poor circulation in the extremities. Regular neck massage and massage of the lower back with the Circulation Blend will significantly improve this condition.

- Poor circulation is a central issue in osteoarthritis and rheumatoid arthritis. Frequent use of the Circulation Blend for back and abdominal massage will help significantly.

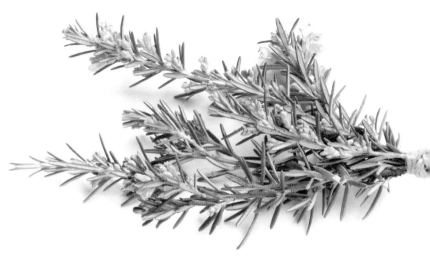

- Abdominal and back massage for improved circulation will benefit sexual and kidney performance as well. When massaging the abdomen, remember to move in a clockwise direction with the directional flow of food through the bowels. Avoid genital areas.

- Use the circulation blend in the shower to massage the body while your skin is moist.

Add variety to your massage routines by rotating among these blends: Immune Balancing Blend, Circulation Blend, Liver Blend, and Digestion Blend.

Try these singles to enhance the action of your Circulation blend: basil, lavender, lemon.

Liver Blend

The liver is one of our most important organs. It is an amazing chemical plant for the process we call metabolism. Every minute it processes 30% of the blood circulating in your body. It performs complex chemical reactions to remove toxins and distribute and store vital nutrients. It chooses when to store and release nutrients so you have an even flow of energy. It processes fats, carbohydrates, and proteins so your body can use them safely. It stores and releases vitamins as needed. It constantly filters your blood, removing inhaled toxins, alcohol, harmful hormones, dead cells, and invading bacteria. If health is a priority for you, you'll want your liver to be clean and healthy at all times.

Suggested Recipes for a Liver Blend

Recipe #1: Lemon 25%, grapefruit 25%, rosemary 25%, juniper 20%, thyme 3%, lemongrass 2%

Recipe #2: Roman chamomile 15%, helichrysum 5%, frankincense 10%, lavender 20%, rosemary 20%, clove 5%, thyme 5%, orange 15%, juniper 5%

That's why the liver blend is used. It enhances the quality of bile and plays a role in the prevention of gall stones. It helps clean out the toxin filters in the liver. This helps prevent acne, eczema, and psoriasis. A regular use of the liver blend will help prevent conditions like asthma and hay fever but also the more serious autoimmune diseases. The Liver Blend performs an important support function in virtually every condition—migraines, PMS, flu, hepatitis and even emotional and mental conditions. Working consistently and aromatically to maintain a healthy liver can have a profound influence on every aspect of your health. Dr. Pénoël says that when a certain dependable aromatic procedure stops working, it is often because the liver needs cleansing first.

INSTRUCTIONS

The Liver Blend can be used in the same ways you would use the Digestion Blend.

- Use a toothpick to stir a trace of the blend into water or into an herbal tea. In more medically oriented treatments, it is convenient to mix it 50:50 with carrier oil and take it in a capsule.

- If you had a heavy (fatty) meal on the previous evening and wake up feeling like you have liver congestion, take a capsule.

- The Liver Blend can be diluted at 5% in a carrier oil and massaged on the liver area, on the abdomen, and on the liver reflex points of the right foot.

- The Liver Blend can also be used effectively as one of the layers in Back and Spinal Massage.

Increase the power of the Liver Blend to release liver congestion by adding a few drops of peppermint into the blend. Mix the Liver Blend with the Digestion Blend 33:66 to enhance the action of both blends and create a synergy.

Inflammation Blend

The point of this blend is soothing inflammation. The Soothing blend can be too strong for some inflammatory conditions, so we need an additional blend with a lighter, more calming action to lower inflammation. This blend is applied externally to keep the inflammatory process under control. Adding even an extra drop of pain-relieving peppermint to the blend will add a little pain relief for an inflammatory condition, but it may be too much. The blend is very mild, but it has a wonderfully calming action on inflammation when used over an extended period of time.

Suggested Recipe for an Inflammation Blend

Roman chamomile 25%, ylang ylang 20%, spruce 10%, rosemary 10%, frankincense 20%, basil 13%, peppermint 2%

The blend, though mild, has a deep action over time on inflammation throughout the body. It doesn't just work on the inflamed tissues, but the aromatic molecules penetrate and move throughout the body.

This is indispensable in difficult autoimmune cases. This gives the blend a wonderful long-term effect when it is used consistently.

INSTRUCTIONS

- For inflammatory conditions like rheumatoid arthritis and fibromyalgia, it makes sense to apply a Soothing blend in the morning and the Inflammation blend in the afternoon and evening before going to bed.

- This blend can be used in the same way as the Soothing blend—undiluted on a small area, in gauze or flannel dipped in aromatic water for a larger area, in a green clay compress, or for a still larger area in a lotion or in a mixing oil.

- You can enhance the action by taking it internally. Three to four drops are easily blended in some natural honey and mixed in a cup of hot water for an herbal tea. The taste is rather nice—not too strong. It is always good to inhale the aroma before drinking it.

- For a calming, anti-inflammatory action, you can use it undiluted on insect bites and stings.

Immune Balancing Blend

One of the most important, life-saving parts of an automobile is its brakes. When your immune system loses its brakes, you have autoimmune diseases in which the immune system goes to war with your body creating serious, life-threatening conditions like type-1 diabetes, Crohn's disease, rheumatoid arthritis, etc.

Suggested Recipe for Immune Balancing Blend

Lavender 30%, Roman chamomile 30%, spruce 20%, frankincense 15%, clove 5%

There are also allergies like hay fever, eczema, and asthma where a substance that is normally not sensitizing becomes a source of irritation and brings on inflammation. The immune balancing blend can be useful for both of these types of conditions.

Why you need this blend

Here's the way Dr. Pénoël describes the development of an autoimmune disease.

Medical problems start in infancy and childhood, generally with ear, nose, and throat (ENT) or bronchial infections. Busy doctors and frantic parents turn too often to antibiotic treatments because they don't see that the reason for these repeated infections is due to the formation of abnormal mucous brought about by a poor diet.

Antibiotics can't solve the problem. Instead they aggravate it a little bit more each time. The "bugs" are not really killed. They are pushed a little deeper with each episode. Instead of helping the immune system become stronger and better trained in its defensive function, the immune system becomes weaker and weaker. In the end it loses its capacity to discriminate between enemy bacteria and the body. This results in "the soldiers shooting at the civilians." The immune system starts attacking the cells of the body. The autoimmune process begins.

For some patients the heavy release of mucous seem to recede. For others the heavy mucous becomes chronic. Others develop allergic conditions like eczema, hay fever, or asthma, according to their genetic predispositions.

In more advanced stages, often after an emotional trauma, the immune system becomes so disoriented that it starts manufacturing antibodies against the tissues of the body itself. The disease is given a name according to the organs that are targeted.

When the process attacks the joints, the disease is called rheumatoid arthritis. When the target is the myelin sheath surrounding the nerves, the disease is called multiple sclerosis. When the target is the mucous membrane of the intestine, it is called Crohn's disease. In systemic lupus, the skin, the kidneys, the arteries and other connective tissues are attacked by the antibodies. The list of autoimmune diseases is long.

The current explosion of auto-immune diseases appears to parallel the explosion of new antibiotic treatments. What mankind appears to have "won" on the strictly anti-infectious battlefront appears to be "lost" on a deeper level and later in life when the immune system goes crazy. There is a price to be paid for excessive use or abuse of antibiotics. An autoimmune disease is a high price indeed.

Saddest of all for Dr. Pénoël is the fact that with his therapies, virtually all the common infections can be taken care of with essential oils, healthy nutrition, and natural hygiene. Autoimmune diseases can be avoided entirely or can be much less severe.

Dr. Pénoël's long experience teaches us that, at the root of most autoimmune conditions, there are lingering low-grade infections. They were probably part of the beginning of the cycle, and even though right now they may not be the main problem, they continue to exert their deep and hidden influence.

This is why he recommends taking an Immune Balancing Blend internally and systematically over an extended period of time in the case of all autoimmune diseases.

Internal use is indispensable since we need a systemic action and because the major area of infectious factors are in the digestive system. Dr. Pénoël and many other natural therapists are convinced that candidiasis or candida infections are also a major factor in immune imbalance as a result of too many antibiotic treatments.

In addition to the Immune Balancing Blend, other blends should be used according to the condition. For example, for respiratory autoimmune diseases like hay fever, allergies, and asthma, a Respiratory Blend is important. Autoimmune diseases of the joints like rheumatoid arthritis call for the external application of the Inflammatory Blend as well as the Soothing blend. The Liver Blend can also be helpful in eliminating toxins.

INSTRUCTIONS

This blend is not a quick fix. It is designed to be taken internally over a period of weeks and months in conjunction with other targeted blends like the Protecting blend to help balance and restore the normal immune response.

- Your main results will come from taking alternating immune balancing and antimicrobial capsules. Create a 50:50 blend with a carrier oil. Fill capsules using a dropper and empty single 0 capsules. Take the immune balancing capsules once or twice at two meals each day with food, and the Protecting blend 50:50 with a carrier oil once a day at your third meal. Capsules should always be taken with food.

- You can take a few drops each day in water, juice, or herbal teas. These are best taken in the evening rather than in the morning.

- It can be applied topically in a 20% dilution with carrier oil over the spleen and thymus areas as well as along the spine.

CAUTION: If you have skin or respiratory allergies, use it on the feet only and do not diffuse it.

Digestion Blend

Between the intake and the outgo of our digestive tract lies an amazingly complex alchemical processing system with delicate tolerances that can become easily upset and go out of balance. The Digestion Blend is designed to use with foods. It is made of culinary spices, and as such can be adjusted to your personal tastes to complement the recipes you most frequently enjoy. If you enjoy Mediterranean Cuisine, you will love adding more Mediterranean spices like basil, rosemary, marjoram and a tiny amount of oregano or thyme. If you prefer food that uses citrus and mint flavors like lemon, orange, and spearmint, you'll want to add more of these digestive oils. Perhaps you enjoy Asian cuisine. Then ginger and citrus oils will take a more central role.

Here's a suggested recipe you can use as a basic formula for a great digestive blend. Feel free to adjust this recipe with culinary oils to fit your personal tastes:

Suggested Recipe for Digestion Blend

Basil 35%, Lemon 25%, Peppermint (or Spearmint) 5%, Ginger 15%, Rosemary 20%

Test the blend by using a very small amount in an olive oil and vinegar (or lemon-juice) salad dressing. You may want to add thickening ingredients and other condiments to enhance the texture and flavor. Make adjustments until you have something that tastes just right to you. You may even create interesting recipes for different purposes. Remember that a single drop of essential oil represents a large quantity of the original herb, so dilute accordingly.

Once you have something that can become a delicious addition to a meal, you can use it for other digestive purposes as well.

This blend is designed to improve digestion by introducing more aromatic molecules into foods you serve; the water, juices, and herbal teas you drink; and the simple capsules you take. While the blend can be used for digestive emergencies to calm an upset stomach or overcome a bout of food poisoning, it is designed for frequent or even daily use. This is the holistic way that gently prevents digestive problems rather than correcting them after they escalate.

SAFETY. Because these oils are all culinary oils, you can be sure they will be safe if you adjust them to taste. As long as they taste good, you can be sure you're using safe amounts.

Here are some ways to use your digestive blend:

• Even before you experience the taste, the aroma of the blend could stimulate your appetite, prepare your digestive glands, and get you ready to enjoy a healthy meal enhanced through aroma.

• In France, a small "aperitif" drink is sometimes offered to stimulate the appetite. You can create your own "aperitif" by putting a drop or two of your Digestive Blend in a teaspoon of honey. Blend with a little water and drink it a few minutes before your meal. You can have this aromatic drink in the morning as a cleansing beverage or use it like a warm herbal tea at the end of the meal.

• You can adjust the strength of your Digestion Blend in a glass of water by using a toothpick dipped in the oil instead of a drop. Adjust it by dipping more or less of the toothpick into the blend and stirring it into your water or juice.

• Dilute the digestive blend in a carrier oil (5% Digestion Blend to 95% carrier oil) for an abdominal massage (clockwise direction). You can also use it undiluted on specific points of the feet, hands, or ears in reflexology therapy. The dilution for a child can be as little as 2 or 3%. Begin the massage with a light touch at the navel then slowly and progressively increase both the size of the circles and the pressure. The movement needs to be quite slow.

• The digestive blend can be used undiluted on the ears. Locate the large and small intestine area in this diagram (Guide p. 32). Use your thumb and index finger with the undiluted oil on both the outside and inside of the outer ear. Never pour a drop of oil down the ear canal.

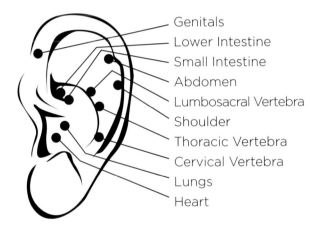

Genitals
Lower Intestine
Small Intestine
Abdomen
Lumbosacral Vertebra
Shoulder
Thoracic Vertebra
Cervical Vertebra
Lungs
Heart

• The diluted oil can also be used for massaging the arch (the digestive area) of the feet.

• If you want to work with the undiluted blend on the back, apply a trace of the Digestion Blend on each thumb and massage downward on each side of the lower spine.

Mental Focus Blend

This blend is a "brain traffic controller" to help regulate and organize the "neurochatter" in the mind that leads to hyperactivity, disorientation, confusion, stress, and overwhelmed feelings. It is designed for use in the daytime where focus and attention are important, not sleep and relaxation. It's a great oil to use when driving, studying, taking exams, or performing tasks that require peak concentration. Using this blend consistently over time whenever you need peak mental ability for difficult tasks can help retard the mental aging process and activate the endocrine command centers of your brain that keep you young and alert.

Suggested Recipe for a Mental Focus Blend

Basil 20%, peppermint 5%, rosemary 20%, bergamot 15%, lemon 20%, Roman chamomile 15%, ylang ylang 5%

INSTRUCTIONS

- When stressed, confused, anxious, or on edge: massage neck, throat, and back with 3-4 drops diluted in 1/2 teaspoon carrier oil.

- Apply undiluted to appropriate reflex points on feet and ears. Also apply undiluted to temples, back of neck, and wrists.

- Diffuse up to 20 drops at a time.

- Put drops on children's pajama collar or pillow case before bed to help calm hyperactivity.

- Put a few drops in your palm, rub palms together, cup over nose and mouth and inhale deeply several times.

- Use 5 to 10 drops in 1/2 cup of Epsom Salts for an aromatic bath.

- Put 4-8 drops on cotton balls or tissues and place them in car vents to help you stay alert while driving.

Intimacy Blend

There are essential oils that claim to prompt a sexual (aphrodisiac) response through (1) relaxation, (2) hormonal activation, or (3) stimulating circulation (Davis, pp. 30-31). A blend created primarily for its aphrodisiac effect could have some limited benefit, but it would need to be used with great care and would not be as useful as a true Intimacy blend.

Suggested Recipe for Intimacy Blend

Orange 20%, ylang ylang 15%, tangerine 20%, bergamot 20%, cinnamon 5%, spruce 15%, lavender 5%

An Intimacy Blend, on the other hand, is designed for doing what essential oils can do better than almost anything else—activate the emotional functions of the limbic brain to create close, intimate memories and build relationships.

Because of their amazing ability to create emotional connections, the oils in an Intimacy Blend can be used for creating all kinds of intimate memories, not just sexual ones. It can be used for the "M" technique in an intimate hand massage between a grandchild and a grandparent. A parent could massage a child's feet with the blend while they watch a heartwarming movie together.

Certainly the blend could be used to create a romantic mood or for "sensate focus" exercises where a therapist assigns a couple to learn non-sexual touching exercises that progressively train them in healthy and satisfying intimate touch.

The main value in this blend is in training the brain to anchor intimate memories that can then be recalled in moments when those same emotions are most needed. We have all experienced fragrance memories when the aroma of our grandmother's perfume or and old boyfriend's aftershave prompted an emotional response. This is the kind of response we are trying to create with this blend.

You have the opportunity to create emotional memories with this blend that will last you a lifetime. Then, whenever you wear it, those memories will instantly fill you with the same emotions of love, caring, pleasure, and connection.

You can start with this basic recipe and adjust it according to the aromatic memories that you and your partner have already acquired. Maybe you have acquired an aversion to lavender but your partner loves it. Maybe bergamot seems too feminine and frilly to you. But blending these into a complex and sophisticated Intimacy Blend can create an entirely new set of emotional responses that will begin to create a cascade of intense intimate responses.

You can begin with this recipe or create your own with your favorite oils. Be sure to involve your partner by asking about the emotional responses that come up as you blend the oils.

INSTRUCTIONS

- Create a beautiful massage oil for "sensate focus" or other intimate massage by mixing a tablespoon of carrier oil with 4 to 6 drops of this blend.

- Diffuse 20 drops of the oil to help capture the happiest most intimate moments of your relationships.

- If you plan to use the oil for occasional sexual dysfunction, be sure to use the blend first under the most positive circumstances to anchor relaxed and open emotions. If you use the oil only during potentially troubling times, the whole process may backfire and the blend will come to be associated with anxiety and frustration.

- You can use this oil for other things too. For example, you can diffuse it while you are calmly, then apply it during the exam to help you relax and remember what you studied. You can use a similar strategy to help you with meditation.

Foot Massage Blend

This blend is not designed for treating any specific ailment or complaint but rather for prevention and helping with any hidden or obvious health problem in your body.

Suggested Recipe for a Foot Message Blend

Balsam fir 20%, frankincense 20%, sandalwood 20%, spruce 20%, juniper 20%

You will see a lot of minor symptoms begin to change and improve with daily foot massage using penetrating aromatic oils. After several weeks of daily therapy, you'll start noticing subtle improvements not only in your overall body functions, but also in your emotions and mental functions. You'll also notice sore or sensitive areas. Then with a little extra massage, the soreness will disappear. Then you may notice improvement in the corresponding areas of your body. This is how Reflexology was developed, by trial and error with careful massage, observation, and note taking.

The oils you'll use for a Foot Massage Blend will be the heavier, thicker bass notes. They are the grounding oils—the resins, the oils that come from roots, wood, bark, twigs, and resins. Conifer oils like fir, spruce, and juniper have been used extensively in emotional healing and spiritual rituals. Frankincense and sandalwood are aromatic treasures used for thousands of years in spiritual rituals for healing and meditation.

Your daily foot massage can be a form of ritual you enjoy each day inhaling these uplifting aromas and working to release any hidden blockages throughout your body—via your feet.

INSTRUCTIONS

- Thorough instructions for simple in-home reflexology and foot massage are found in the "How to Use Essential Oils" chapter.

- You can apply the blend undiluted or diluted 50:50 with a carrier oil.

- You can enhance the action of the Foot Massage Blend by mixing or layering with other blends and single oils according to your personal health goals. For example, during the cold and flu season, you may want to add the Protecting Blend or Respiratory Blend. During hay fever season, you may want to add the Inflammatory Blend or the Immune Balancing Blend.

Immunity-Boosting Blend

Because of the effectiveness of essential oils in support of the immune system, has done a lot of research in this field in his clinical practice. He has seen significant cooperation between aromatic molecules and the immune system that protects us.

Suggested Recipe for a Foot Message Blend

Lavender 30%, Roman chamomile 30%, spruce 20%, frankincense 20%, clove 5%

Dr. Pénoël teaches that there are actually two separate and distinct immune systems. The first is very old. It neutralizes the aggressors through simple immune cells and basic molecular secretions. It is called the innate immune system. It is totally devoid of memory.

The second is the authentic immune system. It has a superior form of intelligence. It has memory and uses highly evolved molecules (called specific antibodies). It has intelligent cells, known as the B lymphocytes. It is an acquired immune system.

In his clinical research, he discovered a type of communication between specific categories of aromatic molecules with the innate immune function on the one hand, and the acquired immune system on the other. This communication has profound significance for our overall health and longevity.

The innate immune system manufactures basic molecules that are needed for our protection. It uses very simple ammunitions to accomplish its primitive task. They are called "leucocytes" or white blood cells. There are three categories of leucocytes. The one that is constantly attacking with its defensive molecules is the neutrophils. Very large defense cells, known as macrophages, also help destroy enemy microbes. As they do their defensive work they leave behind extremely powerful oxidants or free radicals that produce what we call "oxidative stress" in our bodies.

This greatly accelerates the aging process and triggers many inflammatory conditions and degenerative diseases like Alzheimer's disease and even cancerous transformations of the cells. In infectious conditions, the usual production of these damaging substances is increased tenfold! You can imagine what collateral damage this internal war leaves behind. It's like toxic shrapnel that circulates throughout our body lowering our resistance to disease and encouraging inflammation and mutation. Even with our body's antioxidant mechanisms, like superoxide dismutase and similar agents, the damage is extensive. It's much better to prevent these highly damaging oxidative bursts from happening in the first place.

When we take clinical grade essential oils on a daily basis, we're working at the very source of the vast majority of all health problems. We're working on the microscopic aggressors themselves, while still respecting the beneficial bacteria in our bodies.

This means that how quickly we age is directly determined by the activity of our immune system. It's the main factor in our premature decomposition.

But here is the good news. We can take an immunity-boosting blend of clinical quality essential oils into our bodies every day and prevent the aging that comes from our greatest oxidative stress. Because essential oils are so effective against pathogenic bacteria while they respect good bacteria, the need for our immune system and its toxin-producing functions is greatly decreased. And when you reduce the amount of oxidative stress in your body, you get an overall protection against all kinds of degenerative, inflammatory, and cancerous diseases.

Here's another way of putting it. Our immune system is protecting us, but it is also making us sick and old, much more sick and old than we have ever imagined. So, by using powerful, clinical-quality essential oils on a daily basis to minimize the toxic oxidants coming from our immune system, we can greatly reduce this toxic overload, live more disease-free, and age much more slowly.

We not only add years to our lives, but also life to our years. But there is even better news: Clinical quality essential oils also have a critical role to play in the acquired immune system. Whenever our acquired immune system gets overused, we increase our risk of allergies and later from auto-immune diseases. The medical system constantly bombards millions of children with antibiotics from a very young age. Dr. Pénoël believes this is a major factor in the dysfunction of the acquired immune system. He believes it contributes to many unnecessary allergies and auto-immune diseases of all kinds. In this way, allopathic doctors pave the way, from infancy, for diseases to occur later in life. So essential oils allow us to avoid the use of antibiotics, especially in young children, and thus help re-harmonize the craziness and damage done by our second immune system, our acquired immune system.

Dr. Pénoël feels that the most profound role of essential oils is to help, insofar as possible, to reverse entropy or the deterioration of our bodies. Thus, an immunity-boosting blend would be ...

EFFECTIVE for not only fighting but also preventing the extensive free radical damage in the body that we are all subject to daily. It would prevent premature aging and the development of degenerative diseases related to free radicals. Such a blend can also have other functions such as improving the complex digestive and intestinal processes of our bodies.

PLEASING AROMA & TASTE. This blend should have a pleasing flavor and aroma when ingested in small quantities in water, juice, or recipes. You will want to carefully adjust the quantity you're using when flavoring anything with this type of blend.

COMPLEXITY. It will contain a complex blend of oils that boost your antioxidant and cell-protective power. It will be important for you to select a blend with the most highly effective oils that work synergistically together to produce the cell-protective results described here.

SAFETY. It must be safe for ingestion, diffusion, and topical application.

INSTRUCTIONS
Here are a few ways to use the antioxidant blend:

- Mix the blend with an equivalent amount of carrier oil. Fill single 0 capsules using a dropper. Take one a day with food. This will probably be the most efficient way to get the immune protection that your body needs.

- Use a toothpick to adjust the quantity of this oil for adding to your drinking water and various other juices and recipes. Enjoy it in every way that tastes good throughout your day.

- Use 15 drops liberally in a bath with a cup of Epsom Salts.

- Use 10 drops after your daily shower while your body is still damp. The molecules will penetrate immediately even as you are drying yourself with a towel.

- Increase the penetration of this blend by driving the molecules into your body with the heat of a hair dryer to maximize their antioxidant and antimicrobial protection.

- You can also diffuse 10 to 15 drops of this oil in a nebulizing diffuser and breathe deeply to help the oils penetrate your lungs and pass into your blood stream where they will help you accomplish the anti-aging process Dr. Pénoël describes.

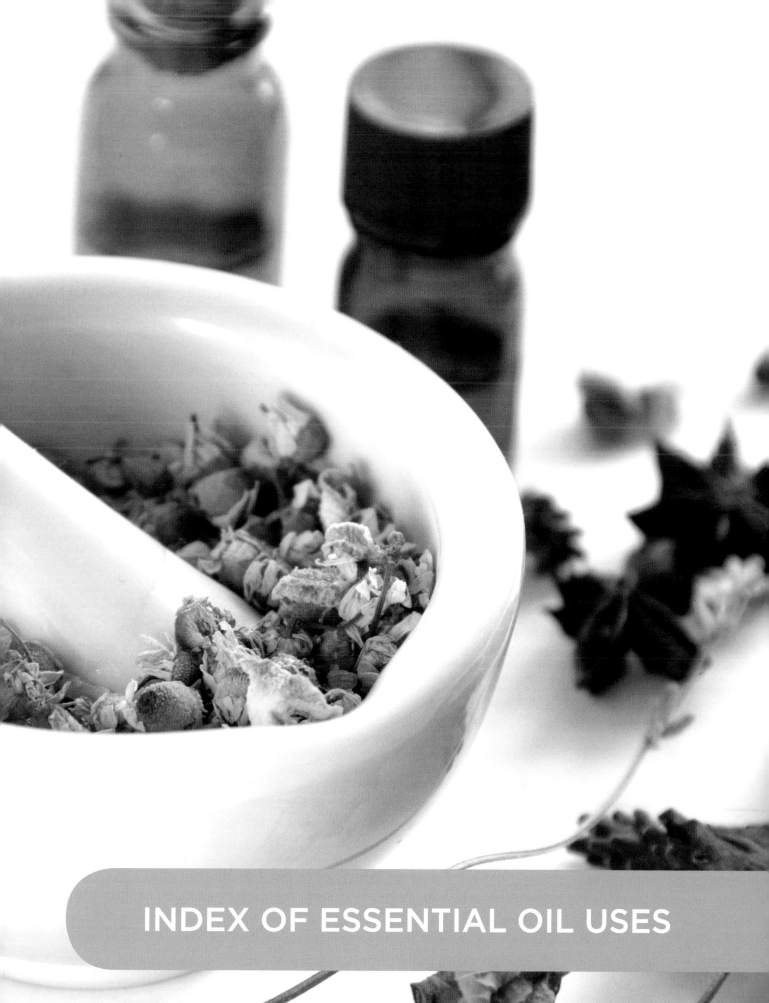

INDEX OF ESSENTIAL OIL USES

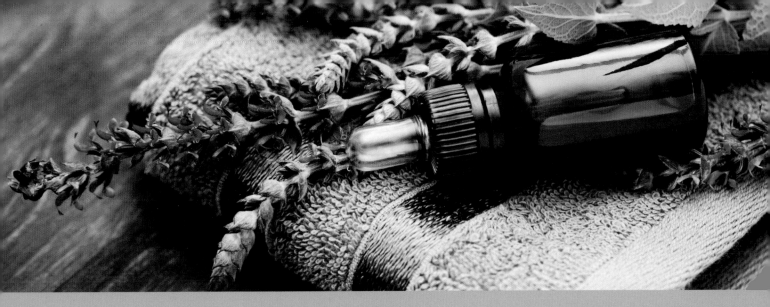

INDEX OF ESSENTIAL OIL USES

 Internal   Topical   Inhalation

Abdominal Discomfort

(See Digestive Conditions)

Acne & Boils

Inflamed or infected sebaceous glands on the skin showing as pimples. More serious infections are boils.

RECOMMENDED SINGLES

Tea Tree		Marjoram	
Juniper		Rosewood	
Bergamot		Basil	
Lavender		Orange	
Rosemary		Cinnamon	
Lemon		Myrtle	
Roman chamomile		Patchouli	

German chamomile	Sandalwood
Helichrysum	Vetiver
Peppermint	Spearmint
Thyme	Oregano
Lemongrass	

RECOMMENDED BLENDS

Protecting blend	Inflammation blend
Liver blend	Purify blend

INSTRUCTIONS:

Dietary improvements will help to minimize infections. Stay away from refined sugar, refined white flour, processed meats, and dairy products until the infections begin to clear. Focus on a diet of vegetables and some fruit.

- Drink more water with a drop of one of the blends—Protecting blend, Digestive blend, or Liver blend—in each quart of drinking water. Or stir a trace of oil in your water using a toothpick dipped in the oil. You can also use tea tree, basil, peppermint, spearmint, orange, cinnamon, or lemon.

- For severe cases, create capsules using the Protecting blend (20%), the Immune Balancing blend (10%), the Liver blend (10%), and carrier oil (50%). Take a capsule with food three times a day. For deep healing take 3 capsules daily for 2 months after the condition has cleared.

- For boils Dr. Pénoël recommends creating capsules with 15% thyme, 15% tea tree, in 70% carrier oil, and taking 3 capsules a day for 10 days (*L'aromatherapie*, p. 300) ++++P.

- For acne Dr. Pénoël recommends peppermint capsules 50:50 with a carrier oil. Take 3 capsules daily for 20 days and extend the use if necessary (*L'aromatherapie*, p. 304). Protecting blend capsules blended 50:50 with a carrier oil are also a great choice.

- Create a blend of rose hip carrier oil (70%) mixed with tea tree (15%) and lavender (15%). Apply 3 times daily until infections clear.

- Apply a trace of tea tree oil or the Protecting blend to individual pimples or boils at least twice daily.

- Create a liniment using 10 drops of the Protecting blend in a 1/2 cup of water, witch hazel, apple cider vinegar, or rubbing alcohol. Soak a cotton ball and tap it twice daily on the infected area.

- Create a facial mask using green clay, water, and 10 drops of a single oil on the list or a combination oils or blends.

CLINICAL SUPPORT

A review of several published studies of tea tree oil reveal effectiveness of tea tree oil in the treatment of acne (Pazyar N et al. "A review of applications of tea tree oil in dermatology." *Int J Dermatol.* 2013 Jul;52(7):784-90).

A randomized, double-blind clinical trial performed on 60 patients with mild to moderate acne vulgaris showed that tea tree oil in a gel was up to 5.75 times as effective as the placebo (Enshaieh S et al., 2007).

"... Antimicrobial resistance has developed in bacterial strains involved in the development of acne. Therefore, alternatives to antibiotic treatment have become necessary." Essential oil formulations were created and their effectiveness was evaluated with 28 volunteers. Evidence of treatment disappeared within minutes, showing little discomfort or side effects after application. The results were good to excellent, especially for the essential oils mixture, which achieved improvements of 75% (Matiz G, et al., 2012).

Addictions & Self-Defeating Behaviors

WHAT THEY ARE:

There are a multitude of seriously addictive as well as less critical self-defeating behaviors that trouble virtually everyone. They can be things like obsessive-compulsive disorders, food addictions, or addictions to drugs or alcohol. There are self-defeating behaviors we all recognize in ourselves that we seem to fall into. They are often the result of some kind of unconscious conditioning.

RECOMMENDED SINGLES

Bergamot		Ylang ylang	
Clary sage		Spruce	
Sandalwood		Rosewood	
Lavender		Juniper	
Balsam Fir		Orange	
Tangerine		Lemon	
Lime		Neroli	
Grapefruit			

RECOMMENDED BLENDS

Focusing blend, Intimacy blend, Calming blend, Stress control blend, Balancing blend, or any other favorite

INSTRUCTION:

The power of aroma to affect behavior is often overlooked. What widow has not been startled by an intense emotional rush when she detects her deceased husband's aftershave in a crowd of people? Who has not instantly jumped into action on smelling natural gas? We can harness the power of aroma to train or re-train behavior. Because aromas go instantly to the brain (unlike other senses, which pass through an interpretation process first), aromas can instantly retrieve signals from a library of unconscious emotions and memories.

Dr. Daniel Pénoël suggests that we can deliberately use aromas to anchor positive behaviors into the library of our unconscious mind. Who knows how many negative responses have been placed there through childhood experiences, highly emotional events, and strong, deliberate marketing indoctrination.

Studies have shown that we can re-train oral dependencies (tobacco, smoking, snacking, coffee, alcohol) that we learned early in life. There are phobias and bad habits that can imprison us and keep us from reaching our potential. These self-defeating behaviors can have an unconscious calming effect on a deeper problem implanted in our unconscious mind, like fear of not having enough to eat, fear of abandonment, etc. Serious addictions and self-defeating behaviors will require intensive therapy beyond the scope of the self-help of aromatic conditioning, but aroma can make a significant contribution.

In aromatic behavioral conditioning, you start by identifying as best you can the origin of the problem. To explore the origins of these habits you can diffuse pleasurable aromas and listen to calming music while you meditate, write in a journal, or visit with a trusted friend or relative. Professional therapy may also help you get to the root of the problem.

- Once you identify the origin of the habit (for example, the need for oral gratification), create a positive replacement (for example, snacking on something delicious and healthy).

- Find an intensely pleasant aroma to associate with your new behavior. It needs to be one you wouldn't grow tired of. It needs to be emotionally associated with the freedom of overcoming your self-defeating behavior.

- Compare the positive feelings of the aroma with the also positive but undesirable feelings associated with the self-defeating behavior.

- Spend 20 minutes using your creative imagination to write your positive new feelings, desires, and habits in a journal while you enjoy the aroma. Again, a relaxed location with relaxing music and healthy, but delicious snacks are important in this anchoring.

- In times of victory over your behavior, diffuse the aroma, put a drop in a tissue, or carry it in a small bottle and bring it out often as you review how well you are doing. Use the oil to anchor your intense desires to enjoy the positive substitute. For example, if weight management is your issue, say to yourself, "nothing can possibly taste as good as healthy feels" as you enjoy the aroma, music, and positive feelings.

- Without leaning on willpower alone (restricting yourself), carry the aroma with you and substitute it as a "treat" whenever you feel a need. The treat will help you emotionally bond with how wonderful "healthy feels," or the freedom from whatever bondage you have been in.

- Create an aromatic treat as a reward for reaching certain goals. Maybe it's a special aromatic potpourri or a relaxing aromatic bath.

- Involve special friends or loved ones with your treat to reinforce the positive emotions associated with your victories.

- CAUTION: This process can work against you if you somehow reinforce a relapse by using your special aromatic experience when you indulge in the behavior you're trying to stop. Your subconscious mind can be just as easily trained to associate undesired behavior with the aromatic experience (Guide, 169-172).

CLINICAL SUPPORT

Jane Buckle reports several findings from studies using essential oils in detoxification from drugs and nicotine. The trials showed only moderate improvement with the recommendation that essential oil therapy could be used to enhance other detoxification methods (Buckle, p. 357-359).

Clary sage and ylang ylang are considered "euphoric" essential oils. They have been used in aromatic baths, diffusion, or inhalation from a tissue to relieve some of the stress that triggers addictive behaviors. (Davis, p. 14)

Allergy (See also specific types like hay fever, eczema, asthma, etc.)

WHAT IT IS

An excessive allergic response or reaction to substances that are not usually harmful. It can be topical or internal. An allergic

reaction may manifest over time, getting worse with each contact.

RECOMMENDED SINGLES

German
chamomile

Roman
chamomile

Helichrysum

Lavender

RECOMMENDED BLENDS

Immune
balancing
blend

Inflammation
blend

INSTRUCTION

Be cautious with using essential oils if you are prone to allergies or are sensitive to skin care products or fragrances. Essential oils could make your allergies worse because they may be related chemically to the very thing you're allergic to.

If you are prone to allergies, be sure to perform a patch test on the inside of your arm before using a significant amount of any essential oil. You are looking for any red, sore, itchy spots or inflammation after topical contact. It may happen within minutes, hours, or even days after applying a particular essential oil. If you are especially allergic, it may even occur after the second contact with the oil. If this is the case for you, apply the oil to the inside of your arm, wait a day, and reapply the oil. If nothing allergic seems to be happening after the second application, then you should be fine for using the oil topically.

Essential oils can cause allergic reactions and they can also calm them. The oils listed above are calming oils that are most likely to ease the symptoms of an allergic reaction both by the calming chemical reaction and also by calming stress. But they can also be allergens in some individuals, especially those who have developed allergies in their professions because of constant exposure to certain chemicals.

After making sure that these oils are not sensitizers themselves, begin gingerly to use them topically, in diffusion, and by ingestion according to the following guidelines and in cooperation with your health care professional if necessary. Try different ones and rotate them until you find one that can be diluted enough to work for you to begin the de-sensitizing process. Read the section on the Immune Strengthening Cleanse for complete details.

Sometimes you can use the oils on the bottoms of your feet or by ingestion when you can't use them topically. In fact, topical application might be the most sensitizing way to use them followed by diffusion. So be cautious and move slowly. A thorough program to rebuild your immune system may take more than a year and may require the assistance of health care professionals skilled in other healing modalities as well.

- For calming relief, use a drop or two on a tissue or handkerchief and breathe through it. Put a drop in the palm of your hand, rub hands together, and inhale the aroma with hands cupped over your nose and mouth.

- Have an aromatic bath using 20 drops of one of the oils in a cup of Epsom Salts.

- Create a 50:50 blend with one of the oils and a carrier oil and fill capsules. Take one with each meal.

- Use a toothpick to put a trace of one of the oils under your tongue or lick a trace off the back of your hand and distribute it around your mouth.

Altitude Sickness

WHAT IT IS

An illness caused by climbing to a high altitude and the resulting shortage of oxygen. Symptoms include hyperventilating, nausea, and exhaustion.

RECOMMENDED SINGLES

Bergamot		Peppermint	
Spearmint		Lemon	
Spruce		Juniper	
Orange		Tangerine	

RECOMMENDED BLENDS

Respiratory blend

INSTRUCTION

- When hiking or in high altitudes, carry one or more of the recommended oils.

- Use a drop in all drinking water. You can use a toothpick to adjust the amount to create a pleasant taste.

- Use a drop or two on a tissue or handkerchief and breathe through it. Put a drop in the palm of your hand, rub hands together, and inhale the aroma with hands cupped over your nose and mouth.

- Put a trace of the oil on your upper lip under your nose.

- Use a toothpick to put a trace of one of the oils under your tongue or lick a trace off the back of your hand and distribute it around your mouth.

Amebiasis

WHAT IT IS:

Intestinal infection that causes diarrhea and may cause severe, life-threatening dehydration and spread to the liver if not controlled. Also called amoebic dysentery.

RECOMMENDED SINGLES

Tea tree		Peppermint	
Spearmint		Thyme	
Oregano			

RECOMMENDED BLEND

Protecting blend

INSTRUCTION:

- Act with the advice of medical professionals to quickly and consistently get this infection under control so it doesn't spread to the liver.

- Use a Protecting blend or an Immune balancing blend singly or together in equal parts.

- Take up to 16 drops daily of any of the recommended oils daily. This can be done by taking 3 capsules a day with food. Mix the essential oils 50:50 with a carrier oil and fill capsules with a dropper.

- Take 1 or 2 drops of one of the recommended oils in an herbal tea with honey, a quart of water, juice, or in recipes. Small children will typically take the oils better in water, juice, or food like applesauce.

- You can also rub the feet of children and even babies with 1 or 2 drops of one the recommended oils diluted in a teaspoon of carrier oil. Do this 3 times a day.

CLINICAL SUPPORT

A recent report on all the literature affirming the effectiveness and in some cases superiority of herbal ingredients and essential oils in treating amoebiasis and other tropical diseases (Pohlit AM et al., 2011).

Angina Pectoris
(See Chest Pain)

Ankle & Leg Swelling (Edema)

WHAT IT IS

Edema is a condition characterized by an excess of watery fluid collecting in the cavities or tissues of the body. It is most common in the legs and ankles, but it can also accumulate anywhere in the body. It can be the result of many causes, but is most commonly due to cardiovascular conditions and inactivity.

RECOMMENDED SINGLES

Birch		Patchouli	
Helichrysum		Cypress	
Grapefruit		Lemon	
Lime		Orange	

RECOMMENDED BLEND

Circulation blend		Massage blend	
Inflammation blend			

INSTRUCTION

- Dilute 4 to 5 drops of one of the recommended oils in teaspoon of a carrier oil and gently massage the feet, ankles and legs upward toward the heart.

- Add a drop of the recommended citrus oil oils to your drinking water to help flush toxins and excess fluids from your body. These oils have some diuretic action, which helps increase the flow of urine and helps flush excess fluids naturally from the body.

- Take an aromatic bath with 20 drops of one of the recommended oils in a cup of Epsom Salts.

- Increase exercise safely to help increase blood flow and normal flow of fluids. Be sure to massage legs and ankles before exercise with a blend of one teaspoon of carrier oil with 2 to 3 drops of the Massage blend. Do stretching and warm-up exercises before beginning and stretching and cool-down exercises after exercising.

- Use the 4 to 5 drops of the Comforting blend for a thorough massage of the legs and ankles after exercise.

Appendicitis (Chronic)

WHAT IT IS

Appendicitis is swelling (inflammation) of the appendix, a small pouch attached to the beginning of the large intestine. You must not confuse acute with chronic appendicitis. Look up the symptoms in a medical diagnostic text or website. Acute appendicitis will require the immediate attention of a health care professional because it is life-threatening. Chronic appendicitis

is a more minor ailment that can be helped with the instructions shown here. It pays to be absolutely sure, so get a diagnosis from a professional if you are uncertain.

RECOMMENDED SINGLES

Grapefruit		Bergamot	
Ylang ylang		Lemon	
Lime		Orange	

RECOMMENDED BLENDS

Inflammation blend		Protecting blend	
Comforting blend			

INSTRUCTION

- As a calming addition to whatever professional care is given, essential oils can help to relieve stress and speed healing from chronic appendicitis. They can also help reduce inflammation and the infection that could come with an inflamed appendix or even a ruptured appendix after surgery or treatment from a health care professional.

- A comforting foot massage using 2 or 3 drops of the Protecting blend or one of the singles on the arch of the foot is comforting. Use the "M" technique on the hands to calm the nerves.

- Take a calming cup of herbal tea with a drop of one of the recommended oils.

- **Do not massage the abdomen** with essential oils or add heat. Refer to advice in an authoritative diagnostic guide or from a health care professional.

- **Diffuse** 20 drops of a calming oil or blend.

Arthritis (Osteoarthritis, rheumatoid arthritis, and rheumatism)

WHAT IT IS

An inflammation, stiffness, and swelling of one or more joints where bones meet. There are many types of arthritis resulting from deterioration of the cartilage, auto-immune inflammation, and many others.

RECOMMENDED SINGLES

Spruce	Helichrysum
Eucalyptus radiata	Sweet basil
Peppermint	Spearmint
Juniper	

RECOMMENDED BLENDS

Inflammation blend	Antimicrobial blend
Immune balancing blend	Comforting blend

As part of an overall plan with the approval of or under the direction of your health care professional:

- For intense pain, use the Soothing blend externally. On a small area, apply a drop undiluted and gently spread it around. For a larger area, mix ten drops in 5 to 10 ml of carrier oil and gently massage. Or you can create a 50:50 blend with a carrier oil and use as needed.

- Here is an anti-inflammatory recipe offered by Dr. Pénoël. It is a blend of 30% Eucalyptus radiata, 20% helichrysum, and 50% carrier oil. Massage painful joints 2 to 4 times a day ++++P. This blend is targeted at rheumatoid arthritis.

- Here is a cortisone-like recipe targeted at rheumatoid arthritis from Dr. Pénoël. It is

a blend of 25% pine, 25% spruce, and 50% carrier oil applied to the spine once or twice daily ++++P.

- Blend 25% peppermint, 25% juniper, and 50% carrier oil to fill capsules you can take three times a day with food ++++P.

- Create a massage blend directed at osteoarthritis of 30% Eucalyptus radiata and 20% thyme with 50% carrier oil ++++P. Massage painful joints 2 to 4 times daily.

- An extremely strong inflammation can be like a burning fire. Even mild oils can sometimes be too strong and add strength to the fire. Create a rough suspension of the Soothing blend in cold water—4 to 5 drops to 1/4 cup water. Shake it well and soak a piece of flannel or gauze in it to create a compress to help the oil penetrate. Apply a little plastic and a cling bandage over it to keep the liquid in contact with the skin. Apply an ice pack to increase the cooling effect.

- Mix 5 to 10 drops of the Soothing blend into green clay to create a poultice for the afflicted area. Protect it with a little plastic wrap and a cling bandage.

- Except in the times of extreme crisis, apply the strong Soothing blend in the morning and then use a soothing inflammation blend in the afternoon, evening, or before bed.

- Use the inflammation blend in the same ways as the Soothing blend above: a few drops applied undiluted on a small area, a few drops diluted in a carrier oil for a gentle massage on a larger area, a gauze or flannel soaked in a cold water suspension to form a compress, or a few drops in a green clay poultice. Especially with the auto-immune aspect, you'll need the inflammation blend or even the immune balancing blend for its deeper, more long-term benefits.

- Use the mild immune balancing blend for rheumatoid conditions as an emergency remedy during a painful crisis when there is a strong allergic reaction. Blend three to four drops in some honey and stir it into a cup of warm water. Enjoy the aroma first, then slowly drink it.

- Dilute 5 drops of the immune balancing blend in a teaspoon of carrier oil. Apply it over the spleen and thymus areas on the abdomen and back and also along the spine.

- Enjoy a bath daily using 5 to 10 drops of sweet basil dispersed in a cup of Epsom Salts.

Here is a more intensive program for arthritis

As part of an overall plan with the CLINICAL SUPPORT of, or under the direction of your health care professional:

- The Protecting blend is anti-infectious and can play a major role in purifying and balancing the intestinal flora inside the body. Ingest at least one drop a day **in** herbal tea or water. Enjoy it preferably in the morning.

- In order to help with liver detoxification, ingest a drop of the liver blend in a soup or juice.

- To improve healing circulation, massage the Circulation blend around painful joints in a larger circle than the other massage oils you use.

- In case of energy blockages use 5 drops of the Comforting blend or Foot Massage blend in a teaspoon of carrier oil for a daily foot massage.

- Control your nutrition strictly according to the dietary guidelines.

- If this complete program seems too complicated or overwhelming, you may give it all up altogether before you experience any permanent benefits. Adapt the program to habits you can maintain consistently and add others as you feel you can.

Essential oils, arthritis pain and stiffness

I have had rheumatoid arthritis for almost a decade. I can't use some tools because the pain is more than I can stand. I can't close my hands enough to hold the tools securely. A friend showed me how to layer four oils on the back of one of my hands. Within a few minutes that hand was able to work like a normal hand while my other hand still had a lot of pain. I was amazed

Asthma (see Hay Fever)

WHAT IT IS

A condition where the airways of the lungs swell and narrow, leading to wheezing, shortness of breath, chest tightness, and coughing. It can result from allergies and/or autoimmune reactions that can be triggered by dust, pollen, exercise, airborne toxins, and viral/bacterial infections.

RECOMMENDED SINGLES

Birch		German chamomile		
Roman chamomile		Lemon		
Balsam fir		Frankincense		
Lavender		Bergamot		
Lime		Myrtle		
Oregano		Peppermint		
Rosemary		Spearmint		
Spruce		Tea tree		

RECOMMENDED BLENDS

Respiratory blend		Protecting blend		
Immune balancing blend		Inflammatory blend		
Comforting blend				

Essential oils can assist in helping you relax (minimizing spasms), breathe more easily (opening bronchial passages) and fight related infections. Because asthmatics' lungs are typically sensitive and respond with spasms to the allergic trigger, avoid inhaling diffused essential oils because they may increase the intensity of the spasms.

CAUTION: if there is any possibility that there may be an allergic reaction to essential oils, use them only on your feet or ingest them. With the involvement of your health care professional, try these procedures:

- For relaxation apply 1 to 2 drops of the most calming oils listed with a carrier oil to respiratory points on the feet. Also use them on the upper back, the nape of the neck, and the upper chest.

- Dr. Pénoël recommends taking a capsule of 25% tangerine, 25% rosemary, with 50% carrier oil 3 times a day with food +++P.

- For openening air passages, apply 1 to 2 drops of Eucalyptus radiata, balsam fir, or the respiratory blend undiluted to the toes and balls of the feet. Also massage them with a teaspoon of carrier oil on the upper back, the nape of the neck, and the upper chest.

- The fingertips are reflex points for the sinuses. Apply traces of Eucalyptus radiata undiluted to your fingertips and tap them together quickly 50 to 100 times to release energy blocks and open air passages.

- To help fight infection apply 1 to 2 drops of the immune balancing blend, the Protecting blend, tea tree, and Eucalyptus radiata undiluted to reflex points on the feet. Blend 3 to 5 drops with a teaspoon of carrier oil and massage the upper back, the nape of the neck, and the upper chest.

- Complete a year of the immune strengthening and balancing cleanse for a deep action against asthma and related autoimmune respiratory diseases like hay fever and other respiratory allergies.

CLINICAL SUPPORT

Patricia Davis suggests that frankincense is sometimes overlooked in asthma treatment, but because it slows breathing, helps overcome respiratory infection, and promotes calmness and meditation, it works on many levels at once (Davis. P. 36).

Marcel Lavabre recommends an aromatic bath with one of the recommended oils (20 drops) blended with Epsom Salts (1 cup) (Lavabre, p. 155).

Atherosclerosis & Coronary Artery Disease

Hardening of the arteries is a common disorder that occurs when fat, cholesterol, and other substances build up inside the walls of arteries and form hard structures called plaques. This is often aggravated by inflammation of the arteries. Over time, this can block the arteries and cause a wide number of cardiovascular conditions.

Coronary artery disease concerns the delicate arteries the supply blood to the heart.

RECOMMENDED SINGLES

Lemon		Tangerine	
Lavender		Thyme	
Ginger		Wintergreen	

RECOMMENDED BLEND

Circulatory blend		Comforting blend	
Liver blend		Foot massage blend	

INSTRUCTION

- Use the following oils in a diluted massage (3 to 4 drops per teaspoon of carrier oil)— lemon, tangerine, lavender, the Comforting blend, and the Circulation blend. These oils can also be applied undiluted or blended with the foot massage blend for calming reflexology massage.

- Ingest one or two drops of the following oils per quart of drinking water or in an herbal tea—the Liver blend, the Digestion blend, tangerine, and lemon. You can also use a toothpick to stir a trace in a glass of water or a cup of hot water or herbal tea.

- Dr. Pénoël recommends a blend of 25% tangerine, 25% lemon, and 50% carrier oil in a capsule taken 2 to 3 times daily for 20 days. It can be started up again after 4 days of rest ++P.

- Diffuse 5 to 10 drops of lemon, lavender, or the Comforting blend for 5 minutes any time during the day for its calming, restorative action.

Athlete's Foot

(See Fungal Infections)

Bad Breath (Halitosis)

WHAT IT IS

An embarrassing condition caused by bacteria and other pathogens that grow in the mouth. Gum, mints, mouthwashes and other products designed to fight bad breath are only temporary cures and may actually compound the problem by feeding the bacteria. Essential oils are particularly helpful in overcoming the root causes of bad breath and thus helping to prevent serious diseases throughout the body that begin in the mouth.

RECOMMENDED OILS

Tea tree	🌀👤	Thyme	🌀👤
Tangerine	🌀👤	Peppermint	🌀👤
Cinnamon	🌀👤	Clove	🌀👤

RECOMMENDED BLEND

Protecting blend	🌀👤

INSTRUCTION

- Brush twice a day with a cinnamon or clove tooth powder mixed with an extra drop of tea tree or tangerine oil. Create your own tooth powder by mixing 2 parts baking soda to 1 part fine-ground, natural salt. Thoroughly mix in drops of peppermint or clove oil to taste. Sprinkle some in your hand, add a drop of tea tree or tangerine oil, wet your toothbrush, and enjoy brushing your teeth without the toxic chemicals.

- Create an aromatic mouthwash using a teaspoon of baking soda, a teaspoon of salt, 10 drops of tea tree, 10 drops of peppermint, and 8 ounces of water. Shake before each use. Swish, gargle, and spit.

- Create an oil pulling mixture with 10 drops of peppermint or a mixture of other oils on the recommended list in a 1/2 cup of olive oil. Take about a tablespoon of oil. Swish and pull the oil back and forth between your teeth for about 20 minutes while you shower. Spit the mixture out. This thicker concoction really gets into the pockets where the bacteria hide in your mouth.

Baldness & Hair Loss

WHAT IT IS

A hereditary condition called male-pattern baldness or female-pattern baldness. This is the most common cause. Other causes of hair loss include hormonal factors, medical conditions and medications.

RECOMMENDED SINGLES

German chamomile	👤🌀👤	Roman chamomile	👤🌀👤
Rosemary	👤🌀👤	Birch	👤🌀👤
Cedarwood	👤🌀👤	Grapefruit	👤🌀👤
Juniper	👤🌀👤	Patchouli	👤🌀👤
Clary sage	👤🌀👤	Ylang ylang	👤🌀👤

RECOMMENDED BLEND

Circulation blend		Immune balancing blend	

INSTRUCTION

- Put 3 or 4 drops in each application of shampoo and conditioner or 20 drops in an 8 oz. bottle.

- Add a few drops of essential oil to each application of hair gel or other mild hair-care products.

- To keep your hair from getting greasy, you can create an aromatic tincture by mixing a few drops (5%) of your favorite essential oils from the list with either rubbing alcohol or vodka (95%) and massage into scalp (Lawless p. 27).

CLINICAL SUPPORT

"[Rosemary essential oil] is used for problems involved in central nervous system, cardiovascular system, genito-urinary conditions, liver treatments, the reproductive system and respiratory system. The volatile oil of the plant is used in oils and lotions for the treatment of various ailments like arthritis, gout, muscular pain, neuralgia, wounds and rubbed into hair for stimulating the hair bulbs to renewed activity, to prevent premature baldness" (Begum A, et al., 2013).

Bell's Palsy

WHAT IT IS

A disorder of the nerve that controls the movement of facial muscles. When this nerve is damaged, the muscles become weak or paralyzed.

RECOMMENDED SINGLES

Helichrysum		Frankincense	
Sweet basil			

RECOMMENDED BLEND

Comforting blend		Stimulating massage blend	
Foot massage blend			

INSTRUCTION

- As part of an overall plan and with the involvement of your health care professional as needed, try these adjunct procedures.

- To release any associated energy blockages, massage the toes, especially the big toe, with a few undiluted drops of frankincense, helichrysum, the Massage blend, the Comforting blend, or the Foot Massage blend.

- If there are spasms involved, massage the toes with sweet basil.

Bladder Infection

(see Urinary Tract Infection UTI or cystitis)

WHAT IT IS

An infection that can happen anywhere along the urinary tract from kidneys to final elimination. They have different names, depending on what part of the system is involved.

RECOMMENDED SINGLES

Tea tree		Lemon	
Bergamot		German chamomile	
Roman chamomile		Lavender	
Sandalwood		Balsam fir	
Cedarwood			

RECOMMENDED BLEND

Protecting blend   Comforting blend

Foot massage blend

INSTRUCTION

- As part of an overall plan and with the involvement of your health care professional as needed, try these helpful procedures.

- On the first day of the infection, prepare as much as a gallon or more of herbal tea (no caffeine) and drink three cups within the first hour and 2 cups each subsequent hour throughout the day. Put one drop of a Protecting blend or tea tree and a little honey in each cup.

- Massage an undiluted drop of the Protecting blend or tea tree on the kidney areas on the back.

- Increase water intake by enjoying a drop or trace of the Protecting blend, tea tree, or any of the other oils and blends recommended. Add a drop or two of lemon or orange to make it more delicious if you wish. Enjoy at least two quarts of this aromatic water a day. Extend your capacity gradually too as much as a gallon of water per day.

- To prevent chronic urinary tract infections, take a drop of any of the recommended oils in a cup of herbal tea once or twice a day.

- Create a lemon juice drink each morning by mixing the juice of 1/2 lemon in a large glass of water with a drop or two of lemon essential oil to buffer the sour taste. This can also help prevent kidney stones.

- Massage your lower arch and heel daily with 2 to 3 drops of undiluted sweet basil, the Comforting blend, or the Foot Massage blend.

- Dr. Penoel suggests that while you are recovering from a urinary tract infection, eliminate all dairy products from your diet.

- To rapidly get a lot of essential oil molecules into your system, try Dr. Penoel's "Live Embalming" therapy found in Chapter 4. Use 5 to 10 drops at a time for a total of 20 or 30 drops of Eucalyptus radiata or ravintsara with a hair dryer to get a large amount of essential oils to penetrate the body in a short amount of time. Be sure to change locations on the body with each application. Be sure to read the instructions in Chapter 4 before trying this therapy.

Blisters

WHAT IT IS

A bubble on the skin filled with clear fluid and caused by friction, a burn, or other skin damage.

RECOMMENDED OILS

Tea Tree   Lavender

Lemon

RECOMMENDED BLEND

Protecting blend

INSTRUCTION

- Do not puncture the blister. Apply an undiluted drop of tea tree to minimize the possibility of infection. If the blister is opened, use an undiluted drop of tea tree oil or the Protecting blend on and around the blister to minimize infection.

- You can put a drop of one of the recommended oils on an adhesive bandage and put it over the blister to protect it.

- If blisters are caused by sunburn, follow instructions under sunburn.

Boils (Abscess)

WHAT IT IS

A boil is an inflamed, swollen, painful lump under the skin. It can look like an extra-large pimple. They can be caused by infected hair follicles. Bacteria from the infection can form an abscess, or a pocket of pus.

RECOMMENDED OILS

Bergamot		Tea tree	
Spearmint		Peppermint	
Lavender		Helichrysum	
German chamomile		Roman chamomile	
Lemon			

RECOMMENDED BLEND

Protecting blend		Digestion blend	
Liver blend			

INSTRUCTIONS

- Personal procedures suggested as part of an overall plan that may involve your health care professional.

- Make any needed changes to your diet that may contribute to infections. Bacteria thrive on refined sugar, refined white flour, processed meats, and some dairy products. Stay away from these foods until infections are cleaned out of your system.

- Add aromatic drinking water to your daily habits with a drop or two of one of the recommended blends per quart of water. Or stir a trace of oil into your drinking water using a toothpick dipped in the oil.

- For severe cases create a blend of 20% Protecting blend, 10% Immune Balancing blend, 10% Inflammatory blend, and 10% Liver blend, and 50% carrier oil and fill capsules. Take a capsule with food three times a day and continue for two months after your skin condition has cleared up.

- Dr. Pénoël recommends a blend of tea tree, (40%), thyme (10%), and a carrier oil (50%). Fill capsules with a dropper and take 3 capsules a day for 10 days ++++P.

- For individual boils or abscesses, apply an undiluted drop of tea tree or the Protecting blend at least twice a day.

- Create a compress. Add four drops of the inflammatory blend or the Protecting blend to a teaspoon of water. Soak a cotton ball or gauze pad and apply it to the infected area. Cover with an adhesive bandage or cling bandage depending on where the boil is located. Add heat to help drive the oils into the skin to help with healing.

- Refer to a medical diagnostic guide or health care professional for any sign that your boils are more serious than personal care should treat.

Broken Bones, Fractures, & Sprains (bones, ligaments, joints)

WHAT THEY ARE

A bone fracture or break is a serious medical condition in which there is a break in the continuity of the bone from a forceful impact or stress. It can also be the result of conditions that weaken the bones, such as osteoporosis or bone cancer. A sprain is a severe wrench or twist in ligaments of an ankle, wrist, or other joint that causes pain and swelling.

RECOMMENDED OILS

Peppermint		Helichrysum	
German chamomile		Roman chamomile	
Marjoram		Lavender	
Rosemary			

RECOMMENDED BLENDS

Soothing blend		Inflammation blend	
Circulation blend			

INSTRUCTION

- You can avoid significant health care issues if you take care of bone, ligament, and joint injuries quickly using essential oils. Carry important oils in your purse or in a handy pouch on a key chain or belt. When you act quickly, you'll relieve a great deal of pain and suffering and prevent other issues that will quickly develop if left untreated. And this can also prevent internal bleeding resulting in bruises and infections, requiring the body to produce its own infection-fighting response

through white blood cells. This puts an enormous strain on the immune system and produces chemicals that promote premature aging and other long-term health problems. With essential oils used quickly and thoroughly, these conditions can be greatly minimized.

- Here are the procedures to use as part of a plan involving your health care professional after a correct diagnosis with the possible help of an authoritative first-aid guide.

- You will want to immediately control pain by using either peppermint or a Soothing blend. If the area is small like a finger or wrist, and not near sensitive skin, simply place a drop on your little finger and touch the area. You can apply a few drops from the bottle directly on a slightly larger area then spread it carefully with your little finger.

- On a larger area, dilute 4 to 5 drops in a teaspoon of carrier oil, and spread it gently on the area.

- Before applying ice, mix 4 to 5 drops of peppermint or the Soothing blend in a 1/3 cup of water and shake the mixture. Soak a gauze, cotton ball, or small cloth in the mixture and apply it to the painful area. Wrap it with a cling bandage. Then apply a cold pack or ice pack.

- When the inflammation and heat from the injury have subsided and when it becomes appropriate to apply heat to aid the healing, use the inflammation blend or the Soothing blend. The inflammation blend will help with inflammation, but will be less effective at controlling the pain. Create a gauze or cotton-ball compress as explained above and apply a heat pack.

- To speed healing, gently massage the area with 4 to 5 drops of the circulation blend in a teaspoon of carrier oil around the area of the injury.

- CAUTION: If you feel the area shows any sign of inflammation—hot, red, swollen, or in acute pain—do not use a hot pack. It would add more heat and worsen the situation! Listen to what your body tells you. If you get relief from cold, use cold. If it feels better with heat, that's what it needs.

Bronchitis

WHAT IT IS

Inflammation of the trachea and bronchial tubes, usually from a viral or bacterial infection—a cold or flu.

RECOMMENDED OILS

Oil		Oil	
Eucalyptus radiata	🔵🔵	Peppermint	🔵🔵🔵
Spearmint	🔵🔵🔵	Tea tree	🔵🔵
Helichrysum	🔵🔵🔵	Balsam fir	🔵🔵
German chamomile	🔵🔵	Roman chamomile	🔵🔵🔵
Frankincense	🔵🔵🔵	Pine	🔵🔵
Marjoram	🔵🔵	Lavender	🔵🔵
Myrtle	🔵🔵🔵	Rosemary	🔵🔵🔵

RECOMMENDED BLENDS

Blend		Blend	
Protecting blend	🔵🔵🔵	Inflammation blend	🔵🔵

INSTRUCTION

When you use essential oils at the earliest signs of a cold or flu before bronchitis even begins, they can help slow or even stop the cycle that leads to inflammation. If you feel a tickle in your throat or feel unusually exhausted, spring into aromatic action. An ounce of prevention will save you days of misery. With the appropriate involvement of your health care professional, use the following procedures:

- Infections thrive and grow quickly on certain foods, so while you have the infection and for 10 days thereafter, avoid eating mucous-producing foods—refined sugar, many dairy products, white flour products, processed meats, etc.

- Stay away from tobacco or industrial pollutants.

- Generally, avoid cough suppressants since normal coughing (not intense coughing spasms) helps to lift and clear the mucous that comes from bronchial inflammation.

- Increase your intake of water to at least 1/2 gallon daily and add a trace or drop of one of the flavorful oils listed above.

- Avoid dry air by using a humidifier. You may add a drop of the respiratory blend or eucalyptus radiate to the humidifier +++++P.

- At the first sign of a bronchial "tickle" telling you that your condition is about to become bronchitis, use your finger to place a drop of tea tree on the back of your tongue and let it stay in your mouth for at least 2 minutes. You can also lick a drop or a trace off the back of your hand. We call this the "lick trick." The tea tree will mix with your saliva to create an antibacterial/antiviral "mouthwash." After two minutes, swallow this saliva mixture slowly. The tea tree will continue its purification action down the esophagus and into the stomach. Repeat this procedure every 5 to 10 minutes for an hour. As the tickle subsides, decrease the frequency gradually. For prevention and to sweeten the breath, some people do this every morning.

- If you suspect a viral infection and you feel the bronchial tubes are restricted and inhibit normal breathing, use Eucalyptus radiata or one of the other recommended oils to open airways and relax your lungs. Apply these oils either diluted (50:50) with a carrier oil or undiluted on appropriate reflex points to maximize their effectiveness:

- Below the outer area of the collarbone, just inside the groove between the deltoid (shoulder) and pectoralis major (breast) muscles.

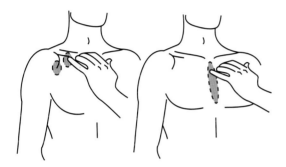

- On the upper part of the breast bone (sternum)

- On the wrist where you take your pulse

- On the balls of your feet

- On each side of the nose (use only a trace). Never put an oil on the mucosal lining inside your nose.

- On the bone behind and under your ear and down to your collar bone.

- These key respiratory points are connected either anatomically or neurologically with your respiratory system +++++P.

- In the early stages of bronchitis, when coughing is often dry and painful, use steam inhalations with Eucalyptus radiata, lavender, balsam fir, frankincense or a respiratory blend. Put 3 – 5 drops of one of the recommended essential oils in a bowl or pan of boiling water. Put a towel over your head and inhale the steam vapors. Reheat and add more oil as needed.

- Take an aromatic bath using 15 drops of one of the recommended oils in a cup of Epsom Salts.

- To strengthen the body's immune system function so you don't get bronchial infections as easily, it may be helpful to do an immune strengthening and balancing cleanse for several months following recovery.

- Create a blend of cinnamon (25%) and carrier oil (75%) or your Protecting blend (50%) and carrier oil (50%). Fill capsules and take one with each meal +++++P. If your bronchitis is asthmatic in nature, a capsule containing rosemary (50:50) with a carrier oil may work better +++P.

- For viral bronchial conditions in young children from 1 to 4 years old, slowly diffuse 20 drops of Eucalyptus radiata two or three times a day for two or three days. You can also dilute the E. radiata 25:75 with a carrier oil and apply the blend to the child's chest several times a day. Massage the feet with the blend as well, focusing on the toes and balls of the feet +++P.

- To rapidly get a lot of essential oil molecules into your system, try Dr. Penoel's "Live Embalming" therapy found in Chapter 4. Use 5 to 10 drops at a time for a total of 20 or 30 drops of Eucalyptus radiata or ravintsara with a hair dryer to get a large amount of essential oils to penetrate the body in a short amount of time. Be sure to change locations on the body with each application. Be sure to read the instructions in Chapter 4 before trying this therapy.

Diffusing helped my husband's bronchitis

My husband used to get two or three cases of chronic bronchitis every winter without fail. He'd be coughing hard for up to three months at a time. He tried every remedy there was. Then we learned about diffusing essential oils. For the last 4 years since he's been using essential oils daily, he's only had one case of bronchitis, and essential oils helped clear that up within a week instead of months.

When he had the one case of bronchitis, he also started taking oils in capsules and aromatic baths with essential oils. But what seemed to work best was using a diffuser. He would actually sit right next to the diffuser for ten to 15 minutes every morning and evening before bed. He didn't have to miss one day of work during the week he had bronchitis, and his coughing was minimal. He was able to keep from coughing at night by using a cold, damp washcloth that had been dipped in a solution of a few drops of peppermint and water. He put it on his neck to decrease the swelling in his bronchial tubes and allow him to go to sleep. It worked wonders.

Bruises, Bumps, Smashed Fingers, & Hematomas

WHAT THEY ARE

Traumas that do not always break the skin, but can cause internal damage, broken capillaries, and leakage of blood and lymph under the skin requiring your body to clean up the injury. A hematoma is a solid swelling of clotted blood inside the body that slowly disperses.

RECOMMENDED OILS

Peppermint   Helichrysum

RECOMMENDED BLENDS

Soothing blend   Protecting blend

Inflammation blend

INSTRUCTION

- When the body has to clean up an injury on its own from a bruise or smashed finger, there is significant collateral damage that most people don't know about. Cleaning up injuries puts an enormous strain on the immune system and produces chemicals that promote premature aging and contributes to other long-term health problems. With essential oils used quickly, these conditions can be greatly minimized. Carry several of these recommended oils with you so you can spring into action when an accident occurs.

- For helping a bruise to quickly heal, use 5 drops of helichrysum undiluted directly on the bruise.

- Apply a drop of either peppermint or a Soothing blend undiluted to your little finger and gently tap around the injured area to quickly relieve pain and prevent the inflammation cycle from beginning, adding even greater and unnecessary pain.

- Keep on hand the following blend: helichrysum (25%), lavender (25%), balsam fir (20%), lemon (15%), and marjoram (15%). Use a few drops of this blend undiluted on small bruises for a deep and synergistic healing. Mix it 50:50 with a carrier oil for larger bruised areas of the body.

- Mix 5 drops of the Comforting blend in a teaspoon of carrier oil on the injured area and massage the surrounding muscles with 5 drops of the Massage blend in a teaspoon of carrier oil.

- If the area is quite large, mix 1/4 cup of water with 4 to 5 drops of peppermint or the Soothing blend, soak a gauze or small flannel piece and apply to the area. Cover it with cling film and apply a cold pack or ice pack as needed.

- Dr. Pénoël recommends applying helichrysum on a hematoma four to six times a day for three or four days +++++P.

CLINICAL SUPPORT

- The effectiveness of tea tree essential oil on injuries and infections seems to be due in part to its ability to activate human white blood cells (Budhiraja SS, et al., 1999).

Bunions

WHAT IT IS

A painful swelling of the joint of the big toe

RECOMMENDED OIL

Peppermint

RECOMMENDED BLENDS

Soothing blend	Foot massage blend
Inflammation blend	

INSTRUCTION

- For pain relief, after soaking your feet after a bath or shower, apply 4 to 5 drops of peppermint or two drops of the Soothing blend mixed with 2 drops of the inflammation blend undiluted on the joint of the toe.

- Do a daily foot massage with 2 - 3 drops of the foot massage blend and 2 - 3 drops of the inflammation mixed in a teaspoon of carrier oil.

Burns and Sunburns

WHAT THEY ARE

A burn can be caused by heat, chemicals, or radiation. Burns come in 3 degrees. First-degree burns are painful, hot, and red, but do not blister. Second-degree burns will blister and swell. Third-degree burns involve seriously damaged skin and a possibly charred surface. Second- and third-degree burns require help from a trained health care professional. All three types, however, can be helped with the use of essential oils.

RECOMMENDED OILS

Lavender		Helichrysum	
German chamomile		Roman chamomile	
Tea tree		Peppermint	

RECOMMENDED BLENDS

Inflammation blend		Soothing blend	
Foot massage blend			

INSTRUCTION

Procedures suggested as part of an overall plan involving your health care professional as needed:

- Where possible, run cold tap water over the first-degree burn for about 10 minutes.

- Use a drop or two of lavender, undiluted, on a small first- or second-degree burn or on a first- or second-degree sunburn. It will decrease the pain quickly and speed healing +++++P. Dr. Pénoël also recommends 3 drops of lavender in 30 drops of a rose hip carrier oil for longer-term healing action +++++P.

- For a second- or third-degree burn, follow the direction of a health care professional, but we suggest using lavender in a sterile water solution sprayed frequently on a healing burn. It cools the burn, helps relieve pain, and speeds up the healing process. Mix 4 to 5 drops of lavender in 1/2 cup of sterile water. You may also wish to add a trace or a drop of peppermint for cooling. Shake and spray frequently.

- You can also soak a sterile gauze in this same solution and place on a first-degree burn. If you cover it for protection, keep it cool by spraying it with cold water or the above lavender/water solution. Apply cold cloths or ice packs as needed.

- For first-degree sunburn, create a blend of 4 to 5 drops of lavender, 1 drop of peppermint, 1 drop of tea tree, and 1 drop helichrysum in a cup of water. Shake and spray on sunburn every 15 or 20 minutes for the first 3 or 4 hours, and then whenever the pain comes back and it starts feeling hot. Then spray it on daily following your shower for 2 or 3 days. You can use a similar solution as a safe deodorant to stop odors before they start by eliminating odor-causing bacteria.

Burn goes away immediately

I have had a lot of experience with routine kitchen burns. I immediately run them under cold water. I usually get blisters and they hurt for days.

Well, the other day I got a serious burn on both hands. I had recently learned that a clinical-grade lavender oil would help. I knew this burn could mean blistering and pain for many days, and I didn't have time to be laid up like that. So after running my hands under cold water for 10 minutes, I tried the lavender oil. To my amazement the pain ceased, the blistering I expected never happened, and I was able to use my hands like normal for the rest of the day.

Cancers & Essential Oils

WHAT IT IS

Cancer is the out-of-control growth of abnormal cells also called malignant cells. There are many types of cancer, each with its own special treatment and therapy. It is not the primary role of essential oils to kill cancer cells. However, essential oils will definitely support the psyche and significantly strengthen the immune system in the best possible way while other therapies tackle the cancer. Essential oils offer unequalled benefits for palliative care of those who are going through radiation, chemotherapy, and recovery from surgery.

RECOMMENDED OILS

Frankincense		Lemon	
Orange		Spruce	
Lavender		Ylang ylang	
Bergam		Neroli	

RECOMMENDED BLENDS

Immune balancing blend		Comforting blend	
Protecting blend		Respiratory blend	
Intimacy blend		Massage blend	
Liver blend			

INSTRUCTION

- Under the direction, and with the involvement of a qualified health care professional, the following therapies will prove valuable.

- You can significantly prevent cancer from taking hold by living a harmonious life, feeding your cells correctly with the right nutrition, and using essential oils quickly in case of injury or infection. Curing cancer, however, is a complex matter that needs to involve competent health care professionals and up-to-date medical procedures. The following will support those interventions.

- Massage the reflex areas of the feet daily with one of the recommended blends.

- Do an Immune Strengthening and Balancing Cleanse.

- Diffuse 20 drops of one of the recommended essential oils or blends to calm you and get more immune-building, aromatic molecules in your body.

- As part of this cleanse with a focus on cancer, create a mixture of the following oils: 20% immunity blend, 15% frankincense, 10% Protecting blend, 5% liver blend, 5% respiratory blend, with 50% carrier oil. Fill capsules with a dropper. Take one capsule 3 to 5 times a day with food.

- Mix 3 to 4 drops of the blend that corresponds to the specific organ or system (for example, a respiratory blend for lung cancer, a digestion blend for colon cancer, etc.) with 3 to 4 drops of frankincense and 3 to 4 drops of the immune balancing blend and apply over the area at least 3 times a day. If in doubt about the blend to use, choose the Protecting blend.

- Massage your feet each morning after your shower with 3 to 4 drops of the Massage blend or 3 to 4 drops of the foot massage blend. Add 2 to 3 drops of frankincense if you choose.

- Massage your feet each evening with 3 to 4 drops of a Comforting blend or the Intimacy blend and 3 to 4 drops of the Foot Massage blend. Add 2 to 3 drops of frankincense if you wish.

Candidiasis

WHAT IT IS

A fungal yeast infection, usually Candida albicans, that most commonly affects only one part of the body but can be serious if it spreads around the body. It is a common reason for vaginal infections in women and may cause mouth infections in people with low immunity or in people taking certain antibiotics. All normal people carry the infection, but it only becomes a problem in a fraction of the population. A strong and balanced immune system is your strongest defense against candidiasis.

RECOMMENDED OILS

Tea tree		Lavender	
Lemongrass		Clove	
Eucalyptus radiata		Oregano	

RECOMMENDED BLENDS

Protecting blend		Respiratory blend	
Stress control blend		Massage blend	

INSTRUCTION

- This condition requires long-term, deep cleansing and may involve consultation with your health care professional.

- Begin with a thorough Immune Strengthening Cleanse combined with parts of the Digestive Cleanse outlined below in the "Cleansing" section. Focus especially on using tea tree and a Protecting blend. A drop or two of the Immune balancing blend daily in water or in an herbal tea will also improve your resistance.

- If candidiasis effects your respiratory system, use a drop of the respiratory blend daily in your drinking water (1 drop per quart), or in your herbal tea (1 drop per cup).

- To calm stress, use the Comforting blend or the Stress control blend in body and foot massages. Mix 4 - 5 drops of the blend you prefer in a teaspoon of a carrier oil.

- If you have a vaginal yeast infection or vaginal candida, create a blend of tea tree (40%), oregano (10%), and a carrier oil (50%). Fill capsules with a dropper and take a capsule three times a day for 30 days. You can use this blend on a tampon as well, but be sure to dilute it more if it feels too hot and change it twice a day ++++P.

- To work out energy blockages throughout your body that inhibit healing, use 3 to 4 drops of the Foot Massage blend in a teaspoon of carrier oil for foot massages. Massage your feet daily if possible, but at least weekly.

- Fungal infections feed on unhealthy foods. So pay special attention to the dietary guidelines. It is fruitless to try a cleanse without making the important dietary and other lifestyle changes including exercise and drinking at least 1/2 gallon of water every day.

Canker Sores

WHAT THEY ARE

Painful sores on the inside of the mouth, usually with a light grayish round area ringed by a reddish area. While their cause is unknown, they may be aggravated by stress, hormones, allergies, or injuries to the tissues of the mouth. They are not infectious. Canker sores are sometimes confused with cold sores caused by the Herpes simplex virus. Cold sores are infectious (see separate instructions for cold sores).

RECOMMENDED OILS

Tea tree		Helichrysum	
Lemon		Clove	

RECOMMENDED BLENDS

Digestion blend		Liver blend	
Protecting blend		Immune balancing blend	

INSTRUCTION

- A **digestive or liver cleanse** will help clear up chronic canker sores.

- **Lick a trace of tea tree or the Protecting blend off the back of your hand** several times a day and distribute it around your mouth to help heal and prevent canker sores. You can also use a toothpick to get a trace. This will also help with bad breath.

- Use **undiluted tea tree or helichrysum** directly on the canker sore to clear it up quickly.

Chappped & Cracked Skin

WHAT IT IS

A common problem, especially during cold, dry weather. It can be aggravated by not having enough natural protection in your skin.

RECOMMENDED OILS

Frankincense		Patchouli	
Sandalwood			

RECOMMENDED BLENDS

Foot massage blend	

INSTRUCTION

- Put a drop or two of the recommended oils in each application of hand lotion, or add 20 drops to an 8 ounce bottle of un-fragranced lotion. Apply lotion while hands are moist after washing them or after your shower or bath.

- **Beware of lotion overuse.** Becoming too lotion-dependent can actually contribute to dryness because even though it moisturizes your skin, it has ingredients that also can dry your skin. You want your skin to do its job naturally as much as possible. Instead of using lotion, simply mix a few drops of one of the oils with jojoba and use it instead of a lotion. It won't absorb as quickly as a lotion, but it will balance and normalize your skin better and allow it to heal.

- Wear protective gloves and mittens in the wintertime.

Chest Pain

(angina pectoris, associated with the heart)

WHAT IT IS

A condition caused by insufficient blood supply to the heart with symptoms of severe chest pain often spreading to the shoulders, arms, and neck.

RECOMMENDED SINGLES

Lavender		Lemon	
Roman chamomile		German chamomile	
Neroli		Marjoram	

RECOMMENDED BLEND

Comforting blend

INSTRUCTION

- Act quickly to get professional medical attention.

- While you are waiting, you may have time to incorporate some of the recommended oils in a diluted massage (3 to 4 drops per teaspoon of carrier oil). They can also be applied undiluted or blended with a foot massage blend for calming foot or hand reflexology massage.

- Use the "M" technique for calming.

- Ingest 2 to 3 drops of lemon in each quart of water. You can also use a toothpick to stir a trace of lemon into a glass of water, a cup of hot water, or an herbal tea.

CLINICAL SUPPORT

"While aromatherapy cannot replace a damaged valve or repair an atrial septal defect, it can be useful for reducing the stress that surrounds a heart attack and may reduce the period of recovery following a heart attack or surgery. Aromatherapy is used in some medical and surgical cardiac units, and many of the essential oils have a history of being supportive to the heart, as well as being generally relaxing" (Buckle, p. 247).

Chickenpox

(See Infant & Child Care)

Chilblains

WHAT THEY ARE

A painful, itching skin swelling, typically on hands or feet, caused by poor circulation in the skin when exposed to cold.

RECOMMENDED OILS

Roman chamomile		German chamomile	
Lemon		Marjoram	
Black pepper		Patchouli	

RECOMMENDED BLENDS

Foot massage blend

INSTRUCTION

- To decrease the pain, apply a drop of one of the oils directly to hands or feet. Dilute if using a hot, sensitizing oil like black pepper.

- Put a drop or two of the recommended oils in each application of hand lotion, or add 20 drops to an 8 ounce bottle of un-fragranced lotion. Apply lotion while hands are moist after washing them or after your shower or bath.

- **Beware of lotion overuse.** Becoming too lotion-dependent can actually contribute to dryness because even though it moisturizes your skin, it has ingredients that also can dry your skin. You want your skin to do its job naturally as much as possible. Instead of using lotion, simply mix a few drops of one of the oils with jojoba and use it instead of a lotion. It won't absorb as quickly as a lotion, but it will balance and normalize your skin better and allow it to heal.

- Wear protective gloves and mittens in the wintertime.

Cholera

WHAT IT IS

A serious intestinal infection that causes vomiting and large amounts of watery diarrhea.

RECOMMENDED OILS

Tea tree   Sweet basil

RECOMMENDED BLENDS

Protecting blend   Digestion blend

INSTRUCTION

- Use the following in-home procedures with the involvement of your health care professional:

- The most effective oils are tea tree, the Protecting blend and sweet basil. They can be used singly or in a blend of equal parts.

- Take up to 16 drops of any of the recommended oils daily. This can conveniently be done by taking 3 capsules a day with food.

Blend an essential oil 50:50 with a carrier oil and fill capsules with a dropper.

- Take 1 or 2 drops of any of the recommended oils, a quart of water, in an herbal tea with honey, a clear juice, or in mild recipes (after taking the recipe off the heat).

- Small children will do better taking the oils in water, juice, or food.

- You can also rub the feet of children and even babies with 1 or 2 drops of the three recommended oils diluted in a teaspoon of carrier oil. Do this several times a day.

- To rapidly get a lot of essential oil molecules into your system, try Dr. Penoel's "Live Embalming" therapy found in Chapter 4. Use 5 to 10 drops at a time for a total of 20 or 30 drops of Eucalyptus radiata or ravintsara with a hair dryer to get a large amount of essential oils to penetrate the body in a short amount of time. Be sure to change locations on the body with each application. Be sure to read the instructions in Chapter 4 before trying this therapy.

Chronic Fatique Syndrome

WHAT IT IS

A medical condition whose cause is unknown. It is characterized by aching, and prolonged exhaustion and depression. It can also involve insomnia, which contributes to the lack of energy. It typically shows up after a viral infection.

RECOMMENDED OILS

Oil		Oil	
Peppermint	🔵🔵🔵	Spearmint	🔵🔵🔵
Rosemary	🔵🔵🔵	Sage	🔵🔵🔵
Sweet basil	🔵🔵🔵	Helichrysum	🔵🔵
Ginger	🔵🔵🔵	Vetiver	🔵🔵
Thyme	🔵🔵🔵	Pine	🔵🔵
Spruce	🔵🔵	Sandalwood	🔵🔵
Frankincense	🔵🔵🔵	Lemongrass	🔵🔵
German chamomile	🔵🔵		

RECOMMENDED BLENDS

Blend		Blend	
Soothing blend	🔵	Massage blend	🔵
Protecting blend	🔵🔵🔵	Immune balancing blend	🔵🔵
Liver blend	🔵🔵	Inflammation blend	🔵🔵🔵

INSTRUCTION

In-home procedures suggested as part of an overall plan with the approval of or under the direction of your health care professional:

- If you have allergies, use oils on feet only.

- For pain apply the soothing inflammation blend and the Soothing blend neat on the feet, hands, or ears to the areas corresponding to the painful areas.

- Also gently massage the affected area with 2 to 3 drops each of the pain and inflammation blends in a teaspoon of carrier oil.

- For an energizing foot massage, apply 1 to 2 drops of the simulating massage blend with 1 to 2 drops of the foot massage blend. Add a little carrier oil if you wish.

- Apply 2 to 3 drops of the Protecting blend, Eucalyptus radiata, tea tree, the Massage blend,

or a combination of any of these in a teaspoon of carrier oil. By doing a regular, invigorating preliminary massage before exercise each day, you will be able to energize yourself and extend your exercise time each day.

- In the 6th bullet: "Create vegetable capsules by mixing a Protecting blend (20%), spearmint (20%), tea tree (10%), and a carrier oil (50%), and filling capsules with a dropper. Take a capsule 3 times a day with food."

- Dr. Pénoël recommends creating capsules containing 40% peppermint, 10% thyme, and 50% carrier oil. Take a capsule 3 times a day with food for 30 days ++++P.

- He also recommends a massage blend of 25% pine, 25% spruce, and 50% carrier oil applied on your back over where your adrenal glands are located. Do this for 3 to 7 days ++++P.

- Use a drop of the Protecting blend, the Exercise blend, Spearmint, or tea tree with honey in an herbal tea once or twice a day.

- See the Immune Strengthening and Balancing Cleanse for more information.

Cleansing with Essential oils

Why do a cleanse?

Cleansing takes away the stress of toxic build-up in the body from pesticides, heavy metals, pollution, excessive hormones, free radicals, and harmful byproducts of undigested food that has fermented inside our bodies because of poor metabolism and irregular elimination. These toxins are associated to many diseases. Periodic cleansing is especially important so that our organs can begin to more completely convert the whole food we eat into energy. Cleansing helps the body more efficiently process the complex constituents from our food and send them to our brain and other organs, allowing us to heal more thoroughly both emotionally and physically.

General advice for cleansing:

- Make the basic dietary and exercise changes first. To start using essential oils or other products such as consuming more fiber in an attempt to cleanse our system without making the necessary dietary, water, exercise, and relationship adjustments, makes no sense. Don't misunderstand. It doesn't mean that it makes no sense to start unless you can "do it all." We have to start somewhere. But sooner or later you need to incorporate all elements to reach a complete cleansing. Why not start now with the simple dietary and exercise guidelines found in this book.

- Use any of the following cleanses depending on what you feel your body needs. Each of them has common elements with the others.

The Liver Cleanse

WHAT IT IS

Use this cleanse to remove internal toxins for the following reasons:

- For skin conditions like psoriasis, eczema, or acne

- For allergic conditions like asthma and hay fever

- For all autoimmune conditions

- It will help prevent possible complications of a viral hepatitis attack

- For headaches and migraines

- To help balance female hormones

- To help mental and physical recovery after an emotional shock

- When other treatments stop working there could be a liver "blockage." Four to six weeks of this cleanse may release the blockage.

RECOMMENDED OILS

Peppermint			Spearmint		
Lemon			Orange		
Roman chamomile			German chamomile		
Rosemary			Cypress		
Thyme			Juniper		

RECOMMENDED BLENDS

Liver blend			Protecting blend		
Digestion blend					

INSTRUCTION

How long?

It depends on how severe your condition is. You may need a year or more. Dr. Pénoël suggests that for every year you have noticed symptoms of a weak or congested liver or inefficient cleansing or metabolism, you may need one month of cleansing. Because it takes time for a deep healing to take place, make sure the habits of this cleanse blend easily into your lifestyle.

Medically-oriented liver cleanse

In a medically-oriented cleanse, you'll want to consume enough essential oils each day. It's most convenient to use the liver blend (50:50) with your choice of carrier oil and fill capsules. Or you can create this blend: liver blend (30%), digestion blend (10%), Protecting blend (10%), and carrier oil (50%). Fill capsules with a dropper and take one 3 times a day with food.

Then choose from among these options:

Ingestion

- Your goal would be to ingest a total of three to nine drops of the liver blend daily.

- Dip a toothpick in the liver blend and stir a trace into your drinking water or into an herbal tea. You may want to add a trace of peppermint, spearmint, lemon, or orange to improve the flavor.

- Stir a drop into a teaspoon of honey and eat it slowly.

- Prepare a **liver-cleansing drink with a** drop of the liver blend (maybe two if you want a more powerful action) in a teaspoon of honey, mix well, add a cup of water and stir for fifteen seconds. Add peppermint, spearmint, lemon or orange to improve the flavor if you wish. Enjoy this aromatic drink in the morning for cleansing or at the end of a meal with warm water, like an herbal tea.

- If you feel sluggish or exhausted from eating heavy, fatty foods, a cup of this drink will help.

- Prepare a sesame spread by mixing a teaspoon of tahini (a sesame paste like peanut butter but much better for you) with a drop of the liver blend. Add a little honey to sweeten it. Use it in moderation.

- Be sure to make healthy changes to your diet by eating more whole fruits and vegetables, preferably raw. Eat more (non-bread) whole grains in hot cereals, salads, soups, etc. You need these foods to build back the complex

minerals and nutrients you need for a complete cleansing.

Aromatic breathing and topical absorption

- Massage a few drops of the undiluted liver blend on the bottom (upper arch area) of your right foot.

- Mix a drop of the liver blend in a teaspoon of carrier oil and massage your chest over the liver area (the lower left part of your rib cage).

- To release energy blockages, apply an undiluted drop on your back in the area where your kidneys are located. The precise spot is "the control point of the liver—one inch on each side of the space between the 9th and the 10th thoracic vertebra as well as on the control point of the gall bladder just one vertebra below—the 11th thoracic vertebra" (Guide p. 50). Don't worry about pinpointing the exact location. Just reach around and apply the oil to the back in the lower rib area on each side.

- On the inside of your legs, apply the liver blend to the spot shown in this diagram. In acupuncture it's the 5th point on the liver meridian.

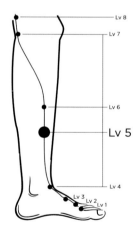

- On each ankle apply the liver blend just in front of the malleolus or ankle bone on the outside of the food (see diagram). This is the 40th point of the gall bladder meridian, "one finger width under and in front of the lateral malleolus" (Guide, p. 50).

This point is useful to know because it is used for alleviating all kinds of pains.

The Digestive Cleanse

WHAT IT IS

A process for cleansing the digestive system so it becomes more efficient and helps the whole body become healthier.

Why do a digestive cleanse?

• Digestion is the source of your energy and well-being

• It reduces the fermentation and putrefaction that can generate gas.

• It helps control and balance intestinal flora and prevent the overgrowth of pathogens and their toxins.

RECOMMENDED OILS

Peppermint	🎮🌀📋	Spearmint	🎮🌀📋
Sweet basil	🎮🌀📋	Ginger	🌀📋
Marjoram	🌀📋	Lemon	🎮🌀📋
Orange	🎮🌀📋	Rosemary	🌀📋
Roman chamomile	🌀📋	German chamomile	🌀📋
Thyme	🌀📋		

RECOMMENDED BLENDS

Digestion blend	🎮🌀📋	Liver blend	🌀📋
Protecting blend	🌀📋	Foot massage blend	🌀

INSTRUCTION

How long should the cleanse go on? Depending on the current condition of your digestion, it may last a year or more. Dr. Pénoël suggests that for every year you have had digestive problems, you may need one month of cleansing. Because it takes time for a deep healing and cleansing to take place, make sure the habits you learn here will easily fit into your lifestyle.

Dr. Pénoël's digestive cleanse

If you want the kind of medically-oriented digestive cleanse Dr. Pénoël recommends to his patients, you will want to consume enough essential oils every day. It is most convenient to make up capsules using the digestion blend. Here is the recipe: digestion blend (30%), liver blend (10%), Protecting blend (10%), and carrier oil (50%). Fill capsules with a dropper and take one 3 times a day with food.

Ingestion

• Prepare a drink that will enhance digestion. Take it before every meal. Mix one drop of the digestion blend (possibly two if you would like it stronger) in a teaspoon of honey, mix well, add a cup of water and mix for fifteen seconds.

• Drink a cup in the morning as a cleansing beverage or at the end of a meal in a cup of hot water, as an herbal tea.

• If you feel a bit heavy in the afternoon because of sluggish digestion, have another cup to pep you up.

• In a restaurant, flavor your drinking water by dipping a toothpick in your digestion blend and then stir your toothpick into a glass of water or a cup of herbal tea. Adjust the flavor by dipping more or less of the toothpick into the oil.

• Mix up a sesame spread using a teaspoon of tahini (a sesame paste similar to peanut butter but better for you) with a drop of the digestion blend. Add honey if you wish. Use it in moderation.

- To improve regularity, you may want to add a little extra safe food fiber or clay drinks to your diet. You can flavor these drinks with your digestive blend, the liver blend, and/or an Protecting blend.

- Make sure your diet has plenty of whole fruits and vegetables, preferably raw. Eat many (non-bread) whole grains in soups, cereals, salads etc. You need whole foods to build back the minerals and nutrients necessary for cleansing your digestion.

Breathing and topical absorption

- Inhale the aroma of the digestion blend from the bottle before a meal to boost your appetite and prepare your digestive glands to digest your food better.

- Mix 2 to 3 drops of the digestion blend in a teaspoon of carrier oil for a general abdominal massage as well as a foot, hand, or ear massage. Use only one drop for children.

- Use clockwise massage in the same direction that food passes through your large intestine. Start just below the navel using slow, spiral movement out to the rib cage and pelvis area. Start gently and increase the pressure slightly the farther out you go.

- Then massage from the outside in. Make it a more aggressive, active massage, starting at the ribs and pelvis and spiraling clockwise into the center. The pressure can be lower but the movement quicker.

- Also massage the back following the same circular bowel pathway but counter-clockwise to follow the normal direction of food through the colon.

- Use the undiluted digestion blend on the upper ear, both in front and behind the ear. The reflex area for the lower bowels is on the upper part of the ear. (show diagram Guide p. 53) The muscular part of the bowels is on the back of the ear. Apply a drop of the undiluted digestion blend to each index finger and thumb. Massage the area where the ear meets the head on the upper part of each ear both in front and back. Don't be too concerned with exact points. Just remember that the diagram the body on the ear is similar to a fetus in a mother's womb (head down and buttocks up). Massage the ear for one or two minutes.

- Massage the digestive area on the feet by blending 2 to 3 drops of the undiluted digestion blend with 2 to 3 drops of the foot massage blend. Massage clockwise. You can then add a little carrier oil for a more general foot massage.

- Massage your back by applying an undiluted trace on each thumb and massaging downward on each side of the spine starting at the lowest lumbar vertebra, an inch on each side of the spine. This creates a strong reflexology action on the small and large intestines. The reflex area that controls the elimination of feces is in the area where the hipbone joins the backbone (the sacral area). Massage downward, starting from where you can feel the hipbone on your back. Massage downward along the sides of the tail bone. It is important to do back massage to help the movement of the feces, especially to help food navigate the angles of the colon. You can do this with abdominal massage, but it is even more effective using back massage.

- Do this massage two to three times a week or more, on yourself or with a partner.

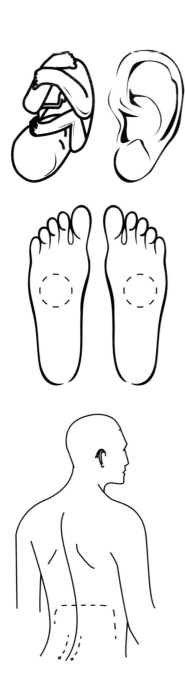

Immune Strengthening Cleanse

WHAT IT IS

A cleanse to stimulate, strengthen, and rebalance your immune system

Why you may need an immune-strengthening cleanse

• If you have any type of autoimmune condition: allergies, asthma, hay fever, Crohn's disease, multiple sclerosis, rheumatoid arthritis, etc.; you need to balance your immune functions. Dr. Pénoël suggests that this process should take you one month for each year you have had your autoimmune issues.

• If you have had a history of using antibiotics that may have destroyed the delicate balance of intestinal flora in your digestive system.

• If you have significant stresses in your life that have resulted in excessive adrenaline and digestive acid in your body, your immune system will have suffered significantly.

• If you have any chronic respiratory, digestive, skin, or other infectious diseases; your immune system may need this cleanse.

RECOMMENDED OILS

Sweet basil		Tea tree	
Sage		Myrtle	
Pine		Orange	
Peppermint		Spearmint	
Rosemary		Thyme	

RECOMMENDED BLENDS

Immune balancing blend		Liver blend	
Protecting blend		Foot massage blend	

INSTRUCTION

How long will you need to be on this cleanse?

- Depending on the condition of your immune system, it may take a year or more. Dr. Pénoël tells his patients that for every year they have had a weakened immune system, they will need a month of cleansing. Because it takes time to perform a deep cleanse, make sure that you master the habits to easily blend into your lifestyle.

- Using the immune balance blend regularly may help all your autoimmune conditions. In many cases, there is also a deeply rooted and often hidden infectious condition that also requires using the Protecting blend over an extended period.

Ingestion

- Prepare a drink to strengthen your immune system. Mix a drop of the Protecting blend with a drop of the immune balancing blend in a teaspoon of honey. Mix well and add a cup of water. Stir for 10 to 15 seconds.

- Enjoy this drink each morning before breakfast or at the end of a meal with hot water, as an herbal tea.

- In a restaurant, flavor your drinking water by dipping a toothpick in the Protecting blend or the immune balancing blend and then stirring it in a glass of water or an herbal tea. Fine-tune the flavor by dipping more or less of the toothpick into the blend.

- Enjoy more whole fruits and vegetables in your diet, preferably raw. Eat more (non-bread) whole grains in cereals, soups, salads etc. You need to build back the minerals and nutrients to complete the cleanse.

- If you have difficulty taking enough of these blends with your food or water, prepare a blend using the immune balancing blend (25%), the Protecting blend (25%), and a carrier oil (50%). Fill capsules with this blend and take a capsule with each meal every day.

- Use the "lick trick" by spreading a trace of tea tree on the back of your hand and licking it off. Distribute it around your mouth as a breath freshener each morning, noon, and evening or whenever you brush your teeth or need fresher breath.

Olfactory and dermal absorption

- Apply Eucalyptus radiata on your chest and back each morning after your bath or shower. Notice the areas on your back and chest that are reflex points where you'll want to concentrate your attention. (Put in illustrations from the Guide, p. 55)

- Each morning while your body is damp coming out of the bath or shower, apply 2 to 3 drops each of tea tree and Eucalyptus radiata to your palms and massage your body where you have the greatest concentration of lymph nodes—sides of neck, under arms, and groin area above genitals. You can add a little carrier oil if you wish. Avoid applying essential oils to your genitals.

- Perform a complete foot massage on yourself or with a partner two or three times a week or more. Use a teaspoon of a carrier oil with 2 to 3 drops of the Protecting blend and 2 to 3 drops of the Foot Massage blend. You can also add tea tree and Eucalyptus radiata if you wish.

- Once a day apply 2 to 3 drops of the Protecting blend or the Immune Balancing blend undiluted over your kidneys on your back. They are located just behind your lowest ribs. The adrenal glands rest on top of the kidneys. Massage this whole area.

Mind & Body Cleanse

WHAT IT IS

- A calming series of procedures using essential oils that may help you release emotional blocks and traumas, and allow you to heal both your mind and your body.

- Many medical professionals are coming to recognize the important relationship between emotional trauma and health. Essential oils offer safe ways to help heal psychological trauma. If you have serious emotional disorders, consult a competent professional. If you are using psychoactive medications, never lower them or stop taking them without consulting with the health care professional who prescribed them. Psychological problems need complete and holistic care over a period of many months.

Why you may need a mind & body cleanse

- If you have any of these emotional or brain disorders: depression, ADHD or ADD, anxiety, obsessive-compulsive disorder, manic-depressive (bi-polar) disorder, etc.; this cleanse may alleviate some symptoms. For serious conditions such as these, however, be sure to work with your health care professional and never adjust medications you are currently taking except under his or her direction.

- If you are not making progress in recovery, try this cleanse to help relax and release hidden emotional blocks.

- If you or someone you love feels you have emotional blockages that may be affecting your health or relationships.

- If you have patterns of anger, resentment, criticism, grief, despair, etc. that you can't shake, this cleanse may help you. If these issues are effecting your employment or important relationships in a major way, be sure to consult a healthcare professional.

RECOMMENDED OILS

Frankincense		Bergamot	
Lavender		Orange	
Neroli		Ylang ylang	
Sandalwood		Valerian	
Vetiver			

RECOMMENDED BLENDS

Mental focus blend		Comforting blend	
Focusing blend		Intimacy blend	
Balancing blend		Foot massage blend	

INSTRUCTION

How long will the cleanse take?

Depending on your condition, it may take a year or more. Dr. Pénoël cautions that for every year you have had this issue, you may need one month of cleansing. It takes time to heal emotional issues. Be sure to master the habits of this cleanse so they blend into your lifestyle. You may find such relief from some of them that you will want to continue using them throughout your life.

Ingestion

- It may be helpful to incorporate elements of the Liver Cleanse or the Digestion Cleanse into this cleanse because they interact.

- As you blend oils for your capsules for a liver or digestion cleanse, you may want to a drop or two of frankincense or another of the recommended calming oils added to your capsules. Simply reduce one of the other essential oils by about 5% to 10% and substitute frankincense.

- If you are not taking frankincense in your capsules, take a drop of frankincense daily under your tongue.

Topical and breathing absorption

- Begin your day by giving yourself a massage using the Massage blend to energize your muscles and your spirits. Massage your joints and muscles each morning with a blend of 4 to 5 drops of the massage blend in a teaspoon of carrier oil.

- You can also massage 3 or 4 drops of these oils undiluted on your feet in the morning after your bath or shower. Focus on your toes, especially "psi" point Dr. Pénoël talks about at the base of the big toe.

- Diffuse 5 to 10 drops of the mental focus blend each morning for about 5 minutes.

- Use the Intimacy blend in the afternoon or evening to help ease the stresses of the day. On the back of your ears, neck, and temples, apply 2 to 3 drops undiluted.

- Diffuse 5 to 10 drops of the Focusing blend, the Intimacy blend, or the Mental Focus blend, for about 5 minutes each afternoon. You can use it in the workplace to celebrate achievements. Use it in times of emotional joy to reinforce positive feelings. Then when low emotions show up, diffusing the blend will bring back feelings of joy and balance. Any blend or single oil that you come to associate with joy can be used to restore positive feelings as well. Sample a wide variety of oils and select the ones for emotional cleansing that you respond to with joyful, positive emotions.

- Before bed for about 5 minutes, diffuse 5 – 10 drops of the Comforting blend.

- Before bed give yourself a calming foot massage with a few drops of the Comforting blend and 3 to 4 drops of the Foot Massage blend undiluted. Focus on the toes, especially the "psi" point at the inside base of the big toe.

- Apply a drop of the Comforting blend along the rim of your ear and in front of the ear where the ear joins the cheek.

- Once a week before bed, soak your feet or bathe for 20 minutes in a cup of Epsom Salts mixed with 5 to 10 drops of frankincense, balsam fir, the intimacy blend, or the Comforting blend.

- Before bed massage a drop or two of sweet basil just below your breast bone (sternum) on your solar plexus. Take a trace of sweet basil on your tongue as well.

- Have someone give you a back massage using balsam fir. Apply 3 to 4 drops undiluted down the center of the spine and ask them to use their knuckles to massage up the spine and feather upward with their fingernails out onto both sides of your back. Start at the lower back and massage upward to the neck.

- Create a blend of 4 drops of balsam fir in a teaspoon of carrier oil and massage the muscles at both sides of the spine from the neck downward.

CLINICAL SUPPORT

"The aim of the present study is to review the available literature to determine if there is evidence for effectiveness of aromatherapy in surgical patients to treat anxiety and insomnia, to control pain and nausea, and to dress wounds. Efficacy studies of lavender or orange and peppermint essential oils, to treat anxiety and nausea, respectively, have shown positive results. Finally, there are encouraging data for the treatment of infections, especially for tea tree oil..."(Stea S, Beraudi A, De Pasquale D., 2014).

Cold Sores

WHAT ARE THEY

They are herpes simplex viral infections that cause painful blisters on or around the lips. Also called fever blisters. A similar virus causes blisters around the genitals (genital herpes).

RECOMMENDED OILS

Oil		Oil	
Bergamot	⊙	Eucalyptus radiata	⊙
Helichrysum	⊙	Tea tree	⊙
Neroli	⊙◉	Clove	⊙◉
Lemon	⊙◉	Peppermin	⊙◉

RECOMMENDED BLENDS

Blend		Blend	
Protecting blend	⊙◉	Balancing blend	⊙◉

INSTRUCTION

Use the following in-home procedures:

- Apply a drop or trace of the Protecting blend undiluted only on the infected spot. Do not apply this blend around the infection on the skin or it may become inflamed. For best results be sure to act quickly at the first sign of a cold sore to stop the spread of the virus. Apply a very small amount by using a dropper or a toothpick. Repeat this treatment several times throughout the day whenever you notice discomfort ++++P.

- After the infection is controlled, do an immune strengthening cleanse for a few months to complete the healing of the infection.

- You can also apply a trace of helichrysum right on the affected spot. If you catch a herpes infection early enough, this application alone will often take care of the trouble quickly, even before it opens into a full-blown infection.

Colds & Flus

WHAT THEY ARE

Viral infections of the ear, nose, and throat that occur frequently with climate changes and when immune function is compromised. Antibiotics are helpful only in preventing secondary bacterial infections, not colds. A cold typically lasts for 6 days unless there are complications and secondary infections, which come from not taking care of a cold properly. The flu can be more severe and last longer.

RECOMMENDED OILS

Oil		Oil	
Ravintsara	⊙	Eucalyptus radiata	⊙
Helichrysum	⊙	Tea tree	⊙◉
Neroli	⊙	Clove	⊙◉
Lemon	⊙◉	Peppermint	⊛⊙◉

RECOMMENDED BLENDS

Blend		Blend	
Protecting blend	⊛⊙◉	Respiratory blend	⊛⊙
Immune balancing blend	⊛⊙◉		

INSTRUCTION

Use these in-home procedures:

- At the first sign of a cold apply a blend of ravintsara (25%), Eucalyptus radiata (25%), and a carrier oil (50%) to your chest and neck at least twice per hour for four hours +++++P. The faster and more frequently you apply essential oils in the earliest stages of your cold or flu, the more successfully you will be at taking care of it quickly.

- At the first tickle of a sore throat or a fever, swipe a trace of tea tree on the back of your hand and lick it off. Spread the antimicrobial molecules around your mouth, especially at the back of your throat. Do this about every minute for 10 minutes, then every five minutes for two hours. Tea tree is both antibacterial AND antiviral. Acting quickly and aggressively can occasionally stop a cold before it ever gets underway.

- Eucalyptus radiata is antiviral in its action. Apply it on your chest (just above the outer clavicle bone) and behind and under your ears. Use it on all the reflex points shown here. These are points you want to get to know well because daily application to these areas will prevent many respiratory infections.

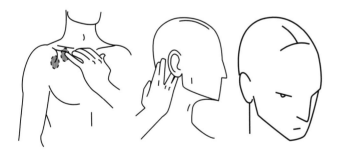

- Apply a drop of Eucalyptus radiata or tea tree on the top of your head on the anterior fontanel. (see above).

- For an effective bedtime treatment (when your cold symptoms are often at their worst), diffuse 20 drops of Eucalyptus radiata or the respiratory blend very slowly. They can be inhaled while you are sleeping.

- To unblock clogged sinuses due to colds or sinusitis, mix a drop of peppermint in a teaspoon of honey. Hold the mixture in the back of your throat until the peppermint vapors start to rise into the sinuses through the back of the throat. This can open clogged airways in a matter of minutes.

- Take a hot aromatic bath using 10 to 15 drops of one of the respiratory oils in a cup of Epsom Salts.

- To rapidly get a lot of essential oil molecules into your system, try Dr. Penoel's "Live Embalming" therapy found in Chapter 4. Use 5 to 10 drops at a time for a total of 20 or 30 drops of Eucalyptus radiata or ravintsara with a hair dryer to get a large amount of essential oils to penetrate the body in a short amount of time. Be sure to change locations on the body with each application. Be sure to read the instructions in Chapter 4 before trying this therapy.

Constipation
(sluggish digestion)

WHAT IT IS

Typically defined as having a bowel movement less than 3 times per week. It is associated with hard stools or difficulty passing stools. It may involve pain while passing stools or the inability to have a bowel movement after straining or pushing for more than 10 minutes. The healthiest elimination is at least once daily with little or no straining.

RECOMMENDED OILS

Marjoram	☯🔵	Orange	☯🔵
Black pepper	☯	Rosemary	☯🔵
Lemon	☯🔵	Sweet basil	☯🔵
Lavender	🔴☯	Balsam fir	🔴☯
Peppermint	☯🔵		

RECOMMENDED BLENDS

Digestion blend	🔴☯🔵	Liver blend	☯🔵
Comforting blend	🔴☯🔵	Massage blend	☯

INSTRUCTION

In-home procedures:

- Increase water intake by adding two to four extra glasses per day. A drop of peppermint, lemon, the exercise, or digestion blend can make water more delightful and also therapeutic. Take a drop of the liver blend in juice or soup daily as well.

- Gradually increase your intake of whole foods containing significant amounts of fiber—raw and dried fruits and vegetables and whole grain cereals and breads. Avoid refined flours, empty prepared cereals, meats (especially processed meats), heavy animal fats, processed sugars, and any overly-processed foods.

- Take calming baths with Epsom Salts mixed with 10 to 15 drops of one of the recommended essential oils.

- Mix 2 to 3 drops of sweet basil in a tablespoo of carrier oil and massage it on your lower back and sacral area below your hip bone on both sides of the spine in a downward motion. (create illustration marking just the sacrum area below the lumbar vertebrae)

- Then give yourself an abdominal massage with the same dilution of sweet basil. Start just below the navel and lightly massage in a clockwise spiral out to the rim of the rib cage and pelvis. Change up this massage by using the Massage blend in the morning and the Comforting blend in the evening. Also try lavender, balsam fir, the Digestion blend, and the Liver blend. It is safest to give these massages 3 hours after a meal or a half hour before a meal.

- Massage the bottoms of your feet (arch area), palms of your hands, and upper part of your ears with an undiluted digestion blend, Comforting blend, liver blend, balsam fir, peppermint, lavender, or sweet basil.

- Use an authoritative medical self-help guide or the advice from a health care professional to check for signs that the constipation is more serious than should be treated with home care alone.

Coronary Artery Disease

(see Atherosclerosis & Coronary Artery Disease)

Cough, Spasmodic

(See Asthma and Bronchitis)

WHAT IT IS

Convulsive coughing sometimes associated with chronic bronchitis, sometimes associated with whooping cough or even emphysema. It involves inflammation of the trachea and bronchial tubes.

RECOMMENDED OILS

Eucalyptus radiata		Cypress	
Thyme		Peppermint	
Spearmint		Tea tree	
Helichrysum		Balsam fir	
Roman chamomile		German chamomile	
Frankincense		Marjoram	
Myrtle		Pine	
Lavender		Rosemary	
Copaiba		Sage	

RECOMMENDED BLENDS

Protecting blend		Inflammation blend	
Immune balancing blend			

INSTRUCTION

- Stay away from tobacco, known allergens, dust, or industrial pollutants.

- Generally, avoid taking cough suppressants since normal coughing (not intense coughing spasms) helps to release the mucous deep in the lungs that comes from bronchial infections.

- Create a blend of cypress (15%), thyme (15%), marjoram (20%), and carrier oil (50%). Apply to both the chest and the back four to six times a day. You can help the oils penetrate better by adding a hot cloth over the application ++++P.

- For a child ages one to four, create a syrup of marjoram (10 drops) in a cup of syrup (agave or another non-honey syrup). Give a teaspoon 4 to 6 times a day ++++P.

- Increase your water intake to at least 1/2 gallon daily and add a trace or a drop of one of the more flavorful oils listed above.

- Use a humidifier to keep the air moist and aid healing. Add a drop of the respiratory blend or Eucalyptus radiata to the humidifier.

- At the first sign of a bronchial "tickle" telling you that coughing spasms are about to start,

  use your finger to put a drop of tea tree on the back of your tongue and let it mix with saliva there for about 2 minutes. Lick a drop or a trace off the back of your hand. We call this the "lick trick." The tea tree mixes with your saliva to create an antibacterial/antiviral "mouthwash." After two minutes, swallow this mixture slowly. The tea tree will continue its antimicrobial action down the esophagus and into the stomach. Do this every 5 to 10 minutes for an hour. As the tickle starts going away, decrease the frequency gradually. For prevention and to sweeten the breath, some people do this every morning.

- If you suspect a viral infection and feel the bronchial tubes are restricting normal breathing, use Eucalyptus radiata or one of the other recommended oils to open airways and relax your lungs. Apply these oils either diluted (50:50) with a carrier oil or undiluted on reflex points of the hands, ears, or feet to maximize their effectiveness. Here are other respiratory reflex areas where you can:

- Below the outer area of the collarbone (clavicle), just inside the groove between the deltoid (shoulder) and pectoralis major (breast) muscles.

- On the upper part of the breast bone (sternum)

- On the wrist where you take your pulse

- On the balls of your feet

- On each side of the nose (use only a trace). Never put an oil on the mucosal lining inside your nose.

- On the bone behind and under your ear, down to your collar bone.

- These key respiratory reflex points are connected with your respiratory system.
- Use steam to inhale healing molecules of Eucalyptus radiata, lavender, balsam fir, frankincense or a respiratory blend. Put 3 – 5 drops of one of the recommended essential oils in a bowl or pan of boiling water. Put a towel over your head and inhale the steam. Reheat and add more oil as needed.

- Take an aromatic bath using up to 15 drops of one of the recommended oils in a cup of Epsom Salts.

Cuts, Scrapes, & Abrasions

WHAT THEY ARE

Breaks in your skin allow infections to enter your body, causing all kinds of possible health issues. Always take care of cuts and injuries quickly using essential oils. Carry small vials or bottles of key first-aid oils in your purse or in a handy pouch on your belt or key chain. By acting quickly you can relieve a great deal of pain and suffering. And this could also help with any internal bleeding, requiring the body to produce a lot of white blood cells. This clean-up effort puts a huge strain on the immune system and produces excessive amounts of chemicals that result in premature aging and other issues that can contribute to degenerative conditions. With essential oils coming to the rescue quickly and thoroughly, these conditions can be greatly minimized. They are more serious than we sometimes think.

RECOMMENDED OILS

Tea tree		Peppermint	
German chamomile		Roman chamomile	
Spearmint		Helichrysum	
Thyme		Lavender	
Sage		Cypress	

RECOMMENDED BLENDS

Protecting blend		Inflammation blend	

INSTRUCTION

In-home procedures:

- After washing a minor cut that doesn't require stitches, use an undiluted drop of tea tree to disinfect it. Apply it again every hour or two for the first 6 hours to minimize any chance of infection.

- If there is excessive bleeding, such as for a cut on the head (but no stitches needed), use a drop of undiluted cypress. At first, bleeding may increase to cleanse the wound, but soon the cypress will help stop the bleeding and start the healing.

- You can put a drop of tea tree and/or helichrysum on the pad of an adhesive bandage. A cloth adhesive bandage will hold up better to essential oil use than a latex bandage.

- You can facilitate healing of stitches by using a drop of undiluted tea tree or the Protecting blend to minimize infection. A drop or two of lavender will also speed the healing.

CLINICAL SUPPORT

"The aim of the present study is to review the available literature to determine if there is evidence for effectiveness of aromatherapy in surgical patients to treat anxiety and insomnia, to control pain and nausea, and to dress wounds. Efficacy studies of lavender or orange and peppermint essential oils, to treat anxiety and nausea, respectively, have shown positive results. Finally, there are encouraging data for the treatment of infections, especially for tea tree oil..." (Stea S, Beraudi A, De Pasquale D., 2014).

> We were on a river trip, and our raft ran into a tree. I got scratched up pretty bad. Since I was carrying my essential oils kit with me, I immediately put on some peppermint. I spent the rest of the day having a lot of fun and watching my scratches heal. There wasn't any pain, redness or inflammation. By the end of the day the scrapes looked like I had them for several days. Within 2 days there wasn't any sign of my accident.

RECOMMENDED BLENDS

Protecting blend

Circulation blend

Inflammation blend

INSTRUCTION

- Use a moisturizing shampoo and a conditioner that contain no harsh, potentially toxic chemicals. Use 10 to 20 drops of lavender, the Circulation blend, or the Protecting blend in 8 ounces of any of your fragrance-free hair care products. You can also mix 2 – 3 drops of any of these recommended oils in a single application of a shampoo or conditioner. Massage the product on your scalp and leave it on for five minutes before washing it out.

- If your scalp is extremely dry, you may also want to mix as much as a tablespoon of carrier oil into 8 ounces of shampoo or conditioner to give it more moisturizing capacity. Mix it thoroughly.

Dandruff

WHAT IT IS

The shedding of dead skin cells in small flakes from the scalp. As skin cells die and are shed from the scalp, a small amount of flaking is normal, and they typically are washed down the drain when we shampoo our hair. Some people experience excessive amount of flaking due to dry weather, the unhealthy condition of the scalp, or irritations of the scalp.

RECOMMENDED OILS

Tea tree

Clary sage

Frankincense

Rosemary

Dehydration

WHAT IT IS

The loss of water in the body affecting the metabolic processes. It usually results from exercise or disease. Moderate dehydration can cause fatigue and dizziness. A loss of over ten percent of body water can cause physical and mental deterioration, accompanied by severe thirst. To lose more than fifteen to twenty-five percent of the body's water is fatal.

RECOMMENDED OILS

Peppermint

Spearmint

Lemon

Sweet basil

Lavender

RECOMMENDED BLENDS

Digestion blend

Respiratory blend

Protecting blend

INSTRUCTION

Use these procedures as part of a plan involving your health care professional when needed:

• Increase water intake as quickly as possible. Mix a drop or two of lemon, peppermint, the Respiratory blend, or the Digestion blend with 1/2 tsp. of salt in a quart of warm or cool water.

• In case the disease was caused by diarrhea or vomiting, stop food all intake for from 4 to 24 hours depending on the severity. Gradually add mild foods such as steamed vegetables or stewed apples. Add a drop of lemon, peppermint, a Respiratory blend, sweet basil, or a Digestion blend after steaming or cooking.

• Take a calming bath with a cup of Epsom Salts mixed with 10 to 15 drops of one of the recommended oils.

• Refer to an authoritative diagnostic guide or medical professional for signs that the dehydration is more serious than you should treat at home.

Detoxification After Poisoning or Addiction

WHAT IT IS

After any initial emergency measures have brought the poisoning under control, it will be necessary to detoxify the body from the deeper effects of poisoning. Poisoning can come from many sources both gradually and suddenly. It can come from overuse of medications, overexposure to industrial chemicals at work, exposure to the substances in your body that come from combatting disease, etc.

RECOMMENDED OILS

Peppermint

Lemon

Spearmint

Sweet basil

RECOMMENDED BLENDS

Liver blend

Respiratory blend

Protecting blend

INSTRUCTION

As a complement to treatment by your health care professional and with his/her approval:

• Regularly use a drop of the Liver blend, peppermint, and/or lemon per quart of drinking water. Try to drink 1/2 gallon or more every day. Do this for several months to help you detoxify.

• If the poisoning is severe, do a Liver Cleanse for up to one year. Refer to specific instructions earlier in this section.

CLINICAL SUPPORT

A study of 10 women suffering from withdrawal after substance abuse showed a significant decrease in cravings when deliberately inhaling ylang ylang essential oil (Caldwell N. "The effects of ylang ylang on craving of women with substance abuse." Hunter, N.Y.: R J Buckle Associates).

"Natural essential oil constituents play an important role in cancer prevention and treatment. Various mechanisms such antioxidant, antimutagenic and antiproliferative, enhancement of immune function and surveillance, enzyme induction and enhancing detoxification, modulation of multidrug resistance and synergistic mechanism of volatile constituents are responsible for their chemopreventive properties. This review covers the most recent literature to summarize structural categories and molecular anticancer mechanisms of constituents from aromatic herbs and dietary plants" (Bhalla Y, et al., 2013).

Diabetes

WHAT IT IS

A group of metabolic diseases characterized by high blood sugar levels over a prolonged period. This produces the symptoms of frequent urination, increased thirst, and increased hunger. Untreated, diabetes can cause many complications including heart disease, stroke, kidney failure, foot ulcers and damage to the eyes.

Diabetes is due to either the pancreas not producing enough insulin, or the cells of the body not responding properly to the insulin produced. There are three main types of diabetes mellitus:

- Type 1 results from the body's failure to produce sufficient insulin. This was previously referred to as "insulin-dependent diabetes" or "juvenile diabetes".

- Type 2 begins with insulin resistance, a condition in which cells are unable to respond to insulin properly. This type was previously referred to as "adult-onset diabetes". The primary cause is likely linked to an unhealthy diet and lack of exercise.

- Gestational diabetes is the third main type and happens when pregnant women without a prior history of diabetes develop a high blood glucose level.

RECOMMENDED OILS

Peppermint		Grapefruit	
Rosemary		Ylang ylang	
Copaiba		Cinnamon	
Lemon		Lemongrass	

RECOMMENDED BLENDS

Liver blend		Digestion blend	
Foot massage blend			

INSTRUCTION

In-home procedures suggested as part of an overall plan involving your health care professional:

- Follow the dietary guidelines given in this book. Medical intervention may only bring the symptoms of diabetes under control with no significant lifestyle changes. If this is the case, there will only be superficial improvement, which can then bring about more serious conditions.

- Enjoy a drop of the Liver Blend, the Digestion blend, peppermint, or lemon in your drinking water or in a cup of herbal tea at least twice a day.

- Create the following blend: liver blend (20%), lemon (10%), peppermint (5%), digestion blend (15%), and carrier oil (50%). Fill capsules with a dropper and take a capsule 3 times a day with food.

- Enjoy a foot massage with 3 to 4 drops of the foot massage blend with the 3 to 4 drops of the liver blend, lemon, peppermint, or the digestion blend in a teaspoon of carrier oil. Massage your feet daily.

- For a deeper action, use important elements of the Liver Cleanse, the Immune Strengthening Cleanse, and the Digestion Cleanse with instructions found earlier in this section.

CLINICAL SUPPORT

The essential oil extract of black pepper could be part of the mechanism by which the essential oil could manage and/or prevent type-2 diabetes and hypertension (Oboh G, et al., 2013).

"Although clinical studies suggest that the use of essential oils may have therapeutic potential, evidence for the efficacy of aromatherapy in treating medical conditions remains poor, with a particular lack of studies employing rigorous analytical methods that capture its identifiable impact on human biology. Here, we report a comprehensive metabolomics study that reveals metabolic changes in people after exposed to aroma inhalation for 10 continuous days. A significant alteration of metabolic profile in subjects responsive to essential oil was found .... This study demonstrates that the metabolomics approach can capture the subtle metabolic changes resulting from exposure to essential oils, which may lead to an improved mechanistic understanding of aromatherapy" (Zhang Y, et al., 2013).

"Significant positive differences between treated and control groups were observed at different aspects of diabetic wound healing process. Results indicated that the essential oil of Rosmarinus officinalis was the most active in healing diabetic wounds and provide a scientific evidence for the traditional use of this herb in wound treatment" (Abu-Al-Basal MA., 2010).

Diarrhea (See also Dehydration)

WHAT IT IS

A medical condition characterized by having at least three loose or liquid bowel movements per day. It typically lasts for a few days and can result in dehydration (see above). The most common cause is from contaminated food or water resulting in a viral, bacterial, or parasite infection. The short duration watery diarrhea may be due to a cholera infection. If blood is present it is also known as dysentery. Some non-infectious causes may also result in diarrhea including: hyperthyroidism, lactose intolerance, inflammatory bowel disease, a number of medications, and irritable bowel syndrome among others.

RECOMMENDED OILS

Peppermint		Spearmint	
Lemon		Sweet basil	
Lavender			

RECOMMENDED BLENDS

Digestion blend

Protecting blend

Intimacy blend

Stress control blend

Respiratory blend

INSTRUCTION

- In-home procedures involving a health care professional as needed.

- Take a teaspoon of green clay powder in 4 oz. of water. Stir and drink it.

- Stop all food intake for as long as 24 hours. Gradually add mild foods such as steamed vegetables or white rice. Add a drop of lemon, sweet basil, or the digestion blend after cooking or steaming the mild foods.

- Increase your water intake. Mix a drop or two of spearmint, lemon, the respiratory blend, or the digestion blend per quart of water.

- If you suspect contaminated drinking water or food, take traces of tea tree on your tongue every few minutes for an hour and prepare capsules with 50:50 tea tree or an Protecting blend and a carrier oil. Take a capsule three times a day with food. This will help prevent illness if you are traveling in places where food and water may be contaminated.

- Take calming baths using 10 to 15 drops of an essential oil in a cup of Epsom Salts. Use the Calming or Stress control blends, lavender, or balsam fir.

- Dilute 2 to 3 drops of carrier oil with one of the following—the Comforting blend in the evening or the Massage blend in the morning for a calming foot massage.

- Use an authoritative diagnostic guide or contact a medical professional to check any signs that the diarrhea is more serious than should be treated at home.

- To treat infectious diarrhea, Dr. Pénoël recommends blending 10% cinnamon, 15% oregano, and 75% carrier oil. Fill capsules with a dropper and take 3 capsules daily with food or in severe cases, take 6 a day with food.

Digestive Conditions, & Necessary Lifestyle Adjustments

WHAT THEY ARE

There are a multitude of conditions associated with digestion and metabolism. They include but are not limited to diarrhea, dehydration, constipation, appendicitis, nausea, heartburn, irritable bowel syndrome, hemorrhoids, ulcers, liver disease, hepatitis, gallstones, pancreatitis, diverticulosis, and gallbladder inflammation. Each of these is discussed separately in this book, but general instructions are given here.

RECOMMENDED SINGLES

Peppermint	Ginger	
Lavender	Grapefruit	
Roman chamomile	German chamomile	
Spearmint	Cinnamon bark	
Lime	Thyme	
Bergamot	Lemon	
Tangerine	Spruce	
Juniper	Ylang ylang	
Orange	Balsam fir	

RECOMMENDED BLENDS

Digestion blend		Liver blend	
Comforting blend		Intimacy blend	
Slimming blend		Focusing blend	
Balancing blend			

INSTRUCTION

- All symptoms associated with abdominal, metabolism, or digestive problems are important signals your body is sending you that you may need to significantly reduce the buildup of toxins, add more whole-food nutrients, and unblock the flow of energy through reflexology massage of the feet, hands, and ears.

- Start by making changes to your dietary habits according to dietary guidelines for cleansing, page. Abdominal problems will almost always come back if good dietary guidelines aren't followed.

- You may need more water (1/2 gallon a day), and exercise at least the equivalent of a 2-mile walk per day.

- Examine your emotional life and reduce toxic buildup of stress, conflicts, resentment, criticism, etc. Calming therapies and massage can help significantly, but problems will recur if emotional problems are not resolved.

- Meditate while diffusing lemon, tangerine, spruce, juniper, ylang ylang, orange, balsam fir, a Comforting blend, or an intimacy blend.

- Use a relaxing massage each day of the feet, hands, abdomen, or ears, with 3 to 4 drops of lavender, geranium, lemon, the Comforting blend, or Intimacy blend, or Children's blend

diluted in a tablespoon of a carrier oil daily

- Eliminate digestion-harming addictions like smoking, drugs, or alcoholism.

- For preventing abdominal problems, enjoy a drop or two of basil, lemon, or a digestion blend daily in your food, juices, herbal teas, etc.

- A drop of basil can add flavor and digestive calming to both sweet and salty foods. Use lemon oil in sweet recipes for a calming effect.

- Put a few drops of peppermint on a tissue and insert it into the air vent of your car to prevent travel nausea.

CLINICAL SUPPORT

"Peppermint has been a classic choice for the treatment of nausea for hundreds of years. However, too much peppermint can cause nausea, so only a few drops are needed. Peppermint was found to relieve colonic spasm within 30 seconds (Leicester & Hunt 1982)" (Buckle, p. 209).

"The effect of peppermint was … found to be effective in reducing the nausea of patients undergoing chemotherapy … (Figuenick 1998)" (Buckle, p. 209).

"Vutyavanich et al (1997) studied 70 expectant mothers over a period of 5 months in a double-masked, placebo-controlled trial. They found baseline nausea and vomiting decreased significantly in the group using ginger" (Buckle, p. 210).

Diverticulitis

WHAT IT IS

A common digestive disease involving the formation of pouches (diverticula) within the bowel wall due to weakness in the muscle lining of the acolon. This process is known as diverticulosis. It can occasionally occur in the small intestine as well. Diverticulitis results when one of these diverticula becomes inflamed.

RECOMMENDED SINGLES:

Single		Single	
Peppermint		Ginger	
Tea tree		Lemon	
Marjoram			

RECOMMENDED BLENDS

Blend		Blend	
Digestion blend		Protecting blend	
Inflammation blend			

INSTRUCTIONS:

In-home procedures as part of an overall plan involving your health care professional:

- Create a blend using the digestion blend (15%), the Protecting blend (15%), and tea tree (20%) and fill capsules with a dropper. Take 3 per day with food to help decrease infection. Continue taking these capsules for 3 to 4 months even after the condition has improved.

- Create a blend using the digestion blend (30%), the Protecting blend (30%), and tea tree (40%) and use 3 or 4 drops undiluted with a drop or two of the foot massage blend and massage the colon area (arch) of the foot.

- Mix the 2 to 3 drops of this blend with a teaspoon of carrier oil and gently apply to the abdomen in a clockwise motion starting just below the navel and moving out to the rib cage and the pelvis (do not massage vigorously).

- Mix a drop of the same blend in a quart of water or a cup of herbal tea and take at least twice a day.

- For a deep healing, do a Digestive Cleanse according to instructions found in this section.

Dry & Sensitive Skin

WHAT IT IS

Skin that lacks sufficient moisture or sebum to keep it from developing fine lines, scaling and cracking. It comes from insufficient natural moisture defenses in the skin. It can be a hereditary condition or be the result of dry weather, too much washing, too many harsh chemicals, too much abrasion, etc. People with sensitive skin break out in rashes easily and are extra sensitive to chemicals in products, cold weather, or other harsh conditions like too much sun or wind.

RECOMMENDED OILS

German chamomile		Roman chamomile	
Sandalwood		Lavender	
Lavandin		Frankincense	
Patchouli			

RECOMMENDED BLENDS

Stress control blend		Comforting blend	
Foot massage blend		Circulation blend	
Focusing blend			

INSTRUCTION

- Focus extra attention on your diet. Add more raw fruits and vegetables, whole grains, and heart-healthy oils such as cold-pressed olive oil. Even a little extra dietary oil can make a difference in your skin. Drink at least a half-gallon of water daily. Exercise the equivalent of least a 2-mile walk every day to increase circulation. Get some sunshine to keep your vitamin D high enough.

- A liver cleanse can often help with a dry skin condition.

- Combine 10 to 20 drops of your favorite recommended oil along with an extra teaspoon of a carrier oil like jojoba to your fragrance-free lotion. Mix well. Apply this lotion after your bath or shower, whenever you wash your hands, and when your skin feels excessively dry.

- Take short, warm (not hot) baths with 10 to 15 drops of one of the recommended oils dispersed in a cup of Epsom Salts.

- After your bath or shower, add a little extra moisture by applying 4 to 5 drops of one of the listed oils mixed in a tablespoon of a carrier oil to your dry skin areas. Try different carrier oils until you find the one that works best for you.

Ear Infections

WHAT THEY ARE

Inflammations of the middle ear that are most common in childhood, but may happen at any age. Most ear infections are caused by a blockage of the Eustachian tube. This is most often caused by a respiratory infection or an allergy. This blockage can cause a vacuum in the middle ear. When materials from the nasal cavities are sucked into this space, they can become infected and pressure is put on the ear drum. Ear infections can be painful with discharges and fever. Treatment with antibiotics is no longer recommended.

RECOMMENDED OILS

Tea tree		Thyme	
Eucalyptus radiata		Sweet basil	
Orange		Lemon	
Spearmint		Lavender	

RECOMMENDED BLEND

Protecting blend	

INSTRUCTION

Never pour an essential oil down the ear canal.

- Dr. Pénoël suggests this remarkable home remedy. Grate or blend a raw onion and press it to release the juice. Mix it half-and-half with olive oil and bring it to body temperature. Soak a small cotton ball in the mixture and insert it into the outer area of the ear canal. Place some dry cotton over it and keep it in place overnight.

- Dr. Pénoël suggests this treatment for babies and children as well as adults. It will help both with pain and infection. Put 2 drops of tea tree on a cotton pad that can be placed in the ear and changed two to three times a day for 4 to 7 days +++++P.

- Apply a few drops of undiluted tea tree and/ or the Protecting blend on the prominent bone behind the ear and under the ear and down the side of the neck to the collar bone. Apply tea tree every 5 minutes for two hours.

- Mix 2 or 3 drops of tea tree or the Protecting blend in a teaspoon of carrier oil and massage the area on the bottoms of the feet under the 3rd and 4th toes.

- For babies and young children, dilute 4 to 5 drops of the oil in a teaspoon of mixing oil if topical application shows any redness or discomfort.

- Create antimicrobial drinking water by adding a drop of the Protecting blend in a quart of water. You can also add a drop to whatever food you may be eating like a flavorful spaghetti sauce or a mild applesauce. Flavor all the foods you can with a drop of the best tasting oils such as lemon, orange, sweet basil, or spearmint.

CLINICAL SUPPORT

This study compared the effects of basil essential oil to a placebo when placed in the ear canal of rats with middle ear infection. The treatment cured or healed 56%-81% compared with 5.6%-6% in the placebo group. Essential oils placed in the ear canal can provide effective treatment of acute middle ear infections (Kristinsson KG, et al., 2005).

Eczema
(also Psoriasis, an autoimmune disease)

WHAT IT IS

Eczema is a broad term that involves many types of red, inflamed skin conditions that range from extremely serious to simply bothersome. Psoriasis is a serious autoimmune disease of the skin. While the manifestations of the two may be similar, the treatments will vary. Eczema stems from an allergic reaction; psoriasis is where the immune system actually attacks the body, causing chronic inflammation.

RECOMMENDED OILS for ECZEMA
(may or may not be an allergy)

Lavender		Bergamot	
German chamomile		Roman chamomile	
Patchouli		Helichrysum	
Rosemary		Sage	

RECOMMENDED OILS for PSORIASIS
(auto-immune)

Stress control blend		Comforting blend	
Foot massage blend		Circulation blend	

RECOMMENDED BLENDS

Inflammation blend

Immune balancing blend

Liver blend

Foot massage blend

INSTRUCTION

- Because recommendations can vary according to the seriousness of skin condition, make sure you have a correct diagnosis from a health care professional according to the type and seriousness of the condition, and then follow these recommendations according to what you learn.

- CAUTION: anyone who suffers from allergies or autoimmune conditions may have a much stronger reaction to essential oils applied on the skin, even those who are of the highest quality. The best ways to manage this condition may be through internal cleansing programs like the Liver Cleanse, the Digestion Cleanse, or the Immune Balancing Cleanse. Use extreme caution when applying oils topically for allergic or autoimmune conditions. Do a 2-day patch test for even the gentlest essential oils before using them generally. Apply a drop of the oil to a small area on the inside of the arm one time each day and wait to see if you get an inflammation on the area.

- For those who may possibly be allergic or sensitive, follow these instructions first on your feet, then on a small part of the infected area for at least 24 hours before you begin to use them generally.

- If you suspect that your eczema or psoriasis is caused by an allergy or autoimmune response, do a Liver Cleanse or an Immune Balancing Cleanse first as shown earlier in this section. This may take up to a year to

complete—one month of cleansing for every year you've had the condition.

- Begin by making sure you have a healthy diet focused on fruits, vegetables, whole grains, heart-healthy oils, and drinking at least a 1/2 gallon of water every day. Exercise the equivalent of walking at least 2 miles daily to increase circulation.

- If you find that an oil does not create a reaction during a 2-day patch test, mix 20 to 40 drops of lavender, the inflammation blend, or a Comforting blend in a mild, fragrance-free and non-toxic lotion. Apply the lotion to the affected areas after each bath or shower and whenever you wash your hands. You can also mix 4 to 5 drops of the oil into each application lotion.

- Take warm (not hot) baths with 5 to 10 drops of lavender, Roman chamomile, the inflammation blend, or the Comforting blend dispersed in a cup of Epsom Salts.

- After your bath or shower, apply 4 to 5 drops of lavender, the Protecting blend, the inflammation blend, or the Comforting blend mixed in a tablespoon of mixing oil to the affected areas.

CLINICAL SUPPORT

This study shows experimentally that tea tree oil can reduce histamine-induced skin inflammation (Koh KJ, et al., 2002).

Edema

WHAT IS IT

The accumulation of fluids in the body typically as a result of cardiac failure or the inability of the heart to pump fluids through the body effectively. It can engorge the limbs and organs of the body. It can also be a sign of a serious liver or kidney condition.

RECOMMENDED OILS

Patchouli		Cypress	
Helichrysum		Ginger	
Black pepper		Cinnamoni	
Rosemary		Sage	

RECOMMENDED BLENDS

Circulation blend		Stimulating massage blend	

INSTRUCTION

• The underlying cause of the condition must be recognized and treated with the assistance of a health care professional. To assist with the symptoms, you can use the following:

• Dr. Pénoël suggests creating a gentle massage blend using helichrysum (25%) and cypress (25%) in a carrier oil (50%) to apply over the areas of accumulation and the veins +++P.

• For a more stimulating massage, use ginger, black pepper, cinnamon, rosemary, sage, or the Massage blend.

• He also suggests taking a capsule of 25% patchouli and 25% cypress with 50% carrier oil. Fill capsules with a dropper and take 3 a day for 30 days +++P.

• Take aromatic baths mixing 10 to 15 drops of your oil of choice with a cup of Epsom Salts.

Emphysema
(Smoker's Cough)

WHAT IT IS

A chronic, long-term lung disease, which makes it difficult to breathe in or out. Smoking is the most common cause. This a serious condition that requires the attention and care of a health care professional.

RECOMMENDED OILS

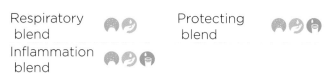

Eucalyptus radiata		Tea tree	
Roman chamomile			

RECOMMENDED BLENDS

Respiratory blend		Protecting blend	
Inflammation blend			

INSTRUCTION

• With the involvement of your health care professional, the following supplemental procedures may help.

• The most important thing to do is to stop smoking as soon as possible. Other efforts are largely wasted if you don't stop smoking.

• Emphysema means you are highly susceptible to many respiratory infections. Be sure to take extra precautions to protect yourself against all infections. Diffuse 5 to 10 drops of the Respiratory blend, the Protecting blend, or Eucalyptus radiate daily in your home or work area. You can do this safely for 5 minutes 4 or 5 times a day.

• Adjust your diet to one that is high in fresh, raw (uncooked) vegetables to provide extra clinical support and protection for your lungs.

- Exercise as often and regularly as you can. While you may be short of breath, if you exercise carefully and prudently, a moderate exercise program can greatly increase your ability to breathe as normally as possible.

- Inhale steam mixed with the Respiratory blend: add 3 to 6 drops to 2 cups of hot or boiling water. This may help improve the oxygenation within your lungs.

Endometriosis

WHAT IT IS

A female disorder that happens when cells from the uterus lining grow in other areas of the body leading to pain, infertility, and irregular menstrual periods and unpredictable bleeding.

RECOMMENDED OILS

| Sweet basil | | Cypress | |
| Helichrysum | | | |

RECOMMENDED BLENDS

| Foot massage blend | |

INSTRUCTION

- With the approval of your health care professional, try the following in-home procedures:

- Under the direction of a well-informed health care professional, use a natural progesterone cream.

- For reducing the pain of menstrual cramps, massage your heel and ankles with 3 or 4 drops of undiluted sweet basil and a foot massage blend.

- To reduce the pain of menstrual cramps, do a lower abdominal massage by mixing 3 to 4 drops of sweet basil in a teaspoon of carrier oil. Massage your abdomen in a clockwise circular motion on the lower abdomen and a counter-clockwise motion on the corresponding area of the back.

Epilepsy

WHAT IT IS

Epilepsy is a neurological brain disorder characterized by repeated seizures or convulsions. Seizures are episodes of disturbed brain activity that can cause loss of consciousness, abnormal electrical activity in the brain, and other changes in attention or behavior.

RECOMMENDED OILS

| Lavender | | Ylang ylang | |
| Bergamot | | Neroli | |

RECOMMENDED BLENDS

| Comforting blend | | Foot massage blend | |
| Stress control blend | | | |

INSTRUCTIONS

Use the following suggestions under the direction of your health care professional:

- For a calming daily foot massage, use 1 or 2 drops of any of the oils listed mixed with 2 to 3 drops of the Foot Massage blend. Focus on the toes.

- For calming the brain functions, diffuse 5 to 10 drops of one of the recommended oils for 5 minutes whenever you need it throughout the day. CAUTION: Calming aromas are sometimes unpredictable. Some will actually trigger an epileptic reaction in some people, while they will greatly help others. Check your own reaction to the oils while you are in a situation where you can receive help should you have a negative reaction.

- Take a bath with 5 to 10 drops of one of the Comforting blends dispersed in a cup of Epsom Salts.

- Do a full-body massage with 3 to 4 drops of one of the calming oils mixed with a teaspoon of mixing oil.

Fibromyalgia

WHAT IT IS

A syndrome characterized by long-term pain all over the body and tenderness in the joints, muscles, tendons, and other tissues. Symptoms include fatigue, depression, sleep problems, headaches, and anxiety.

RECOMMENDED OILS

Eucalyptus radiata		Tea tree	
Frankincense		Vetiver	
Copaiba		Wintergreen	
Peppermint		Balsam fir	

RECOMMENDED BLENDS

Inflammation blend		Soothing blend	
Protecting blend		Massage blend	

INSTRUCTIONS

- In-home procedures suggested as part of an overall plan with the approval of or under the direction of your health care professional:

- For pain apply 2 to 3 drops of the inflammation blend and 2 to 3 drops of the Soothing blend undiluted on the feet and ear reflexology points corresponding to the painful area.

- Also gently massage painful areas of the body with 2 to 3 drops of any of the recommended oils in a teaspoon of mixing oil.

- Apply the 2 to 3 drops of the Protecting blend, Eucalyptus radiata, tea tree, or the Massage blend in a teaspoon of the mixing oil. Massage the affected areas regularly.

- Create a blend using the Protecting blend (20%), Spearmint (10%), tea tree (10%), and a carrier oil (50%). Fill capsules with a dropper and take one capsule 3 times a day with food.

- Use a drop of the Protecting blend or tea tree with honey in an herbal tea once or twice a day.

- Use the habits in the Immune Strengthening Cleanse to help in recovery.

CLINICAL SUPPORT

Essential oils produced a significant reduction in chronic non-inflammatory muscle pain in an animal model, which remained for 24 hours demonstrating its possible use in the treatment of fibromyalgia (Nascimento SS, et al., 2014).

Fluid Retention

(see Edema)

Food Poisoning

WHAT IT IS

Various types of illnesses caused by bacteria, parasites, viruses or other toxins in food, typically accompanied by vomiting and diarrhea.

RECOMMENDED OILS

Peppermint		Ginger	
German chamomile		Roman chamomile	
Lavender		Sweet basil	
Tea tree		Spearmint	
Lemon		Eucalyptus radiata	

RECOMMENDED BLENDS

Protecting blend		Digestion blend	

INSTRUCTION

• Mix a drop of either the Protecting blend or the Digestion blend in a quart of drinking water, or use a trace of one of these oils on a toothpick stirred into a cup of hot or cold water. Drink about 1/2 gallon of water per day to help flush the offending toxins out of the body.

• To alleviate nausea, take a drop of any of the ingestible oils listed in an herbal tea or warm water.

• Use a drop or two of either of the Antimicrobial or Digestion blend in mild recipes—steamed vegetables or vegetable bouillon (after they are taken off the stove).

• If you suspect that you may be continuing to take contaminated food or drinking water, use the "lick trick" to take traces of tea tree oil every few minutes for about an hour and whenever you feel it may be needed throughout the day.

• Create a blend with tea tree (20%), Rosemary (20%), peppermint (10%), and a carrier oil (50%). Fill capsules with a dropper and take a capsule 3 times daily with food. Use this for prevention if you are traveling in areas where there may be contaminated food and water.

• Refer to a medical diagnostic guide or a health care professional to understand if there are signs that your symptoms are more serious than you should be treating by yourself.

• To get rid of intestinal parasites associated with food poisoning, create a blend containing spruce (15%), tea tree (20%), and thyme (15%) with a carrier oil (50%). Fill capsules and take a capsule 2 or 3 times a day with food ++++P.

Frostbite

WHAT IT IS

Damage to the skin and tissues caused by exposure to extreme cold. It typically affects the nose, fingers, or toes, and left untreated, can result in gangrene.

RECOMMENDED OILS

Lavender		Thyme	
Cypress		Rosemary	

RECOMMENDED BLENDS

Inflammation blend   Circulation blend

INSTRUCTION

- Create a compress by mixing 2 to 3 drops of lavender, cypress, the circulation blend, or the inflammation blend in a small bowl of warm water. Soak a cloth in the mixture and put it on the frostbitten area. Cover it with a plastic film to help the aromatic molecules to penetrate and keep the area warm with a hot water bottle for a few hours.

- Then massage the area gently several times a day with 2 to 3 drops of any of the recommended oils mixed in a teaspoon or less of the a carrier oil.

- Soak feet in a warm bath with 3 or 4 drops of one of the recommended oils mixed with a half cup of Epsom Salts.

Fungal Infections
(of the skin & feet)

WHAT IT IS

Athlete's foot and ringworm are types of fungal infections that attack the skin, nails, and hair follicles of the feet, hands, and typically folds of skin all over the body. They are common during pregnancy and with diabetes. They produce itching, burning, redness, and sometimes cracked areas of skin. The microscopic fungi hide in crevices in nails and moist skin folds like the groin area.

RECOMMENDED OILS

Tea tree		Frankincense	
Lavender		Lemon	
Oregano		Cinnamon	
Thyme		Lemongrass	
Eucalyptus globulus		Eucalyptus radiata	

RECOMMENDED BLENDS

Protecting blend   Immune balancing blend

Inflammation blend

INSTRUCTION

- Use these suggestions as part of an overall plan involving your health care professional as needed for more serious fungal infections.

- Fungal infections can keep coming back if they are not deeply eliminated. Do a Liver Cleanse and an Immune Strengthening Cleanse that last about a year to clear fungal infections completely out of your body.

- Create a blend of equal parts tea tree, thyme, and Eucalyptus globulus. You can initially apply 3 or 4 drops of the blend in a teaspoon of rubbing alcohol to dry the area out, and then add 3 or 4 drops to each application of lotion or simply mix them with the little water so the area stays completely dry and clean. Apply this blend to the infected area 3 or 4 times a day ++++P.

- Use any of the milder recommended oils undiluted to the infected area 3 or 4 times a day. Dilute the stronger oils (lemongrass, thyme, oregano) 25:75 with a carrier oil or a few drops mixed in a teaspoon of lotion before application.

- Soak feet in a warm bath with 3 or 4 drops of one of the recommended oils mixed with a half cup of Epsom Salts.

- Do a foot massage daily with a 50:50 blend of frankincense and a carrier oil or any of the milder recommended oils to restore the skin and nails to their best condition over time.

Chronic athlete's foot cleared up with clinical-grade tea tree

I've had a fungal infection from athlete's foot in my toenail for years. I tried tea tree from an aromatherapy shop or health food store because I heard that it might help. It made no difference. When I heard about high-quality clinical grade oils, I decided to try it again. The discoloration I had lived with for so long started going away, and within a month the infection I had lived with for decades went completely away.

CLINICAL SUPPORT

This was a test of the treatment of athlete's foot in a foot bath using essential oils. The order of the fungicidal activity among the 11 essential oils tested was oregano, thyme, cinnamon bark, lemongrass, clove, peppermint, lavender, geranium, and tea tree. (Inouye S, et al., 2007).

Gallbladder Inflammation

(Cholecystitis often associated with gallstones)

WHAT IT IS

Inflammation of the gallbladder, usually because of blockages caused by gallstones. The resulting inflammation and swelling of the gallbladder can lead to infections and cell death due to insufficient oxygen. More than 25% of people who get this conditions require surgery or develop complications.

RECOMMENDED OILS

German chamomile		Roman chamomile	
Peppermint		Juniper	
Lemon		Pine	

RECOMMENDED BLENDS

Immune balancing blend		Foot massage blend	
Liver blend		Protecting blend	

INSTRUCTION

In-home procedures suggested as part of an overall plan involving your health care professional for this potentially serious condition:

- Be sure to follow instructions by your health care professional for dealing with gallstones if you suspect that they may be part of the reason for the inflammation you are experiencing.

- Immediately start a Liver Cleanse and make sure that the immune balancing blend is an important part of your cleanse.

- Blend one or two drops undiluted of three blends: the immune balancing blend, the liver blend, and the foot massage blend and massage the oils on the gallbladder area on the foot every day.

- Apply 3 to 4 drops of any of these 3 blends over the gallbladder area of the abdomen 3 times a day. It is behind the lower ribs 3 inches from the center of the body. (see diagram)

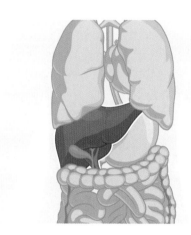

Gallstones

WHAT THEY ARE

Hard, pebble-like deposits that can form inside the gallbladder. They can be as small as a grain of sand or grow as large as a golf ball and cause serious damage to the ducts of the gallbladder.

RECOMMENDED OILS

Lemon		Peppermint	
Juniper		Grapefruit	
Helichrysum			

RECOMMENDED BLENDS

Liver blend		Digestion blend	
Protecting blend			

INSTRUCTION

Follow these procedures as part of a plan involving your health care professional:

- Do a thorough Liver Cleanse as described earlier in this section to help keep your gallbladder in peak condition.

- Massage the central abdominal area of your feet every day with 3 to 4 drops of the foot massage blend mixed with lemon essential oil.

- For a least two days ingest one drop each of lemon and peppermint in a quart of vegetable juice each day.

Genital Herpes

WHAT IT IS

Viral Herpes simplex infections are sexually transmitted, and cause painful blisters on or around the genitals.

RECOMMENDED OILS

Tea tree		Lemon	
Helichrysum		Thyme	
German chamomile		Roman chamomile	
Ginger			

RECOMMENDED BLEND

Protecting blend		Immune balancing blend	

INSTRUCTION

Use the following in-home procedures with the agreement of your health care professional as needed:

- Apply the Protecting blend undiluted only to

the infected spot. Do not apply it around the spot on the skin or the skin may become inflamed. Do this as early as possible to stop the spread of the virus. Use a small amount of oil by using a small dropper, a pipette, or even a toothpick. Do this several times a day.

- After you have controlled the infection, do an Immune Strengthening Cleanse for several months to completely clear up the infection, or it may spring up again and spread. Instructions for the cleanse are given earlier in this section.

- If you have helichrysum, apply a trace right on the affected spot. If you catch it early, it will often take care of it even before it opens.

CLINICAL SUPPORT

Genital herpes is a chronic, persistent infection spreading as a sexually transmitted disease. Thyme oil, ginger oil, chamomile oil and sandalwood oil were tested against the virus that causes the disease. A clearly dose-dependent activity against the genital herpes virus could be demonstrated for all essential oils tested. Chamomile oil seems to be a promising candidate for topical therapeutic application as an antiviral agent for the treatment of genital herpes (Koch C, et al., 2008).

Giardia

WHAT IT IS

An intestinal infection with a protozoal parasite, often leading to diarrhea with potentially serious dehydration complications.

RECOMMENDED OILS

Lavender		Peppermint	
Lemon		Tea tree	

RECOMMENDED BLENDS

Protecting blend		Digestion blend	

INSTRUCTION

As a complement to the advice of your health care professional and with his/her approval, follow these suggestions:

- Create a mixture of the Protecting blend (25%), lavender (25%), and a carrier oil (50%). Fill capsules and take 3 capsules a day with food.

- Take 1 or 2 drops of the Protecting blend or lavender in an herbal tea with honey. Mix a drop of the Protecting blend in a quart of drinking water, in juice, or in recipes (after taking the recipe off the stove).

- When traveling in locations where there may be water contaminated with giardia, use a drop of tea tree or lemon to purify all drinking water. One drop per quart is sufficient. Also take one or two of the capsules for prevention when traveling in these areas.

CLINICAL SUPPORT

Giardia is one of the most important worldwide causes of intestinal infections. Essential oils or some of their constituents may be useful in the clinical management of giardia infections (Machado M, et al., 2010).

There are many plant-derived agents that are more effective against human tropical diseases than the synthetic alternatives. Tropical diseases studied include: amebiasis, Chagas disease, cholera, cryptosporidiosis, dengue, epidemic typhus, filariasis (elephantiasis), giardia, human African trypanosomiasis (sleeping sickness), isosporiasis, leishmaniasis,

Lyme disease, malaria, onchocerciasis, plague, recurrent fever, sarcocystosis, scabies, spotted fever, toxoplasmosis, West Nile fever, and yellow fever. Essential oils exhibiting noxious or toxic activity are comparable or superior to the synthetic control agents of choice for many tropical diseases (Pohlit AM, et al., 2011).

Gingivitis (Inflamed gums)

WHAT IT IS

A periodontal disease of the gums. It comes from a biofilm called plaque that sticks to the surface of the teeth. Left untreated, it may progress to a more serious form of periodontal disease where inflammation and tissue destruction lead to bone destructions, which can ultimately lead to the loss of teeth.

RECOMMENDED OILS

Tea tree		Thyme	
Helilchrysum		Tangerine	
Peppermint		Cinnamon	
Clove			

RECOMMENDED BLEND

Protecting blend	

INSTRUCTION

• Mix 2 to 3 drops each of helichrysum and lavender in about the same amount of carrier oil, and apply it to your infected gums 2 or 3 times a day ++++P.

• Brush twice a day with a cinnamon or clove tooth powder mixed with an extra drop of tea tree or tangerine oil. Create your own tooth powder by mixing 2 parts baking soda to 1 part fine-ground, natural salt. Thoroughly mix in drops of peppermint or clove oil to taste. Sprinkle some in your hand, add a drop of tea tree or tangerine oil, wet your toothbrush, and enjoy brushing your teeth without the toxic chemicals.

• Create an aromatic mouthwash using a teaspoon of baking soda, a teaspoon of salt, 10 drops of tea tree, 10 drops of peppermint, and 8 ounces of water. Shake before each use. Swish, gargle, and spit.

• Create an oil pulling mixture with 10 drops of peppermint or a mixture of other oils on the recommended list in a 1/2 cup of olive oil. Take about a tablespoon of oil. Swish and pull the oil back and forth between your teeth for about 20 minutes while you shower. Spit the mixture out. This thicker concoction really gets into the pockets where the bacteria hide in your mouth.

CLINICAL SUPPORT

An essential-oils mouthwash was compared against an alcohol vehicle solution and a water-based control on plaque and gingivitis. After 6 months, the studies showed that the essential oils mouth wash provided significantly better plaque control and gingival inflammation reduction. Essential oils provided a significant oral health benefit during the 6 months of use (Van Leeuwen M, Slot D, Van der Weijden G., 2014).

Gout

WHAT IT IS

A painful disease caused by a chemical imbalance in the body, which makes it unable to eliminate uric acid. This acid forms into painful crystals, often around a joint. The joint becomes hot, red, and inflamed.

RECOMMENDED SINGLES

Spruce

Eucalyptus radiata

Peppermint

Spearmint

Helichrysum

Sweet basil

Juniper

RECOMMENDED BLEND

Inflammation blend

Immune balancing blend

Antimicrobial blend

Comforting blend

INSTRUCTION

As part of an overall plan with the approval of or under the direction of your health care professional:

- An extremely strong inflammation can be like a burning fire. Even the mildest oils can sometimes be too strong and add strength to the fire.

- Here is a recipe Dr. Pénoël suggests for gout. Mix 5 drops of juniper and 2 drops of peppermint in an 8 oz. glass of water and stir. Dip a small piece of gauze in the mixture, press it to keep it from dripping, and apply it to the painful area. Put a piece of plastic over it and secure it with a cling bandage. Use an ice pack over the bandaged area to keep it cool.

- Here is another anti-inflammatory recipe offered by Dr. Pénoël. It is a blend of 30% Eucalyptus radiata, 20% helichrysum, and 50% carrier oil. Lightly apply this blend to the painful joint 2 to 4 times a day ++++P.

- Here is a cortisone-like recipe from Dr. Pénoël. It is 5 drops of pine and 5 drops of spruce in a cup of water. Soak a gauze as described above and add an ice pack.

- Blend 25% peppermint, 25% juniper, and 50% carrier oil to fill capsules you can take three times a day with food.

- Create a rough suspension of the Soothing blend in cold water—4 to 5 drops to a half cup of water. Shake it well and soak a piece of flannel or gauze in it to create a compress to help the oil penetrate. Apply a little plastic and a cling bandage over it to keep the liquid in contact with the skin. Apply an ice pack to increase the cooling effect.

- Mix 5 to 10 drops of the Soothing blend into green clay to create a poultice for the afflicted area. Protect it with a little plastic wrap and a cling bandage. Use an ice pack over it to keep it cold.

- Except in the times of extreme crisis, apply the strong Soothing blend in the morning and then use a soothing inflammation blend in the afternoon, evening, or before bed.

- Use 4 to 5 drops of the Inflammation blend in the same ways as the Soothing blend above. Use a gauze or flannel soaked in a cold water suspension to form a compress, or a few drops in a green clay poultice. You may need the inflammation blend or even the immune balancing blend for its deeper, more long-term benefits. Apply an ice pack to keep it cool.

- To improve healing circulation, massage the circulation blend around the painful joint.

- In case of energy blockages use 5 drops of the Comforting blend or Foot Massage blend in a teaspoon of carrier oil for a vigorous daily foot massage.

- Control your nutrition strictly according to the dietary guidelines given in this book.

- The Protecting blend is anti-infectious and can play a major role in purifying and balancing the intestinal flora inside the body. Ingest at least one drop a day in herbal tea or water. Enjoy it preferably in the morning.

- In order to support liver detoxification, ingest a drop of the liver blend in a soup or juice once a day.

HIV Infection & Aids

WHAT IT IS

A chronic infection that can result in severely reduced immunity. This is an important case where a holistic approach is important. If the whole body and the immune system in particular is healthy, the HIV virus is not as serious a problem. When the immune system is weak, the virus can do serious damage. Those who improve their nutrition, learn to manage stress, and use essential oils to stimulate their immune response, can have a much greater chance of avoiding the full-blown AIDS syndrome.

RECOMMENDED OILS

Tea tree		Peppermint	
Lemon		Ravintsara	
Thyme		Marjoram	
Eucalyptus radiata		Rosewood	
Bergamot		Clary sage	
Roman chamomile		German chamomile	
Frankincense		Grapefruit	
Neroli		Sandalwood	

RECOMMENDED BLENDS

Immune balancing blend		Foot massage blend	
Liver blend		Antimicrobial blend	

INSTRUCTION

Use the following in-home procedures with the approval of your health care professional:

- Create a blend in equal parts of any of these oils: tea tree, peppermint, lemon, the Protecting blend, the Liver blend, and frankincense. Half of the blend should be essential oils, the other half a carrier oil of your choice. Use a dropper to fill capsules and take 3 a day with food.

- Take 1 or 2 drops of any of the recommended oils in an herbal tea with honey. Put a drop in a quart of drinking water, juice, or recipes (after taking the recipe off the stove).

- Use any of the recommended oils or a blend of several of them to prepare a foot massage oil. Use 3 to 4 drops of the oil in 3 to 4 drops of the foot massage blend. Add a teaspoon of a carrier oil if you desire for a more general massage. The blend can be used undiluted on the feet.

- To strengthen immunity and avoid infections, diffuse 5 to 10 drops of any of the recommended oils for 5 minutes twice a day.

- Use 3 to 5 drops of any blend of the recommended oils mixed with a teaspoon of a carrier oil for massage of joints or localized areas that may be affected. Because each case of this disease is so unique, be sure to work with your health care professional for specific and unique ideas that could be helpful.

- Gentle, calming massage using the most aromatically pleasing oils can be remarkably helpful. Use the gentle "M" technique for calming and lowering anxiety.

CLINICAL SUPPORT

"The aim of the present study is to review the available literature to determine if there is evidence for effectiveness of aromatherapy in surgical patients to treat anxiety and insomnia, to control pain and nausea, and to dress wounds. Efficacy studies of lavender or orange and peppermint essential oils, to treat anxiety and nausea, respectively, have shown positive results. Finally, there are encouraging data for the treatment of infections, especially for tea tree oil..." (Stea S, Beraudi A, De Pasquale D., 2014).

Hay Fever

(see also Asthma)

WHAT IT IS

Like asthma, hay fever (allergic rhinitis) can be triggered by an allergen: pollens, dust, airborne chemicals, etc. Hay fever symptoms are manifest mostly in the sinuses (runny nose, sneezing, watery eyes, etc.) rather than in the lungs (asthma). Asthma is a chronic inflammatory autoimmune disease whereas hay fever is an allergy.

RECOMMENDED OILS

Oil		Oil	
Thyme	🌿🍃	Balsam fir	🌿
Cypress	🌿	Cajuput	🌿
Clove	🌿🍃	Frankincense	🌿🍃
Lavender	🌿	Lemon	🌿🍃
Lime	🌿🍃	Marjoram	🌿🍃
Peppermint	🌿🍃	Spearmint	🌿🍃
Myrtle	🌿🍃	Rosemary	🌿🍃
Sage	🌿	Clary sage	🌿
Tea tree	🌿🍃	Spruce	🌿
Helichrysum	🌿		

RECOMMENDED BLENDS

Blend		Blend	
Respiratory blend		Protecting blend	
Immune balancing blend		Inflammation blend	

Essential oil applications for hay fever would be much the same as those for asthma. *Anyone with allergies needs to exercise extra caution in using essential oils because of the potential of triggering an allergic response.* Use them mainly by ingesting them or using them on your feet. Do not diffuse them or inhale them. And do not use them on your skin without first testing a small area on your back or the inside of your arm. Use them only with the approval of your health care professional.

- Do a 24-hour test of Eucalyptus radiata on a small area of the back or the inside of the arm to see if the oil creates a red, inflamed, itchy reaction. If it does, use essential oils only on the feet and through ingestion. Make sure they are well diluted.

- After checking for an allergic reaction and finding that they are safe to use topically, Dr. Pénoël recommends creating a blend of thyme 10%, lavender (40%), and carrier oil (50%); and applying it on the chest and back over the lung and bronchial area 3 times a day for 4 to 7 days +++++P. Use this blend only on the feet if your test showed an allergic reaction. You may want to dilute even more than what is recommended.

- Try this blend on your tongue: 10 drops of sweet basil, 3 drops of balsam fir, and 2 drops of peppermint. Take a drop on your tongue and mix it with your saliva for 2 minutes before swallowing. Use it as often as needed to help control hay fever.

Headaches

(Tension, migraine, and cluster)

WHAT IT IS

The brain itself cannot feel pain because it doesn't have sensory nerves. There are sensory nerves, however, in the membranes covering the surface of the brain as well as all over the head and face.

Prolonged periods of stress or tension are responsible for most headaches. Headaches typically develop slowly. Some are inconvenient, lasting an hour or less; others are severe and debilitating, lasting for days. Causes are numerous: too little or too much sleep, overeating, allergies, alcohol consumption, prolonged loud noise, poor air circulation, eyestrain, too many hours in front of the computer screen, fluctuating hormone levels, sinus infections, TMJ, and fever. A severe headache can also be the result of an aneurysm or a brain tumor.

RECOMMENDED OILS

Peppermint		Lavender	
Frankincense		Lemon	
Sweet basil		Rosewood	
Spearmint		Citronella	
German chamomile		Roman chamomile	
Clary sage		Valerian	
Lavandin		Lemongrass	
Rosemary		Sage	
Thyme			

RECOMMENDED BLENDS

Respiratory blend		Comforting blend	
Intimacy blend		Mental focus blend	
Stress control blend		Focusing blend	
Inflammation blend			

INSTRUCTION

As part of a complete program involving your health care professional's recommendations as needed, essential oils can help eliminate headache pain. They accomplish this by stimulating circulation and improving oxygen transfer in the blood and the brain. Here are suggested remedies.

- Diffuse two or three different essential oils in succession. (Note: people with serious emotional and physical blockages and accumulated toxins from poor diet and poor elimination may find that inhaling diffused essential oils aggravates rather than relieves their headaches. In these cases it is best to start with applications on the feet, specifically on the toes.)

- For headaches that originate from digestive conditions, Dr. Pénoël suggests a blend of peppermint (25%), lemon (25%), and carrier oil (50%) for filling capsules. Take a capsule when you feel a headache coming on, as many as 3 times a day +++P.

- For headaches that can be treated with more circulatory action, he recommends this blend: marjoram (30%), lemon (20%), and a carrier oil (50%). Fill capsules with a dropper and take a capsule 3 times a day with food +++P.

- He recommends this topical blend: peppermint (75%) and sweet basil (25%). Apply 2 – 3 drops undiluted to the forehead, temples, and ear lobes +++P.

- When pain relief is urgent, apply 2 to 3 drops of peppermint to the nape of the neck and temples. This may not entirely eliminate the headache, but it can make it more tolerable.

- For relief that lasts longer, apply 2 to 3 drops of lavender undiluted on the temples, then massage 2 to 3 drops of lavender on the back of the neck stroking downward. You can dilute the lavender in a teaspoon of carrier oil if you wish to help it glide more freely. Then apply 1 to 2 drops of undiluted frankincense or lemon to your temples.

- For stress headaches, use the Comforting blend. Apply a drop or two to the back of the neck and the temples. Also place a drop under the nose. The aroma alone can stimulate and oxygenate your brain. If this particular aroma on the head and neck doesn't seem to help, apply a few drops of the Comforting blend with the Foot Massage blend on the toes. Do not apply the Comforting blend before driving or any activity that requires keen attention.

- Any of the most pleasing blends can help with headache pain when applied topically according to the instructions above. Try the Focusing blend, the Balancing blend, the Mental Focus blend, the Stress control blend, and the Intimacy blend.

- Regular aerobic exercise releases endorphins and helps bring oxygen to the brain. These will both help control pain. Exercise at least 3 times a week for 30 minutes. This will almost always help with simple headaches.

- Drinking more water (at least 1/2 gallon a day) will help. Use a drop of your favorite oil or blend in the water.

- Try eliminating any the most common food allergy triggers, such as wheat (gluten), chocolate, dairy (especially cheese), MSG, nitrates (in processed meats), alcohol, vinegar, or marinated foods.

- A cool, damp, aromatic compress on the forehead or the back of the neck may help a lot. Mix 3 drops of lavender and 3 drops of peppermint (or 6 drops of Comforting blend) in 1/2 cup of cool water and shake it vigorously. Soak a cloth in it, wring it out slightly, and apply to your forehead or the back of your neck. Change and replenish it when it warms up from your body heat. Lie down with a compress in place in a dark room for 30 to 60 minutes. A dry cloth and a cold pack might help.

- A good night's rest, a nap, going on a walk with deep breathing, or getting some fresh air can often relieve a simple tension headache and offer temporary relief from a more serious one.

- Avoid coffee, tea, caffeine sodas, tobacco, and alcohol.

How to identify and treat the type of migraine headache you have

Migraines can be related to hormones, digestion, stress, or even the electrical impulses of your nervous system.

- A migraine associated with electrical frequencies will respond to inhaling peppermint or spearmint. Rub a few drops into the palms of your hands, cup hands over the mouth and nose, and breathe deeply several times. You can also inhale these aromas a few drops in a tissue, handkerchief, or cotton ball. Then use a drop on the back of the neck.

- Migraines that relate to hormones respond well to natural progesterone creams, a drop clary sage, or a drop of the digestion blend in a cup of herbal tea or water. Inhaling these aromas also helps.

- Stress related migraines respond to the Comforting blend or lavender massaged into the toes or the ear lobes (the area corresponding to the head).

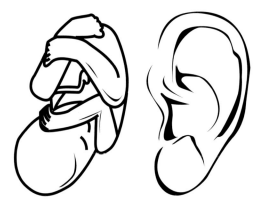

- Migraines that result from digestion issues respond well to ingesting a drop or trace of peppermint, sweet basil, the digestion blend, or the liver blend in a cup of herbal tea or warm water (with a little honey if desired). Try a massage with a few drops of any of these oils on the abdomen, the arches of your feet, or the upper area on your ears. If this works.

- Chronic headaches require a deeper action, such as digestive cleansing. See the instructions under Cleansing earlier in this section.

- Once you identify which types of headaches are most common for you, try diffusing 20 drops of the oils that correspond to your most common headache types.

CLINICAL SUPPORT

"... Results suggest that antioxidant and antiapoptotic activities of the lavender essential oils are the major mechanisms for their potent neuroprotective effects against scopolamine-induced oxidative stress in the rat brain (Hancianu M, et al., 2012).

"The present study suggests that inhalation of lavender essential oil may be effective and safe treatment modality in acute management of migraine headaches" (Sasannejad P, et al., 2012).

Peppermint helps my headaches

I've never tried anything like essential oils before. One night a friend put two drops of peppermint on my hands and asked me to rub my hands together, cup them over my nose and mouth and inhale. WOW. Then she told me to put a little oil on my forehead, temples and on the back of my neck. I noticed that I immediately felt calm and relaxed, so I decided to try it the next time I got a headache. I was taking a lot of pain medication for headaches. I knew all the over-the-counter headache medication wasn't good for me. I was amazed at how well the peppermint worked. Now I use peppermint instead of pills.

Heart & Cardiovascular Conditions

Cardiovascular conditions usually result from lifestyle habits followed for decades. These habits must be changed for any significant improvement to take place. Follow the dietary guidelines and exercise habits recommended in this book. Make sure you involve a competent health care professional in the treatment of all serious cardiovascular symptoms and conditions.

Chronic Progressive Heart Failure

WHAT IT IS

Insufficient pumping action of the heart. The associated swelling that comes with fluid retention can create cellulite and other symptoms.

RECOMMENDED OILS

Lavender			Marjoram		
Peppermint			Rosemary		
Neroli			Ylang ylang		

RECOMMENDED BLENDS

Comforting blend		Balancing blend	
Focusing blend		Stress control blend	
Mental focus blend			

INSTRUCTION

• Some of the oils listed are heart tonics with stimulant action (peppermint, rosemary, and marjoram) and the others, including the recommended blends are more calming. Under the direction of a health care professional:

• For associated fluid retention, gently apply 2 to 3 drops of lavender diluted in a teaspoon of carrier oil over areas of fluid retention. Massage toward the heart.

• Diffuse 5 to 10 drops of any of the calming oils list at any time during the day for their calming, restorative action.

• To help with fluid retention and cellulite, Dr. Pénoël suggest a blend of Eucalyptus radiata (10%), lemon (10%), cedarwood (10%), sage (10%), cypress (10%), tea tree (10%), and carrier oil (40%). Gently massage this blend into the affected areas three times a day for 30 days +++P. You can use clear plastic to help the oils penetrate. Wrap the area for a half an hour, put your feet up, and relax.

Heart Attack
(Myocardial infarction)

WHAT IT IS

When blood flow to a section of the heart is blocked long enough for the heart muscle to be damaged or die. Also called coronary thrombosis.

RECOMMENDED OILS

Lavender			Helichrysum		
German chamomile			Roman chamomile		
Tangerine			Bergamot		
Neroli			Ylang ylang		

RECOMMENDED BLENDS

| Comforting blend | | | Stress control blend | | |
| Foot massage blend | | Balancing blend | |

INSTRUCTION

Get professional medical help as quickly as possible. These suggestions are part of an overall plan in cooperation with your health care professional:

• Create a Comforting blend of lavender (25%), helichrysum (25%), and a carrier oil (50%). Fill capsules and take a capsule 3 times a day with food as a calming, settling help for serious heart conditions.

- To decrease anxiety while waiting for health care professionals to arrive or accomplish what they need to do, perform the "M" technique on the hands using one of the recommended calming oils like lavender.

- An undiluted or diluted lavender massage (3 to 4 drops per teaspoon of mixing oil) for the feet can be calming and reassuring.

- Diffuse 20 drops of any of the calming oils listed two or three times daily.

CLINICAL SUPPORT

Report on 7 scientific studies of essential oils used for calming following a heart attack—lavender, Roman chamomile, neroli, marjoram, and German chamomile (Buckle, p. 251).

"The aim of the present study is to review the available literature to determine if there is evidence for effectiveness of aromatherapy in surgical patients to treat anxiety and insomnia, to control pain and nausea, and to dress wounds. Efficacy studies of lavender or orange and peppermint essential oils, to treat anxiety and nausea, respectively, have shown positive results. Finally, there are encouraging data for the treatment of infections, especially for tea tree oil..." (Stea S, Beraudi A, De Pasquale D. et al., 2014).

Heart Rhythm Disorders

WHAT IT IS

An abnormal variation from a normal heart rhythm showing up in one or more of these: speed of heart rate, regularity of the beats, sites where the electrical impulses come from, or the sequence of the activation of heartbeats.

RECOMMENDED OILS

Lavender		Frankincense	
Lavandin		Tangerine	
German chamomile		Roman chamomile	
Ylang ylang		Neroli	
Bergamot		Cypress	
Spruce		Balsam fir	
Pine			

RECOMMENDED BLENDS

Comforting blend		Focusing blend	
Stress control blend		Mental focus blend	

INSTRUCTION

Suggestions that are part of an overall plan involving your health care professional as needed:

- Use lavender, any of the other calming oils, or the Comforting blend applied undiluted or diluted (3 to 4 drops with a teaspoon of carrier oil) for a reflexology foot massage to relieve stress.

- Ingest 2 to 3 drops of the Comforting blend in a quart of drinking water or a drop or trace in your herbal tea. You can also use a toothpick to adjust the amount of your favourite calming essential oil in a glass of water, a cup of hot water, or an herbal tea.

- Diffuse 5 drops of lavender, the Comforting blend, ylang ylang, or any of the other calming oils for 5 minutes at any time during the day for their stress-reducing action.

High Blood Pressure

(Hypertension)

WHAT IT IS

A chronic medical condition in which blood pressure stays higher than normal. It has two measurements: systolic and diastolic. Normal systolic pressure (the first number) ranges between 100 – 140; normal diastolic (the second number) is between 60 – 90. High blood pressure is defined as something consistently over 140/90. It puts a strain on the heart and arteries if not treated. It's a major risk factor for stroke, aneurysms (ballooning) of the arteries, and is a cause of chronic kidney disease. Symptoms include headaches (especially at the back of the head in the morning), lightheadedness, dizziness, buzzing or ringing in the ears (tinnitus), and fainting.

RECOMMENDED OILS

Tea tree		Lavender	
Helichrysum		Juniper	
Lavandin		Patchouli	
Rosewood		Vetiver	

RECOMMENDED BLENDS

Circulation blend		Comforting blend	
Stress control blend			

INSTRUCTION

Suggestions as part of an overall plan under the direction of your health care professional as needed:

- Use 2 or 3 drops of one of the recommended oils, undiluted, for a regular reflexology foot massage to help control stress.

- Avoid using a lot of peppermint, cinnamon, rosemary or other highly stimulating oils over an extended period of time if you have high blood pressure. Occasional use for indigestion or a painful bump is fine.

- Diffuse 5 to 10 drops of the recommended oils, for 5 minutes at any time during the day for its calming effect.

- Have a calming aromatic bath using 10 – 15 drops of any of the recommended oils mixed with a cup of Epsom Salts.

CLINICAL SUPPORT

To evaluate the hypertensive effects of a massage with essential oils, the experimental group received a massage with essential oils weekly. The placebo group received a massage using an artificial fragrance weekly. BP, pulse rate, sleep conditions, and 24-hour ambulatory BP were monitored before and after the experiment. There was a significant improvement in blood pressure and sleep quality (Ju MS, et al., 2013).

This study identified the effects of essential oil inhalation on blood pressure in prehypertensive and hypertensive subjects. There were significant decreases blood pressure. Authors concluded that essential oils may have relaxation effects for controlling hypertension (Kim IH, et al., 2012).

Low Blood Pressure

(Hypotension)

WHAT IT IS

A low force of blood pushing through the arteries. The systolic blood pressure (first number) is less than 90 and the diastolic pressure (second number) less than 60. People in top physical health can have a low blood pressure, therefore, in actual practice, blood pressure is only considered too low if there are symptoms like dizziness and fainting.

RECOMMENDED OILS

Peppermint 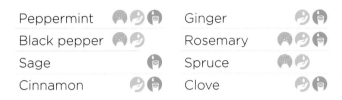		Ginger	
Black pepper		Rosemary	
Sage		Spruce	
Cinnamon		Clove	

RECOMMENDED BLENDS

Massage blend

INSTRUCTION

- Incorporate more of the stimulating and energizing oils listed into your daily life.

- Use any of the recommended oils in a diluted massage (3 to 4 drops per teaspoon of carrier oil). They can also be applied undiluted or blended with the foot massage blend for an energizing reflexology foot massage.

- Put 2 to 3 drops of peppermint in each quart of drinking water or add a trace to your herbal tea. You can also use a toothpick to stir a trace of lemon into a glass of water, a cup of hot water, or herbal tea.

- Diffuse 5 to 10 drops of any of the recommended oils at any time during the day for their energizing action.

Pericarditis

WHAT IT IS

Inflammation of the covering of the heart. This is a condition that requires the attention of a health care professional. With his or her involvement, add this helpful therapy recommended by Dr. Pénoël.

RECOMMENDED OILS

Eucalyptus radiata		Tangerine	

RECOMMENDED BLENDS

Circulation blend

INSTRUCTION

Apply any of the oils listed to the chest right over the heart every 15 minutes during a crisis ++++P.

Heartburn (Acid reflux & GERD)

WHAT IT IS

A painful burning just below or behind the breastbone, usually coming from the esophagus. The pain seems to rise in the chest from the stomach and can spread to the neck or throat. It can be so severe—especially in the evening and at night—that people have to sleep in a semi-upright position. Chronic conditions can damage the tissues of the digestive system and create more serious conditions.

RECOMMENDED OILS

German chamomile		Roman chamomile	
Lavender		Marjoram	
Lemon		Peppermint	
Spearmint		Black pepper	
Sweet basil			

RECOMMENDED BLEND

Digestion blend

INSTRUCTION

- Many cases of heartburn can be helped with the following dietary adjustments: more whole foods (especially raw foods), fewer highly-processed foods (sodas, sugar, white flour), more dietary fiber, sufficient prebiotics and probiotics, paying attention to the way you mix foods, and the amount of food you eat at one time.

• Drink a cup of hot or cold water with a trace or drop of sweet basil, peppermint, spearmint, lemon, or the digestion blend before or after a meal. Add honey if needed. Use a toothpick to adjust the flavor.

• Refer to diagnostic guide or medical professional for signs that your heartburn is lasting too long or is more serious than should be treated by home remedies alone.

Heat Stroke (Sunstroke)

WHAT IT IS

The most serious form of heat injury. The most obvious symptoms are fainting and a body temperature over 105 degrees Fahrenheit. Other signs include a throbbing headache, dizziness, light-headedness, dry skin (not sweating), red skin, muscle weakness, cramps, nausea, vomiting, fast heartbeat, rapid breathing, shallow breathing, confusion, disorientation, staggering, seizures, or unconsciousness. Call 911 immediately because this is a medical emergency and any delay can prove fatal or cause serious brain damage.

RECOMMENDED OILS

Peppermint		Spearmint	
Birch		Wintergreen	

RECOMMENDED BLEND

Mental focus blend	

INSTRUCTIONS

• Call 911 and while waiting for paramedics, perform these first-aid procedures: If a thermometer is available, the goal is to cool the body temperature to at most 101 or 102 degrees Fahrenheit as quickly as possible. If no thermometer is available, cool the body temperature so it feels more like the temperatures of those who are not experiencing heat stroke.

• Try these strategies: Fan yourself while wetting your skin with water from a sponge, cloth, or garden hose.

• Drink whatever safe liquid you can find (preferably water). Adding a trace of peppermint in the water will help bring a "cooling energy" quickly into the body.

• Apply ice packs (or bags of frozen foods) to the armpits, groin, neck, and back— areas where blood vessels are close to the skin.

• Get in a cool shower, a tub of cool water, or a bath with some ice to cool it. A few drops of peppermint on a damp body can enhance the cooling action.

• After recovering from heat stroke, a person will be more sensitive to high temperatures during the week following a heat stroke, so it will be important to drink plenty of liquids with a little peppermint for cooling, stay out of the heat, and avoid heavy exercise until a health professional confirms that it's okay to perform normal activities.

Hemorrhoids

(See constipation)

WHAT THEY ARE

Swollen veins in the anal canal that are painful, but not usually serious. They can swell inside the anal canal to form internal hemorrhoids or near the opening to bulge out and form external hemorrhoids. You can have both types at the same time. They are caused by too much pressure on the veins from straining due to constipation. Pregnancy can also contribute to hemorrhoids. Signs of hemorrhoids include bleeding during bowel movements or seeing red blood on toilet paper, itching, and pain in the anal area.

RECOMMENDED OILS

Lavender		Sweet basil	
Helichrysum		Cypress	
Tea tree			

RECOMMENDED BLENDS

Inflammation blend		Liver blend	
Digestion blend			

INSTRUCTION

- Refer to a medical guidebook or website for an accurate diagnosis, then use the following remedies with the involvement of a health care professional when appropriate.

- Follow instructions given in the constipation section (above) to relieve the pressure that leads to or aggravates hemorrhoids.

- To relieve itching and prevent infection, create a blend of 3-4 drops of lavender oil in a half teaspoon of carrier oil and apply to the affected veins.

- Ingest a drop of the liver and digestion blends three times a day in water or juice.

- Enjoy a warm bath with 5 to 10 drops of lavender or tea tree oil mixed in a cup of Epsom Salts.

- Defer to your health care professional to make sure that the signs associated with hemorrhoids are not more serious than home care alone should treat.

- Dr. Pénoël suggests using an equal blend of patchouli and cypress 50:50 with a carrier oil for hemorrhoids ++++P.

CLINICAL SUPPORT

A double-blind, placebo-controlled clinical trial tested a topical formulation including tea tree oil for an anti-hemorrhoidal treatment. Anal pain, pain during defecation, visible bleeding, pruritus and irritation/inflammation were recorded. Safety and tolerability of the treatments were also recorded. The treatment significantly reduced all the symptoms compared to placebo (Joksimovic N, et al., 2012).

Hepatitis (VIRAL)

WHAT IT IS

A liver inflammation caused by a viral infection. The condition can heal on its own, or it can progress to fibrosis (scarring) and cirrhosis of the liver, a serious, life-threatening condition. You may have hepatitis with few or no symptoms; but jaundice, a poor appetite, and unexplained physical and emotional exhaustion may be signs. It is most often caused by viruses, but it can also be caused by toxic substances including alcohol and some medications, autoimmune diseases, and some industrial solvents and plants.

RECOMMENDED OILS

Sweet Basil		Ravintsara		
Peppermint		Cypress		
Roman Chamomile		German Chamomile		
Eucalyptus Radiata		Lemon		
Rosemary		Thyme		

RECOMMENDED BLENDS

Liver blend		Protecting blend	

INSTRUCTION

In-home procedures suggested as part of an overall plan involving your health care professional:

- Your goal is to ingest 5 to 10 drops of the Protecting blend, peppermint, lemon, sweet basil, or the Liver blend daily. You can do this in your drinking water, capsules, or herbal teas. Mix 1 drop per quart of water or a trace per cup of herbal tea.

- An easier way to take oils internally is to blend 2 or three of the oils in equal parts. Here's a sample recipe: sweet basil 25%, peppermint 25%, and carrier oil 50%. Fill capsules with a dropper and take a capsule three times a day with food. Any of the oils on the list oils for ingestion would work in a blend.

- Massage the liver area of the feet and the part of the chest over the liver with 2 or 3 drops of any of the recommended oils undiluted. The only oil on the list you will want to always dilute is thyme. Dilute thyme 25:75 with a carrier oil before topical application.

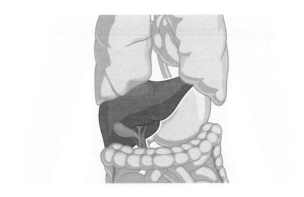

Hiccups

WHAT THEY ARE

Involuntary repetitive contractions of the diaphragm that may repeat several times. The rhythm and time between hiccups tends to be relatively constant. They usually resolve themselves without any treatment, although many remedies are suggested to help shorten the duration.

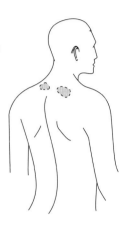

RECOMMENDED OILS

Sweet Basil		Lavender	

RECOMMENDED BLENDS

Comforting blend	

INSTRUCTION

In-home procedures:

- Apply a trace of sweet basil undiluted on the back on either side of the 5th cervical vertebra as shown.

- Lick a trace of sweet basil or lavender off the back of your hand and hold it in your mouth for 2 minutes.

- Place a drop of sweet basil or lavender on the back of your neck.

- Place a few drops of any of the recommended oils in your palm. Rub hands together, cup hands over mouth and nose, and breathe deeply several times, holding your breath for 10 seconds each time.

Hives & Rashes

WHAT THEY ARE

Hives vs Rash

Hives (urticaria) is a skin condition characterized by visible red bumps that are raised and itchy. A rash is a change in the skin causing discoloration and an unusual texture and look. Hives typically result from a serious allergic reaction caused by an allergic trigger. Rashes, on the other hand, are the result of a number of causes including, allergies from medicines, foods, metals, dyes, etc.; fungal infections; anxiety; a viral or bacterial infection; chafing; a reaction to immunization; or menstruation. Rashes itch less than hives.

RECOMMENDED OILS

Roman chamomile	German chamomile
Lavender	

RECOMMENDED BLENDS

Immune balancing blend	Liver blend
Digestion blend	Inflammation blend

INSTRUCTION

- Add these home remedies as part of an overall plan involving your health care professional as needed.

- For chronic conditions do an Immune Strengthening Cleanse that lasts at least one year.

- For rashes, mix this blend. In a teaspoon of carrier oil, mix 3 to 4 drops of the inflammation blend and apply to the affected area two or more times daily. If the rash area is large, be sure to patch test the blend on a small area for 24 hours before applying it to the whole area.

- With hives, be cautious of skin applications because of likely allergic reactions. The immune balance blend would be safer taken internally accompanied by the liver blend and possibly even the Digestion blend. See instructions in the Immune Strengthening Cleanse under Cleanses listed earlier in this section.

Hypoglycemia
(Low blood sugar)

WHAT IT IS

A metabolic condition resulting from excess insulin in the body due to medications, a complication of diabetes treatment, insufficient carbohydrates, etc. Most people can treat it themselves by regulating their diet, typically by having more frequent meals. It is characterized by disorientation, depression, and cloudy thinking.

RECOMMENDED OILS

Sweet basil	Lemon
Grapefruit	

RECOMMENDED BLENDS

Liver blend	Ingestion blend

INSTRUCTION

- Suggestion as part of an overall plan involving your health care professional as needed:

- First of all, adjust your diet to avoid quick sugars found in candy, sodas, breads, pasta, and most processed and other highly refined food products. This is an extremely critical component. Your body's metabolism needs a diet of slow sugars found in whole foods: steamed vegetables, legumes, whole raw fruits, non-bread whole grains, nuts, seeds, etc. The dietary guidelines in this book suggest this type of diet. Have more frequent meals or healthy snacks between meals to provide a steady flow of nutrients.

- Add a drop of the liver blend to each quart of your drinking water or a trace in each cup of herbal tea at least twice a day.

- You can also mix the liver blend with a carrier oil (50:50) and fill capsules. Take 3 capsules a day with food.

- For a deeper resolution of this condition, do a Digestion Cleanse for a year. You'll see instructions earlier in this chapter.

Hypothermia

WHAT IT IS

A dangerously low body temperature, under 95 °F (35 °C).

RECOMMENDED OILS

Sweet basil		Black pepper	
Rosemary		Marjoram	

RECOMMENDED BLENDS

Massage blend

INSTRUCTION

Follow instructions from a first-aid guide on warming your body with fluids, clothing, blankets, etc. In addition, follow these suggestions using essential oils:

- Use 3 to 5 drops of the Massage blend undiluted with a warm, damp cloth on areas where you can warm the body quickly: wrists, elbows, ankles, knees, or armpits.

- Drink a cup of herbal tea or warm water with a drop of any of the stimulating oils.

- Massage your body with a 50:50 blend of the Massage blend and a carrier oil.

- Create a warming bath or foot bath with 5 – 15 drops of a stimulating essential oil in a cup of Epsom Salts.

Impetigo

WHAT IT IS

Impetigo is a highly contagious, infectious skin condition.

RECOMMENDED OILS

Tea tree		Thyme	
Lemongrass			

RECOMMENDED BLENDS

Circulation blend		Protecting blend	
Liver blend		Foot massage blend	

INSTRUCTION

- Because recommendations can vary according to the type of skin condition, make sure you have a correct diagnosis of impetigo from a health care professional, and then follow these recommendations according to what you learn.

- Begin by making sure you have a healthy diet focused on fruits, vegetables, whole grains, heart-healthy oils, and drinking at least a 1/2 gallon of water every day. Exercise the equivalent of walking at least 2 miles daily to increase circulation.

- If you are certain this is infectious impetigo, Dr. Pénoël recommends an equal blend of thyme, tea tree, and Eucalyptus globulus applied in a 25:75 dilution with a carrier oil. Apply it 3 or 4 times a day for 8 to 10 days ++++P. The same blend can be made into capsules to be taken 3 times a day with food.

- Mix 20 to 40 drops of lavender, the inflammation blend, or a Comforting blend in a mild, fragrance-free and non-toxic lotion. Apply the lotion to the affected areas after each bath or shower and whenever you wash your hands. You can also mix 4 to 5 drops of the oil into each application lotion.

- Take warm (not hot) baths with 5 to 10 drops of lavender, Roman chamomile, the Protecting blend, the inflammation blend, or the Comforting blend dispersed in a cup of Epsom Salts.

- After your bath or shower, apply 4 to 5 drops of lavender, tea tree, or the Protecting blend mixed in a tablespoon of mixing oil to the affected areas.

- Take a capsule three times a day with a strong Protecting blend mixed 50:50 with a carrier oil or a blend of thyme (10%), cinnamon (5%), lemongrass (10%), and carrier oil (75%). Fill capsules and take one capsule 3 times daily with food.

Infant & Child Care

For all symptoms relating to children, be sure to have a home health care guide handy online or in print to answer questions and give guidelines. Be sure your child's pediatrician or health care professional is comfortable with alternative therapies like using essential oils. He or she should be familiar with the safety rules and be confident that you understand them as well. Invite your health care professional to look through this guide. Be sure your health care provider is cautious about prescribing antibiotics when there are safer and gentler ways to deal with childhood infections using essential oils.

Here is a list of the most common childhood conditions and ways you can use essential oils to treat them safely and effectively.

Chicken Pox

WHAT IT IS

A viral childhood infection that causes a fever and widespread crops of extremely itchy blisters all over the body. It is highly contagious. It sometimes occurs in adults, and although there is usually a lifetime immunity to the disease following the childhood infection, it can recur in the form of painful shingles.

RECOMMENDED OILS

Tea tree		Lavender	
Lemongrass		German chamomile	
Roman chamomile			

RECOMMENDED BLENDS

Digestion blend	Liver blend
Protecting blend	Immune balancing blend

INSTRUCTION

- Mix 50 to 100 drops of tea tree in a half cup of talc. Stir well. Put the antimicrobial mixture in a shaker and shake it over the infected area so you don't even have to touch the skin.

- Create capsules by mixing 50:50 the Protecting blend and a carrier oil. Take 3 capsules a day with food.

- Take a drop of the Protecting blend in an herbal tea with honey, drinking water, juice, or recipes (after taking the recipe off the stove). Small children will do better taking the Protecting blend in juice, water, or food.

- Make a topical paste using 3 or 4 drops of any single oil or a mixture of any the following: the Protecting blend, Eucalyptus radiata, tea tree, and lavender. Drop them in a tablespoon of corn starch or green clay powder and add enough carrier oil to make a paste you can manage easily. Apply it on the chickenpox lesions.

- You can also massage the feet of children and even babies with 1 or 2 drops of the Protecting blend diluted in a teaspoon of carrier oil. Do this several times daily.

- If there is a high fever with the chickenpox, mix a drop of peppermint in a cup of tepid water. Soak a cloth in the mixture and wipe the child's back. This will cool the child safely and quickly. Remember to not put peppermint on the neck of children under 30 months.

Colic

WHAT IT IS

Regular episodes of inconsolable crying, usually at the same time every day. It's caused by intestinal gas or obstruction in the intestines.

RECOMMENDED OILS

Lavender	Sweet basil
Roman chamomile	German chamomile
Tea tree	

RECOMMENDED BLEND

Comforting blend

INSTRUCTION

With the approval of your health care professional as needed, try the following safe, in-home procedures:

- Massage your baby's feet with a drop of one or more of the following oils blended in a half teaspoon of mixing oil: children's blend, the Comforting blend, or topical basil.

- Use a toothpick to gather only a trace of sweet basil and mix it with the baby's food or formula.

- Create a tummy blend and keep it on hand for multiple uses when an extremely mild blend is needed. Lavender (20%), Roman chamomile (20%), tea tree (10%), and a carrier oil (50%). Use this blend for a gentle foot and possibly abdominal massage.

Cradle Cap

WHAT IT IS

A thick, scaly rash that appears on the scalp during first months of life.

RECOMMENDED OILS

Lavender

Roman chamomile

Marjoram

Tea tree

German chamomile

INSTRUCTION

After reviewing a home health care guide or an authoritative online resource to be sure your diagnosis is correct, use this in-home procedure:

- Massage a drop of lavender diluted in 1/2 teaspoon of carrier oil on the baby's head.

Croup

WHAT IT IS

Inflammation and narrowing of the main airway—larynx—due to a viral infection.

RECOMMENDED OILS

Lavender

Roman chamomile

Tea tree

Cypress

Myrtle

Helichrysum

German chamomile

Marjoram

Rosemary

RECOMMENDED BLEND

Comforting blend

INSTRUCTION

After a review of a home health care guide and with the approval of your health care professional, try the following in-home procedures:

- Prepare a warm and damp towel soaked in aromatic water created by mixing 10 drops of tea tree and 10 drops of lavender in a cup of warm water. Squeeze out excess water. Place the towel all around the neck and nape of neck of the child. Place a dry towel over it. The damp towel with help reduce the dryness in the lungs.

- Create an all-purpose children's blend and keep it on hand for multiple uses when an extremely mild blend is needed for childhood respiratory conditions. Lavender (20%), Roman chamomile (30%), tea tree (25%), marjoram (10%), cypress (5%), rosemary (5%), and myrtle (5%). For all infants and children, mix the blend 25:75 with a carrier oil.

- Massage 1 to 3 drops of the blend undiluted on the balls of the baby's feet two or three times a day.

- If there is no discomfort or redness when applying the blend topically (try it on a small area of skin first). Try using 2 to 3 drops in a teaspoon of carrier oil. Massage it on the baby's chest and back.

- Mix a teaspoon of Epsom Salts with 2 to 4 drops of this blend and mix them in the baby's bath water.

- Diffuse 5 to 10 drops of the children's blend for 5 minutes before bed and whenever the condition seems most prominent.

Diaper Rash

WHAT IT IS

Irritation of an infant's skin in the area covered by a diaper. It's usually caused by too-long contact with urine.

RECOMMENDED OILS

Lavender		Tea tree	
Roman chamomile		German chamomile	
Tangerine		Helichrysum	

INSTRUCTION

- Dilute a drop of tea tree and a drop of lavender with 1 teaspoon of mixing oil. Apply to rash area as needed.

- Try a drop of helichrysum with a drop of tangerine mixed with a teaspoon of carrier oil for a topical application to the rash area.

> I have been working with essential oils in massage for several years. I frequently use lavender with my children for diaper rash, poison ivy and cuts. They enjoy the smell, it doesn't linger a long time on them, and everything seems to clear up quicker than other things I've used.

Diarrhea & Vomiting in Children

WHAT IT IS

A common condition usually due to a short-term childhood infection.

RECOMMENDED OILS

Lavender		Tea tree	
Roman chamomile		German chamomile	
Tangerine		Marjoram	

INSTRUCTION

- Consult a home health care guide or authoritative website for the kinds of liquids and foods to introduce when. Be aware of unusual danger signs related specifically to vomiting and diarrhea in children under 12.

- Create this "tummy blend" for many uses when an extremely mild blend is needed. Lavender (40%), Roman chamomile (40%), tea tree (20%). Mix 2 drops with a teaspoon of carrier oil and gently massage the abdomen.

Fever

WHAT IT IS

A temporary increase in body temperature in response to an illness. A child has a fever when the rectal temperature is above 100.4 °F (38 °C) or 99.5 °F (37.5 °C) measured in the armpit.

RECOMMENDED OILS

Peppermint		Spearmint	

RECOMMENDED BLEND

Protecting blend		Respiratory blend	

INSTRUCTION

A fever is the body's way to help heal a disease. Use wisdom in not lowering a fever too quickly using over-the-counter remedies that may, over time, do more harm than good. After a review of a competent home health care guide and with the approval of your health care professional if necessary, use these in-home procedures:

- Only lower a child's fever if it is over 102 degrees Fahrenheit.

- For children under 6, soak a small gauze or cloth in a solution of 1 cup of tepid water with a drop of Eucalyptus radiata. Place the cloth around the child's ankles, wrists, knees, or elbows to cool a fever.

- For children over 6 and for adults, soak a small cloth in a solution of I cup of tepid water with 1 drop of peppermint. Put the cloth on the wrists, elbows, ankles, or knees. You can gently rub the mixture on the chest and back.

- Mix 2 drops of peppermint in a teaspoon of carrier oil and massage the child's back.

- You can lower a fever by holding a baby in a warm shower or giving an older child a warm shower.

- Blend 3 to 5 drops of peppermint or spearmint in a half cup of Epsom Salts and dissolve in a warm bath.

Heat Rash (Prickly Heat)

WHAT IT IS

A childhood skin disease (Miliaria) that is most common during hot, humid summer months and in the tropics. It is most often seen in children and infants because of their underdeveloped sweat glands. It is also called sweat rash. It manifests as multiple small, raised, itchy area on the body.

RECOMMENDED OILS

Lavender   Roman chamomile

German chamomile

INSTRUCTION

After a review of a home health care guide or authoritative diagnostic website, try the following safe in-home procedures:

- Mix a drop of lavender in a cup of water and spray it on the child's chest and back. Or you can soak a small cloth in the solution and apply it to the chest and back several times a day.

- Put a drop of lavender in a quart of water or juice and drink frequently through the day.

Pinworms

WHAT THEY ARE

An infestation of thin worms that lay eggs around the anus, causing intense itching.

RECOMMENDED OILS

Tea tree   Roman chamomile

Lemon   Lavender

INSTRUCTION

Check with a home health care guide or authoritative website to make sure your diagnosis is correct, then try the following in-home procedure:

- Apply an undiluted drop of tea tree on the affected area 2 to 4 times a day.

- Create a calming herbal tea with a little honey using traces of any of these oils, which help expel pinworms and their toxic effects: lemon, bergamot, and sweet basil.

Infected Wounds

WHAT THEY ARE

Wounds in which microorganisms have colonized, causing either a deterioration of the wound or a delay in healing. Bacteria is usually the cause, but a weakened immune system can allow pathogens to take over. Studies show that 70 percent of the deaths after surgery are caused by surgical site infections. Some infections are remarkably difficult to heal, and essential oils can help.

RECOMMENDED OILS

Tea tree			Lavender		
Lavandin			Helichrysum		
Roman chamomile			German chamomile		
Frankincense			Bergamot		
Rosemary					

RECOMMENDED BLEND

Protecting blend

INSTRUCTIONS

In-home procedures suggested as part of an overall plan involving your health care professional.

- Help reduce infection in a wound by applying a drop or two of tea tree or the Protecting blend undiluted on the wound 3 or 4 times daily. This will begin a deep action that will start clearing up the infection without requiring antibiotics. Visit with your health care professional about substituting tea tree or the Protecting blend for antibiotics.

- Dr. Pénoël recommends this blend for helping overcome infections in hard-to-heal wounds: Five drops of helichrysum and 5 drops of rosemary in two tablespoons of carrier. Apply to the wound twice daily ++++P.

- Here is another blend he recommends: Rosemary (6%), lavender (4%), and a carrier oil (90%). Apply to the wound twice daily ++++P.

- These last two blends can help to reduce scarring in old wounds if applied twice daily over an extended period (3 to 6 months) ++++P.

- Blend Protecting blend diluted 50:50 with a carrier oil and fill capsules. Take a capsule three times a day with food until the wound is healed.

Influenza (FLU)

WHAT IT IS

A respiratory disease caused by the influenza (flu) virus. Strains typically change from year to year, varying in intensity. Symptoms include fever, chills, muscle pain, backache, sore throat, headache, dry cough, and chest pain.

RECOMMENDED OILS

Tea tree			Ravintsara		
Eucalyptus radiata			Eucalyptus globulus		
Pine			Spruce		
Lemon			Thyme		
Peppermint			Balsam fir		
Oregano					

RECOMMENDED BLEND

Antimicrobia blend

Immune balancing blend

Respiratory blend

INSTRUCTION

With the approval of your health care professional as needed, use the following in-home procedures:

- Massage your back and chest with a blend of 5 to 6 drops balsam fir, Eucalyptus radiata, lemon, or the Respiratory blend in a teaspoon of carrier oil.

- Diffuse 20 drops daily of any of the recommended diffusing oils during the cold and flu season. Diffuse tea tree, Eucalyptus radiata, the respiratory blend, the Protecting blend or the Immune balancing blend.

- Create capsules by blending either the Respiratory blend or the Protecting blend 50:50 with a carrier oil. Fill capsules with a dropper and take 3 to 6 capsules a day with food. Continue taking the capsules for at least 7 to 10 days after your symptoms have subsided.

- Every day apply 2 to 3 drops of the Respiratory blend, the Protecting blend, or the Immune balancing blend undiluted to the lung reflexology area of the foot (between the ball and the arch).

- To help relieve infection in the lungs through the chest or upper back, apply hot cloths soaked in a mixture of 1 cup warm water and 6 drops each of tea tree, balsam fir, Eucalyptus radiata, and either the respiratory blend or the Protecting blend. Or you can apply the oils undiluted on the back or the chest and then put a damp cloth over it. This allows for maximum and quick absorption.

- To rapidly get a lot of essential oil molecules into your system, try Dr. Pénoël's "Live Embalming" therapy found in Chapter 4. Use 5 to 10 drops at a time for a total of 20 or 30 drops of Eucalyptus radiata or ravintsara with a hair dryer to get a large amount of essential oils to penetrate the body in a short amount of time. Be sure to change locations on the body with each application. Be sure to read the instructions in Chapter 4 before trying this therapy.

CLINICAL SUPPORT

Tea tree oil exhibits antiviral activity against the influenza virus. This study attempted to show how it is done biologically (Garozzo A, et al., 2011).

Insect Bites & Stings

WHAT THEY ARE

A skin reaction from contact with an insect. The bite of fire ants or the sting from bees, wasps, and hornets are usually painful. Bites caused by mosquitoes, fleas, and mites are more likely to create itching than pain.

RECOMMENDED OILS

Citronella		Lemongrass	
Eucalyptus Globulus		Peppermint	
Lemon		Tangerine	
Lime			

RECOMMENDED BLENDS

Purifying blend		Soothing blend	
Protecting blend			

INSTRUCTION

- As quickly as possible use a trace or drop of the purifying blend, peppermint, or the soothing blend on an insect bite or sting. The oils will work quickly and effectively +++++P.

- A blend of 3 drops each of lime, lemon, and tangerine applied undiluted or blended with a little water will help stop the itching of mosquito bites +++++P.

Bee sting experience

It seems to me that the misery of a bee sting seemed to last for days. So imagine my surprise when I got a bee sting the other day and tried a purifying blend on it. Within ten minutes the pain had vanished—no swelling, no burning, nothing. It was completely gone.
I've since learned that I have to act quickly. If I wait too long before grabbing the oils, it takes longer to stop the pain, and there's still some stinging, but not as bad as before. It's amazing how fast it works when it's used right away.

Insect Repellent

WHAT IT IS

A substance that you spray in the air, diffuse, apply topically, or take internally to repel insects.

RECOMMENDED OILS

Citronella		Lemongrass	
Peppermint		Eucalyptus globulus	

RECOMMENDED BLEND

Purifying blend

INSTRUCTIONS

- Mix 4 – 5 drops of each of the following: tea tree, peppermint, and citronella or lemongrass in a cup of water and either distribute over skin and clothing or put it in a spray ++++P.

- Diffuse any of the recommended oils.

- Take the oils in your drinking water or in 50:50 capsules with a carrier oil (one capsule daily with food) to keep insects at bay.

- Peppermint is a safe and aromatic insect repellent. Create a spray with 4 to 5 drops of peppermint shaken into 1/2 cup water. Spray or spread on skin and clothing. This spray can be used around the house to keep ants and other insects out.

CLINICAL SUPPORT

These recent tests in Thailand demonstrated the effectiveness of citronella and lemongrass as insect repellents (Boonyuan, Wasana et al., 2014).

Essential oils of peppermint, eucalyptus, anise, basil, and bay laurel were tested for their mosquito repellency. All were effective, with basil and anise being the most active (Erler F, Ulug I, Yalcinkaya B. Fitoterapia. "Repellent activity of five essential oils against Culex pipiens." 2006 Dec;77(7-8):491-4).

Insomnia

(See Emotional Disorders Leading to Insomnia)

WHAT THEY ARE

Difficulty falling asleep, staying asleep, or both

RECOMMENDED OILS

Lavender		Lavandin	
German chamomile		Roman chamomile	
Neroli		Orange	
Bergamot		Tangerine	
Balsam fir		Clary sage	
Sandalwood		Vetiver	
Ylang ylang			

RECOMMENDED BLENDS

Comforting blend		Foot massage blend	
Balancing blend			

INSTRUCTION

If you have severe, chronic issues with insomnia, work with a health care professional and incorporate these suggestions as part of an organized effort to control your symptoms.

- Apply a drop of lavender or any of the other recommended oils undiluted to the outer ear daily.

- Have a balsam fir Layer Therapy treatment weekly. See instructions in the How to Use Essential Oils, Chapter Four. Begin by applying a drop of the Balancing blend to the sternum on the chest. Drip 4 to 5 drops of balsam fir neat up the spine, feather it out with your fingertips, the use your knuckles to work it into both sides of the spine. Then massage a blend of 3 to 4 drops of balsam fir with a teaspoon of the mixing oil on the muscles at the sides of the back in a downward direction. Lie still for about 20 minutes following this massage with a warm, damp compress over the spine.

- Enjoy an aromatic bath before bed using 10 to 15 drops of one of the suggested oils in a cup of Epsom Salts.
- Diffuse 20 drops of one of the calming oils or the Comforting blend while preparing for bed.

- Enjoy a few drops of the calming oil with a few drops of the foot massage blend in a teaspoon of mixing oil massaged on the feet several times a week before bed.

CLINICAL SUPPORT

"The aim of the present study is to review the available literature to determine if there is evidence for effectiveness of aromatherapy in surgical patients to treat anxiety and insomnia, to control pain and nausea, and to dress wounds. Efficacy studies of lavender or orange and peppermint essential oils, to treat anxiety and nausea, respectively, have shown positive results. Finally, there are encouraging data for the treatment of infections, especially for tea tree oil..." (Stea S, Beraudi A, De Pasquale D., 2014).

A calming blend on my feet for a good night's sleep

If I've had a really stressful day, then I know I'm going to have trouble sleeping, so I give myself a complete foot massage with a calming blend and I fall right asleep and wake up feeling so much better.

Irritable Bowel Syndrome

(IBS abdominal bloating, gas pain, flatulence, etc.)

WHAT IT IS

A disorder characterized by abdominal pain and cramping, bloating, gas, diarrhea, constipation, changes in bowel movements, and other aggravating symptoms. It is associated with stress, depression, anxiety, or a previous infection of the digestive system.

RECOMMENDED OILS

Peppermint		Juniper	
Lemon		Ginger	

RECOMMENDED BLENDS

Digestion blend		Comforting blend	
Stress control blend		Mental focus blend	

INSTRUCTION

- Increase your water intake by 2 – 4 extra glasses a day. A drop of spearmint, peppermint, lemon, or the digestion blend can make water more delightful to drink as well as therapeutic.

- Gradually increase your dietary intake of whole foods containing natural fiber—raw and dried fruits and vegetables, as well as whole-grain cereals and breads. Avoid refined flours, processed meats, prepared cereals, animal fats, sugars, and overly processed foods.

- Evaluate your stress. Schedule time for calming meditation, prayers, and exercise, especially calming exercise like walks and yoga. Use frankincense and other calming oils during meditation. Diffuse 20 drops or apply a few drops undiluted topically before meditation.

- Diffuse the mental focus blend for increased energy or focus and the Comforting blend for relaxation.

- Take a calming bath daily with a cup of Epsom Salts mixed with 10 to 15 drops of one of the calming essential oil. Try these blends: Comforting blend, intimacy blend, and Stress control blend. Also try lavender and balsam fir.

- Mix 2 to 3 drops of sweet basil, lavender or the Comforting blend in a tablespoon of carrier oil and massage on the lower back on the sides of the spine in downward motions.

- Do an abdominal massage with the same dilution of oils above starting just below the navel and lightly massaging in a clockwise spiral out to the edge of the rib cage and the pelvis. You can also use the Massage blend (a.m.), Comforting blend (p.m.), or children's blend. Also try the Liver blend and the Digestive blend.

- Massage the bottoms of your feet (especially the arch area), the palms of your hands, and the upper part of the ear with the undiluted Digestion blend, Liver blend, Comforting blend, Stress control blend, peppermint, or sweet basil.

- Refer to a medical diagnostic guide or a health care professional for signs that your symptoms are more serious than personal care alone should treat.

CLINICAL SUPPORT

"The aim of the present study is to review the available literature to determine if there is evidence for effectiveness of aromatherapy in surgical patients to treat anxiety and insomnia, to control pain and nausea, and to dress wounds. Efficacy studies of lavender or orange and peppermint essential oils, to treat anxiety and nausea, respectively, have shown positive results. Finally, there are encouraging data for the treatment of infections, especially for tea tree oil..." (Stea S, Beraudi A, De Pasquale D., 2014).

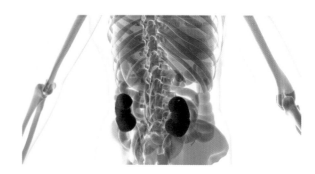

Kidney Stones

WHAT THEY ARE

Solid pebbles formed from dietary minerals in the kidneys or urinary tract. Eighty percent of those with kidney stones are men. Most stones are formed and passed without causing symptoms, but if they grow large enough they can cause a painful obstruction of one of the tubes of the kidney or ureter. This leads to extreme pain, most commonly felt in the back, the lower abdomen, and groin. Symptoms include nausea, vomiting, fever, blood in the urine, pus in the urine, and painful urination. Pain comes in waves lasting 20 to 60 minutes.

RECOMMENDED OILS

Lemon		Lavender	🌀💧
Roman chamomile	🌀💧	Juniper	
Orange		Peppermint	🌀💧
Birch	🌀	Wintergreen	🌀

RECOMMENDED BLEND

Soothing blend	🌀

INSTRUCTION

Suggestions as part of an overall plan involving your health care professional:

- For prevention, have a lemon juice drink daily by mixing the juice of 1/2 lemon in a cup of water with a drop of lemon essential oil +++P.

- To help relieve the pain and help prevent the formation of kidney stones, create an equal blend of cedarwood (25%), juniper (25%), and a carrier oil (50%). Massage to the kidney area of the back (just under the lowest ribs) 3 to 4 times a day +++P.

- Take a lemon oil and carrier oil blend (50:50) in a capsule 3 times a day +++P.

- To help with the pain, massage the back with the Soothing blend undiluted as needed.

- Increase your water intake by adding a drop of lemon oil per quart of drinking water. Enjoy at least two quarts of this aromatic water a day. Extend your capacity gradually to as much as a gallon of water per day.

Laryngitis

WHAT IT IS

An inflammation or infection of the vocal cords usually associated with a respiratory infection. The cords swell, changing the sound they produce. In severe cases, the sound becomes a hoarse whisper.

RECOMMENDED OILS

Peppermint	🖐️🌀💧	Eucalyptus radiata	🖐️🌀
Lemon	🖐️🌀💧	Frankincense	🖐️🌀
Juniper	🖐️🌀	Spruce	🖐️🌀
Thyme	🌀💧		

RECOMMENDED BLENDS

Respiratory blend

Antimicrobial blend

INSTRUCTION

- Prepare a warm and damp towel soaked in aromatic water created by mixing 10 drops of tea tree and 10 drops of lavender in a cup of warm water. Squeeze out excess water. Place the towel all around the neck and nape of neck. Place a dry towel over it. The damp towel with help reduce the dryness in the lungs.

- Create an antibacterial mouthwash using 2 drops of tea tree oil in 1/2 cup of water. Shake vigorously, gargle, and swallow.

- Lick a trace of tea tree, the Respiratory blend, or the Protecting blend off the back of your hand. Mix it in your mouth with saliva for a minute then swallow it. Do this often throughout the day.

- For deep healing, use a drop of the Respiratory blend in each quart of your drinking water for a month after your symptoms have subsided.

- Use 3 or 4 drops of any of the respiratory essential oils dropped into steaming water. Place a cloth over your head and inhale deeply many times. You can reheat the water, add more oil and continue this therapy as long as you need to help break up the encrusted mucous on your vocal cords.

- Take a hot bath with 15 drops of any of the respiratory oils mixed with a cup of Epsom Salts.

- Apply 3 to 4 drops of Eucalyptus radiata undiluted to your throat several times a day.

Leprosy (Hansen's disease)

WHAT IT IS

An infection affecting the nerves and skin, causing numbness and disfigurement.

RECOMMENDED OILS

Lavender

Tea tree

RECOMMENDED BLENDS

Immune balancing blend

Protecting blend

INSTRUCTION

Use the following in-home procedures with the approval of your health care professional:

- The most effective oils are lavender, tea tree, the immune balancing blend, and the Protecting blend. They can be used singly or in a blend of equal parts.

- Apply any of the recommended oils undiluted directly on lesions.

- Take up to 16 drops of the recommended oil(s) each day. This can conveniently be done by taking 3 capsules a day with food. Blend any one or a mixture of the oils 50:50 with a carrier oil and fill capsules with a dropper.

- Take 1 or 2 drops of any of the recommended oils in an herbal tea with honey. Add a drop to a quart of drinking water. Add them to juice or to recipes (after taking them off the stove).

Lice Infestations

WHAT THEY ARE

Populations of tiny parasites that feed on human blood. There are three types: head lice, body lice, and pubic lice. All three forms are passed along easily and can spread quickly through a family or a classroom. Itching from the bites is a common symptom.

RECOMMENDED OILS

Eucalyptus globulus		Myrtle	
Tea tree		Thyme	
Bergamot		Lavender	
Rosemary			

RECOMMENDED BLEND

Protecting blend

INSTRUCTION

- Essential oils are a much safer alternative to the toxic treatment that is commonly prescribed for lice infestations.

- Mix 10 to 15 drops of any of the recommended oils into a single application of your shampoo or conditioner. Massage into scalp. Put a disposable shower cap over your hair and let it sit for 30 minutes.

- After rinsing your hair, add 4 to 5 drops of one of these oils to a half cup of water, massage it into your scalp and leave this solution on your hair for another 10 minutes before rinsing.

- You will want to repeat these procedures every 48 hours for a week to make sure the infestation is completely gone. Be sure to wash and disinfect bedding, coat collars, furniture, and anywhere lice may be lurking.

Liver diseases

WHAT ARE THEY

The symptoms related to liver disease are legion—physical, emotional and mental. There are digestive problems, blood sugar problems, immune disorders, abnormal absorption of fats, gallstones, vomiting, bloating, constipation, and multiple metabolism problems. Nervous disorders linked to liver disease include mood changes, anger, foggy thinking, headaches, migraines, and nausea. There are also a host of cardiovascular problems leading to heart attacks and strokes. A sluggish metabolism and an inability to lose weight even when dieting have far-reaching effects. Certainly anything we can do to overcome liver diseases will have a major impact on our quality of life. An ongoing Liver Cleanse could be among our most important habits to help ensure future health.

RECOMMENDED OILS

Birch		Peppermint	
German chamomile		Roman chamomile	
Rosemary		Cypress	
Lemon		Thyme	
Juniper		Sweet basil	
Helichrysum		Cinnamon	

RECOMMENDED BLENDS

Liver blend		Digestion blend	
Immune balancing blend		Circulation blend	

INSTRUCTION

In-home procedures suggested as part of an overall plan involving your health care professional for all serious conditions:

- In water or herbal teas, take 5 to 10 drops of the liver blend, peppermint, or lemon daily. Mix 1 drop per quart of water or one drop per cup of herbal tea. Adjust with a toothpick to get the quantity right.

- You may prefer to take the oils internally by filling capsules with a 50:50 blend of an essential oil or blend and a carrier oil. Take a capsule three times a day with food for 20 days.

- Massage the liver area of the feet and the part of the chest over the liver with 2 or 3 drops of any of these oils undiluted.

- Do a Liver Cleanse according to the instructions found earlier in this section.

- Cirrhosis (alcohol-related)

- In-home procedures suggested as part of an overall plan involving your health care professional:

- In water or herbal tea take 5 to 10 drops daily of any of the following oils: the liver blend, peppermint, lemon, the immune balancing blend, and the circulation blend. Mix 1 drop per quart of water or one drop per cup of herbal tea.

- You may prefer to take the oils internally by mixing a 50:50 blend of one of these essential oils with a carrier oil, filling capsules with a dropper, and taking 3 capsules a day with food.

- Massage the liver area of the feet and the part of the chest over the liver with 2 or 3 drops of any of these oils or a mixture of them—undiluted.

Lower Back Pain

(Lumbago) & SCIATICA

WHAT IS IT

A common chronic or temporary disorder involving the spine, muscles, nerves, cartilage, and bones of the back. It affects about 40% of us. It can stem from muscle weakness or joint strain from poor posture alignment or insufficient exercise of the appropriate types. Much of it is caused by damaged intervertebral discs. Sciatica is related to lower back pain in that it results from spinal nerves, but the symptoms manifest not only in the back but down the leg as well—numbness, pain, weakness, tingling. Symptoms typically only manifest on one side of the body.

RECOMMENDED OILS

Birch		Wintergreen	
Lavender		Marjoram	
Rosemary		Black pepper	
Ginger		Balsam fir	
Peppermint			

RECOMMENDED BLENDS

Soothing blend		Massage blend	
Circulation blend		Inflammation blend	
Immune balancing blend			

INSTRUCTION

- Lower back pain, like neck pain, can be caused by a many things—muscle tension, structural alignment, poor circulation, bone pain, nerve damage, or tendon or cartilage inflammation. Try different oils and blends the inside arch of the foot to see which ones reduce the discomfort most effectively.

- Those will be the oils to use for back massage. You'll be selecting oils to use for Layer Therapy—a massage for the back and spine described in the chapter on How to Use Essential Oils.

- For muscle tension, use the Comforting blend and rotate between warm and cool compresses with a damp cloth and either an ice pack or a hot water bottle.

- For structural alignment, use the Soothing blend and/or the Inflammation blend with warm compresses. Also add the foot massage blend. Use warming single oils like black pepper and rosemary for this therapy with warm, damp compress and a heat pad or hot water bottle to help the oil penetrate.

- For poor circulation, use the Circulation blend or stimulating oils like rosemary. Also use a warm, damp compress and a heat pad or hot water bottle to help the oils penetrate.

- For nerve damage, use helichrysum or geranium with a warm, damp compress and a heat pad or hot water bottle to help the oils penetrate.

- For bone pain, try birch, balsam fir, or peppermint. This can be a cool compress with a damp cloth and an ice pack. Or you can rotate between warm and cool.

- For tendon or cartilage inflammation, try the Massage blend (cool or rotate warm and cool).

- When you have determined the oil(s) that are most effective, use it (them), undiluted, two or three drops down the spine. Use your knuckles to knead the oils in on both sides of the spine. Then use the nail side of your fingertips to feather out the oils onto the back. Add a carrier oil if the oils become too hot. Then add a warm or cool compress and heat or ice according to the reason for the therapy you're using.

- Apply damp towel compresses at the end of the therapy while the oils are being absorbed. For muscle tension, bone pain, or tendon or cartilage inflammation, apply a cool compress at first, then rotate between cool and warm compresses on subsequent days. Apply a warm compress for the all the others.

- Add the all-important stretching and back strengthening exercises according to instructions given by your health care professional. Listen to your body, and don't do any stretching or exercise, including yoga, that creates more pain or makes the back feel worse over time.

Lung Cancer

Treatment options for cancer vary depending on the type and progression of the cancer. It absolutely requires a physician's care. Cancer treatments are necessarily aggressive, and essential oils have been shown in many studies to complement but not replace conventional treatment. See Cancer Section.

Lyme Disease

WHAT IT IS

Infection transmitted by ticks that causes flu-like symptoms. Lyme disease begins as an infectious disease. If neglected it will become inflammatory and progress to an autoimmune disease. It starts at first with a rash, headache, fever, and chills, but later becomes similar to arthritis or neurological and cardiac disorders.

RECOMMENDED OILS

Tea tree		Clove	
Cinnamon		Thyme	
Oregano		Lemongrass	
Frankincense		Ylang ylang	

RECOMMENDED BLENDS

Protecting blend

INSTRUCTION

Use the following in-home procedures with the approval of your health care professional:

- In its first stage, treat it in an intensive way with the Protecting blend using 50:50 capsules taken with food 6 times a day. If you can bring down the infection quickly enough, it will not progress to the later stages.

- The most effective oils for Lyme disease in the early stages are tea tree and the Protecting blend. They can be used singly or in a blend of equal parts: tea tree (25%), the Protecting blend (25%), and a carrier oil (50%) for massage or filling capsules for ingestion.

- In the early stages of the disease, if you are filling capsules with the exceptionally strong oils mentioned (clove, cinnamon, oregano, thyme, or lemongrass), be sure to dilute them in a ratio of 25% strong essential oils with 75% carrier oil.

- You can also massage the feet of children and even babies with 1 or 2 drops of tea tree or the antimicrobial diluted in a teaspoon of carrier oil. Do this several times daily to help with this stubborn infection.

- If Lyme disease becomes chronic, you will want to use the immune balancing blend combined with the Protecting blend. Dilute

them 50:50 with a carrier oil and make up capsules. Take 1 or 2 of each daily with food.

- If the disease has progressed to become an autoimmune disease, do an immune balancing cleanse for a least a year to try to restore your immune system to its proper equilibrium. See cleansing earlier in this chapter.

- Try taking 1 or 2 drops of any of the recommended oils in an herbal tea with honey. Adjust the flavor by adjusting the quantity of oil used from a couple of drops down to a trace. Do the same in a quart of drinking water, juice, or recipes (after taking the recipe off the stove).

- Small children will typically do better taking essential oils in water, juice, or food rather than in a capsule. If you are treating small children, dilute these oils down to 10% or even less. A little of the strongest oils goes a long way with children. They also respond to a lot less essential oil in their drinking water or foods than adults, so involve them in deciding the flavors they enjoy.

Lymph Nodes & Vessels

(lymphadenitis) (swelling & infection)

WHAT THEY ARE

Lymph node infections or lymphadenitis occurs when bacteria, viruses, fungi, and parasites infect lymph nodes (also called glands) and vessels causing swelling and pain.

The lymphatic system is a network of lymph nodes, ducts, vessels, and organs that produce, filter out and overcome pathogens, and move a fluid called lymph from tissues to the bloodstream. It is an important part of your immune system. The glands, or nodes, are small structures that filter lymph fluid. These glands contain many white blood cells to help fight infection. They can become swollen, red, hard, and tender from a bacterial, viral, parasitical, or fungal infection. Swollen nodes are often found near another infection, tumor, or inflammation. The nodes that are most likely to be infected are in the neck, the armpits, and the groin.

RECOMMENDED OILS

Tea tree		Bergamot	
Lavender			

RECOMMENDED BLENDS

Protecting blend

INSTRUCTION

• Apply a drop or two of tea tree or the Protecting blend undiluted on the area where the glands are swollen.

• Lick a trace of tea tree off the back of your hand, distribute it around your mouth, and swallow. Do this frequently throughout the day to help with swollen glands in your neck and throat.

• Create a blend of 25% tea tree, 25% Protecting blend and 50% carrier oil. Fill capsules with a dropper and take a capsule 3 times a day with food.

• Put a drop of the Protecting blend in 1/2 teaspoon of honey, then stir it into a cup of water. Take this drink once or twice a day.

Lymphedema

WHAT IT IS

The blockage of the lymph nodes, causing lymph to build up and swell a specific portion of the body. It is not to be confused with swelling (edema) due to other causes like cardiovascular problems. Lymphedema is usually not generalized swelling as in the swelling in your legs on a long plane trip or after sitting too long at the computer.

RECOMMENDED OILS

Lavender		Lemon	
Myrtle		Balsam fir	
Juniper		Rosemary	
Birch		Patchouli	

RECOMMENDED BLENDS

Circulation blend	Protecting blend
Immune balancing blend	

• All conditions involving liquid retention and swelling may receive some help by gently applying lavender, lemon, balsam fir, or the circulation blend either neat on the feet or in dilution (3 to 4 drops per teaspoon of mixing oil) on the affected areas or on an overall body massage. Always massage from the extremities toward the center of the body.

• Gently apply the same blend to affected areas or generally on the body for its calming effects.

• Consult with a certified health care professional to understand which type of swelling should be treated with massage and what kinds of massage would be beneficial for lymphedema.

General lymphatic massage

- For generalized and highly beneficial lymphatic massage to stimulate healthy, normal drainage and strengthen the immune system, use juniper, rosemary, birch, patchouli, and the Massage blend as individual oils or in a blend 25% essential oil and 75% carrier oil. This would be for a more vigorous kind of massage, not the gentle kind you would use for lymphedema.

Meningitis or Viral Encephalitis

WHAT IT IS

Acute inflammation of the membranes that cover and protect the brain and spinal cord. It is usually caused by an infection but occasionally by drugs or an autoimmune response. It can be life-threatening medical emergency because it is so close the brain and spinal cord. Symptoms in adults are headache and a stiff neck associated with fever, confusion, vomiting, and an inability to stand light or loud noises. Children with meningitis may not exhibit all these symptoms, but may merely be irritable or drowsy. Viral encephalitis is inflammation of the brain caused by a virus. Both can be fatal or can have long-term consequences—seizures, behavioral changes, memory and speech problems, etc. Both conditions require that you be rushed to the hospital because they can move very quickly and be extremely aggressive.

RECOMMENDED OILS

Eucalyptus radiata   Ravintsara

Tea tree

RECOMMENDED BLENDS

Comforting blend   Soothing blend

Protecting blend   Massage blend

INSTRUCTION

Because these are medical emergencies, do not try to treat them without the help of a qualified health care professional. But with professional diagnosis and treatment and in cooperation with your health care professional, use these suggestions:

- For headaches apply the Comforting blend and the Soothing blend neat on the feet or ears on the areas corresponding to the most painful areas of the body.

- Also gently massage the affected area with 2 to 3 drops of the Soothing blend and the Comforting blend in a teaspoon of carrier oil.

- For an energizing foot massage, apply 1 to 2 drops of the Massage blend with 1 to 2 drops of the Foot Massage blend.

- Apply the 2 to 3 drops of the Massage blend, the Protecting blend, Eucalyptus radiata, tea tree, or a combination of any of these in a teaspoon of a carrier oil. Do regular whole-body massages. Energize yourself with massage and try to extend your exercise time each day with a little preliminary massage.

- Create a blend using the Protecting blend (20%), Rosemary (15%), tea tree (15%), and a carrier oil (50%). Fill capsules with a dropper and take one capsule 3 times a day with food.

- Use a drop of the Protecting blend, the Massage blend, Spearmint, or tea tree with honey in an herbal tea once or twice a day.

- If autoimmune conditions are involved, use the Immune Strengthening Cleanse for a deep action.

Menopause
(and related conditions)

WHAT IT IS

The time in a woman's life when her reproductive ability ceases because the ovaries stop functioning and menstruation ends. It usually occurs between her late 40s and early 50s. The transition is normally not sudden or abrupt, but occurs gradually over a number of years. Signs of oncoming menopause include lack of energy, hot flashes, insomnia, vaginal dryness, and mood changes. These changes can significantly hamper daily activities and a woman's sense of well-being.

RECOMMENDED OILS

Roman chamomile		German chamomile	
Bergamot		Clary sage	
Sweet basil		Lavender	
Neroli		Sandalwood	
Ylang ylang		Cypress	
Peppermint		Frankincense	

RECOMMENDED BLENDS

Comforting blend		Foot massage blend	

INSTRUCTION

With the involvement of your health care professional as needed, try the following procedures:

- Use a natural progesterone cream under directions of a health care professional.

- If you have insomnia, enjoy an evening foot massage with 2 to 3 drops of lavender, the Comforting blend, and the Foot Massage blend undiluted.

- Also to help you sleep, diffuse 10 drops of the Comforting blend or lavender for 5 minutes each evening. And take warm baths with 5 to 10 drops of lavender or the Comforting blend dispersed in a cup of Epsom Salts.

- For headaches related to hormones, use a drop of peppermint or frankincense in a cup of herbal tea with a little honey or a quart of drinking water. Also apply a trace of frankincense or peppermint on your forehead, temples, and the back of your neck. Use a drop of sweet basil in herbal teas and many recipes (after taking the food off the stove). Use sweet basil in dips, salad dressings, and everything you can think of while you are experiencing your most difficult symptoms.

- For hot flashes, Dr. Pénoël suggests creating a blend of cypress (25%), peppermint (25%), and a carrier oil (50%). Fill capsules with a dropper and take 3 a day with food from the 7th to the 21st day of your menstrual cycle +++P.

- Also for hot flashes, Dr. Pénoël suggests a blend of cypress (25%), helichrysum (25%), and a carrier oil (50%). Apply this oil topically to the base of the spine for 20 days +++P.

- For headaches and emotional challenges, give yourself foot massages with 2 to 3 drops of frankincense, 2 to 3 drops of peppermint, and the foot massage blend. Concentrate your massage under the ankle bones and in the center under the heel of the foot.

- For cramps massage the same spots on the heel and ankles with 3 or 4 drops of sweet basil.

- For cramps have a lower abdominal massage using 3 to 4 drops of sweet basil mixed in a teaspoon of carrier oil. Massage in a clockwise circular motion on the lower abdomen and a counter-clockwise direction on the lower back and hip area.

- For swelling in feet, ankles, legs, and arms, gently massage the swollen areas in the direction of your heart. Use a mixture of 3 to 5 drops of the circulation blend with a teaspoon of carrier oil.

- For varicose veins, read the instructions later in this section.

- For dry skin add 10 to 20 drops of lavender to 8 ounces of unscented, non-toxic lotion and apply it regularly.

- For dry skin, exfoliate once a week with a salt scrub. Add 1/2 cup of a light carrier oil like grapeseed to a cup of fine-textured sea salt (or sugar if your skin is extra sensitive). Add 5 to 15 drops of one of the recommended essential oils.

Mental & Emotional Health

Mental and emotional health are influenced by the limbic brain where aromatic signals are instantly processed. You can harness the enormous power of pleasing aromas to anchor new ways of thinking, feeling, and acting. You can also replace self-defeating behaviors that may have caused unhealthy mental and emotional problems in your life.

Using the power of aroma, you can train your limbic brain to enjoy new, liberating, healthy emotions by linking them to a specific aroma, and then later using those aromas to trigger positive, uplifting feelings and emotions.

For some reason, when you cleanse the systems of the body using essential oils, you also experience residual benefits in your mental and emotional health. Therefore, we will offer suggestions for cleanses and procedures which may appear to be totally physiological, yet they have proven to be remarkably effective at clearing the mind and spirit.

With every disease we attempt to treat, it is essential to correct any lifestyle choices that contributed to the disease. Review the dietary guidelines in this book as well as exercise habits, drinking plenty of water, and enjoying fresh air and sunshine. These are all amazingly therapeutic. No permanent healing can happen without them.

Living a life of purpose and building great relationships are also fundamental to good health. It is impossible to do bad and feel good. Evaluate carefully your priorities and goals. Then eliminate as much as possible, with the help of psychological or spiritual counselors if necessary, any vengeful, critical, spiteful, unkind, unfeeling, angry, anxious, arrogant, bitter, fearful, or despairing emotions in your life. Negative feelings like these need to be constantly released and replaced with positive emotions. Essential oils can be highly effective in helping you relax and release your emotions, embrace positive new emotions, and associate them with the healthier emotional lifestyle you are trying to develop.

Patricia Davis suggests that for emotional and sleep work, you need to have a good selection of oils to choose from because, though a particular oil may work extremely well for a couple of weeks, its effectiveness then may taper off. If you replace it for two weeks and then return to the original, it may work just as well as before. It's important to rotate oils and have a fair selection to choose from (Davis, p. 169).

Use Aromatic Behavioral Conditioning described under Addictions and Self-Defeating Behaviors in this chapter to replace those emotions that keep you from enjoying the life you would like to have. With the possible help of your health care or psychiatric professional, try some of the following for the conditions listed:

Anger & Hostility
(tantrums)

WHAT IT IS

Anti-social, emotionally charged, and aggressive behavior.

RECOMMENDED OILS

Roman chamomile		German chamomile	
Lavender		Frankincense	
Ylang ylang			

RECOMMENDED BLENDS

Comforting blend		Stress control blend	
Focusing blend		Digestive blend	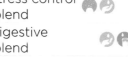
Liver blend			

INSTRUCTIONS

- Identify from all the oils you have those that settle your emotions and make you feel less angry and hostile. These are the ones you will start with.

- Enjoy a trace of the Comforting blend, the Stress control blend, the Focusing blend, lavender, or frankincense or any oil you find emotionally calming or pleasurable in drinking water, herbal tea, or by taking a trace on the tongue as often as you think about it during the day. Enjoy it especially at times when you are successful at controlling anger and hostility to help you emotionally connect with the good feelings of freedom from these destructive emotions.

- Diffuse 5 to 10 drops of any of your most pleasurable for 5 minutes whenever you would be most likely to slip into angry or hostile feelings.

- In the chapter on how to use essential oils, identify for you personally all the most pleasurable ways to use essential oils— aromatic baths, diffusing, massage, etc.— and rotate those therapies to reinforce the victories you are having over your antisocial tendencies.

- Review the aromatic behavioral conditioning system in the Cleansing section of this chapter to help you replace the self-defeating behaviors that lead to anger and hostility.

Anxiety, Stress, Depression, Bipolar Disorder (Manic-Depressive)

WHAT THEY ARE

These three conditions range from mild symptoms all the way to severe clinical and chronic states of mental illness. Anxiety can range from a little frustration and stress all the way to a debilitating mental disorder of excessive uneasiness and apprehension, typically with compulsive behavior or panic attacks. Depression ranges from simply feeling sad and blue all the way to severe, persistent despondency and dejection, with suicidal tendencies. Bipolar or manic-depressive disorder is a mental illness characterized by elevated moods (mania) followed by periods of severe depression ranging from mild to severe.

RECOMMENDED OILS

Bergamot		Cedarwood	
German chamomile		Roman chamomile	
Clary sage		Cypress	
Lemon		Lime	
Peppermint		Rosemary	
Spearmint		Frankincense	
Lavender		Marjoram	
Neroli		Patchoulii	
Sandalwood		Ylang ylang	

RECOMMENDED BLENDS

Comforting blend		Focusing blend	
Stress control blend		Balancing blend	
Liver blend		Intimacy blend	
Foot massage blend		Mental focus blend	

INSTRUCTION

If you have severe, clinical mental illness, be sure to work with a trusted mental health professional and incorporate these suggestions as part of an organized effort to control the symptoms and move toward recovery.

- Enjoy the any of these recommended oils that are for ingestion (8) in water, herbal tea, or by licking a trace off the back of your hand several times a day. Enjoy them especially happy, emotionally-balanced times when you are enjoying a reprieve from the most negative emotions so they can help you anchor the good emotions of freedom from these conditions.

- Diffuse 5 to 10 drops of your favorite oils for 5 minutes during your best times so you can use them as positive triggers to put you into a healthy state when you would be most likely to slip into your negative emotions.

- Use Aromatic Behavioral Conditioning described under Addictions and Self-Defeating Behaviors in this chapter to replace those emotions that keep you from enjoying the life you would like to have.

- Follow the Liver Cleanse for a year to clear your body of the toxins that may contribute to the state of mind that encourages these brain disorders.

- Create a 50:50 blend with frankincense and a carrier oil. Fill capsules with a dropper and take a capsule three times a day with food.

- Apply a drop of frankincense on the crown of your head, temples, forehead, and base of the neck many times throughout the day to help you with emotional clearing.

- Enjoy foods rich in complex nutrients and life-giving minerals such as green leafy vegetables. Have at least one meal a day with a large salad. Cruciferous vegetables (cabbage, broccoli, cauliflower, and Brussel sprouts) are also helpful for healing these conditions.

- Massage your feet two or three times a week with the foot massage blend with added frankincense and a few drops of the calming or intimacy blend.

CLINICAL SUPPORT

"The aim of the present study is to review the available literature to determine if there is evidence for effectiveness of aromatherapy in surgical patients to treat anxiety and insomnia, to control pain and nausea, and to dress wounds. Efficacy studies of lavender or orange and peppermint essential oils, to treat anxiety and nausea, respectively, have shown positive results. Finally, there are encouraging data for the treatment of infections, especially for tea tree oil..." (Stea S, Beraudi A, De Pasquale D., 2014).

I use peppermint to de-stress and energize myself

I put a drop of peppermint on my hand and rub it on the back of my neck. Then I cup my hands over my nose and mouth and breathe deeply. This simple habit is amazing for relieving the tension in my neck. I've noticed that it also de-stresses me and energizes my brain. It's something quick I can do several times a day. It has made my stressful life so much nicer.

Emotional Disorders Leading to Insomnia

WHAT THEY ARE

Almost everyone with mood and anxiety disorders have insomnia either chronically or during the height of their distress. Insomnia also increases the risk of future relapses or additional conditions, so the cycle needs to be broken.

RECOMMENDED OILS

Oil		Oil	
Lavender	🙂🙂	Frankincense	🙂🙂
German chamomile	🙂🙂🙂	Roman chamomile	🙂🙂🙂
Lavandin	🙂🙂	Neroli	🙂🙂
Orange	🙂🙂🙂	Bergamot	🙂🙂
Tangerine	🙂🙂🙂	Balsam fir	🙂🙂
Clary sage	🙂🙂	Sandalwood	🙂🙂
Vetiver	🙂🙂	Ylang ylang	🙂🙂

RECOMMENDED BLENDS

Blend		Blend	
Comforting blend	🙂🙂	Foot massage blend	🙂
Balancing blend	🙂		

INSTRUCTION

If you have severe, clinical mental illness leading to sleeplessness, be sure to work with a trusted mental health professional and incorporate these suggestions as part of an organized effort to control the symptoms and move into recovery.

- Apply a drop of lavender or any of the other recommended oils undiluted to the outer ear daily.

- Have a balsam fir Layer Therapy treatment weekly. See instructions in the How to Use Essential Oils, chapter four. Begin by applying a drop of the Balancing blend to the sternum on the chest. Drip 4 to 5 drops of balsam fir neat up the spine, feather it out with your fingertips, the use your knuckles to work it into both sides of the spine. Then massage a blend of 3 to 4 drops of balsam fir with a teaspoon of the carrier oil on the muscles at the sides of the back in a downward direction. Lie still for about 20 minutes following this massage with a warm, damp compress over the spine.

• Enjoy a few drops of the calming oil with a few drops of the foot massage blend in a teaspoon of carrier oil massaged on the feet several times a week before bed.

Eating Disorders

(Anorexia/Bulimia)

WHAT THEY ARE

Abnormal eating habits involving either too much or too little food intake causing physical or mental harm. The most common disorders are anorexia nervosa (food restriction) and bulimia nervosa (bingeing and vomiting). Other characteristics include over-exercise and starvation. The condition may be linked to a cultural idealization of thinness and youthfulness. While treatment can be effective, the consequences of allowing the behaviors to continue can be fatal.

RECOMMENDED OILS

Bergamot	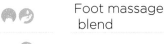	Clary sage	
German chamomile		Roman chamomile	
Lavender		Neroli	
Ylang ylang			

RECOMMENDED BLENDS

Comforting blend		Foot massage blend	
Balancing blend			

INSTRUCTION

These are serious, life-threatening conditions that often require the help of professionals trained in effective treatment. With the involvement and consent of such professionals, these suggestions may prove helpful.

• Patricia Davis suggests that you need to choose your own oils from among the most calming and soothing based on your personal pleasure. Bergamot, in particular, is recommended by a number of authors as an oil that is not only relaxing but also increases the appetite and is uplifting to the spirits—an important aspect for those caught in self-loathing emotions (Davis, p. 26).

• Create an aromatic bath by using 10 to 15 drops of the chosen essential oil or blend with a cup of Epsom Salts. Pampering and nurturing in this way can be an important part of therapy.

• Self-massage and foot massage using a 50:50 or 25:75 blend of a favorite essential oils with a carrier oil or lotion may be helpful in anchoring emotions of self-approval.

• Diffusing 10 to 20 drops of favorite oils in moments of clear thinking can also help.

• Be sure to look through the section on Aromatic Behavioral Conditioning described under Addictions and Self-Defeating Behaviors in this chapter to help guard against inadvertently anchoring the wrong behaviors and emotions.

Trauma Release

WHAT IT IS

A trauma is an event, events, or circumstances that are physically or emotionally harmful or threatening with lasting adverse effects on normal functioning whether physical, social, emotional, or spiritual. Trauma release is helping to separate the debilitating response from the events or circumstances and thus returning to normal functioning.

RECOMMENDED OILS

Lavandin		Roman chamomile	
Lavender		Neroli	
Bergamot			

RECOMMENDED BLENDS

Comforting blend		Mental focus blend	
Focusing blend		Balancing blend	
Foot massage blend			

INSTRUCTION

This kind of therapy can require the assistance of a professional. Here are some suggestions that may be helpful additions to what a professional may recommend.

- Apply an undiluted drop of one of the recommended oils on your breast bone (sternum). Massage your feet with the same oil according to the reflexology instructions.

- Follow the instructions on Layer Therapy in Chapter 4. Use 4 to 5 drops of balsam fir and other calming oils undiluted up the spine. Use your knuckles to work it into both sides of the spine and feather it out on the sides of the back with the fingernail side of your hand.

Apply a damp compress and lie still for about 20 minutes following the massage.

- An aromatic bath using 20 drops of one of the recommended oils in a cup of Epsom Salts can help to calm symptoms.

- Diffusing 20 drops of one of the oils can also be helpful.

Moles

WHAT THEY ARE

Clusters of pigmented cells, also called nevi, that appear as dark brown spots. They come in a range of colors and can develop virtually anywhere on you're the body. The most common are skin tags, raised moles and flat moles. Most moles are benign and do not develop into life-threatening skin cancer (melanoma). But it is wise if you have moles to be watchful of signs that a mole may be changing or a new, cancerous melanoma may be appearing. Dermatologists suggest that we learn the signs that a mole may be cancerous. They suggest the mnemonic device using the letters A, B, C, and D, standing for asymmetry, border, color, and diameter. If a mole begins changing size, color, or shape; or, if the border of a mole develops uneven edges or becomes larger than a pencil eraser, it becomes important to contact a health care professional.

RECOMMENDED OILS

Frankincense		Tea tree	
Oregeno			

INSTRUCTION

If you have multiple moles (more than 100) or a genetic history of skin cancer, follow these instructions.

- Eat a healthy, plant-based, whole-food diet with plenty of helpful antioxidant protection to prevent moles from becoming cancerous and melanomas from forming.

- Do an Immune Strengthening Cleanse of at least one year.

- Apply a trace of tea tree or frankincense oil twice daily on any moles you suspect may become cancerous.

Mononucleosis

(Mono or Epstein-Barr)

WHAT IT IS

A viral infection transmitted through saliva—coughing, sneezing, kissing, or sharing utensils. Signs and symptoms may include fatigue, sore throat, fever, swollen lymph nodes and tonsils, headache, and skin rash. It has an incubation period of four to six weeks, though in young children it may be shorter. Signs and symptoms such as fever and sore throat usually lessen within a couple of weeks, although fatigue, enlarged lymph nodes and a swollen spleen may last for a few weeks longer.

RECOMMENDED OILS

Bergamot		Ravintsara	
Lime		Neroli	
Rosewood		Eucalyptus radiata	
Thyme			

RECOMMENDED BLENDS

Protecting blend		Respiratory blend	

INSTRUCTION

If, after following these instructions including rest and a healthy diet, the symptoms have not cleared up within two weeks, be sure to contact your health care professional.

- Apply 2 or 3 drops undiluted of any or a blend of the following oils: Eucalyptus radiata, tea tree, the Protecting blend, and the Respiratory blend. Apply it on the sides of your neck where the concentration of lymph nodes is greatest.

- Create a 50:50 blend of the Protecting blend and a carrier oil. Fill capsules and take one three times a day with food.

- Create a blend using rosewood (30%), thyme (15%), bergamot (5%), and carrier oil (50%). Apply it to your chest and abdomen 3 or 4 times a day for 20 days ++++P.

- Do an Immune Strengthening Cleanse (see Cleansing) for at least one year, even after the infection is under control to make sure you have healed the root of the infection.

Muscles/Bones/ Joints

Possible causes of bone, muscle, joint, and back problems and necessary lifestyle adjustments

- Bone, joint, and muscle symptoms are significant signals that you may need to improve your exercise program, reduce the toxins, add important whole-food nutrients, and unblock painful areas of your body through reflexology and other massage.

- Begin with dietary changes according to suggestions in this book. Pay greatest attention to reducing the toxins coming from too much meat and dairy protein, especially from processed meats. If there is an autoimmune component like rheumatoid arthritis, reduce your proteins and try eliminating the most likely allergens—dairy, eggs, meat, wheat (gluten), and things that encourage toxin buildup like refined sugars and soft drinks.

- You may need to be drinking more water (1/2 gallon a day), and exercise (the equivalent of a 2-mile walk per day). If you have any serious medical condition, follow the advice of a competent health care professional in setting up a personalized graduated exercise program that involves aerobic, weight-bearing, and flexibility training.

- Look into your emotional life and reduce any toxic emotional buildup of unresolved conflicts, resentments, criticism, etc. Calming therapies can help, but your issues will recur if emotional problems are not brought under control and resolved.

RECOMMENDED OILS

Lemon		Helichrysum	
Balsam fir		Lavender	
Marjoram			

RECOMMENDED BLENDS

Comforting blend		Mental focus blend	
Intimacy blend		Stress control blend	
Massage blend		Balancing blend	

INSTRUCTION

- Incorporate stress-reducing activities each day such as meditation while diffusing 20 drops of lemon, balsam fir, the Stress control blend, the Mental Focus blend, the Comforting blend, or the Intimacy blend. Yoga exercises combine relaxation, balance, body awareness, and exercise. Diffuse calming, meditative oils while doing yoga exercises.

- Massage your muscles with a 50:50 blend of the Massage blend and a carrier oil before yoga exercise. You can massage muscles early in the morning just to warm them up. For a single application, dilute 5 or 6 drops in a tablespoon of carrier oil and massage your joints and main muscle groups.

- At the end of the day, treat yourself to a relaxing massage on your feet, hands, abdomen, ears, or joints. Use 3 to 4 drops of lavender, lemon, the Comforting blend, the Intimacy blend, or the Foot Massage blend diluted in a tablespoon of a carrier oil.

- Eliminate all unsafe addictions: smoking, drugs, or alcoholism.

- To disinfect, cleanse, restore healthy intestinal flora, and release toxins in the joints, bones, back, and muscles ingest a drop of tea tree, the Protecting blend, the digestion blend, and/or the liver blend in your drinking water, an herbal tea, juice, or a recipe (after taking it off the heat).

First Aid for Injuries Involving Bones, Muscles, & Joints

WHAT THEY ARE

Sports injuries, sprains, fractures, broken bones, etc. A sprain is a damaged ligament and will involve inflammation, heat, and swelling.

RECOMMENDED OILS

Lavender		Peppermint	
German chamomile		Roman chamomile	
Spearmint		Birch	
Wintergreen			

RECOMMENDED BLENDS

Soothing blend		Circulation blend	

INSTRUCTION

Follow first aid instructions and cautions found in an authoritative health care guide or website or consult a health care professional for advice. If home care is indicated, follow these suggestions:

- Immediately control pain by applying either peppermint or the Soothing blend. If the area is small (finger, wrist, etc.) put a drop of oil on your little finger and dab the area. For a bit larger area (ankle, elbow, or shoulder), use a pipette and apply a few drops undiluted and spread it gently with your little finger. For a larger area (hip, leg, back), dilute the oil, 4 to 5 drops in a teaspoon of carrier oil, and spread it on the area. DO NOT MASSAGE THE MUSCLES OR MOVE THE BONES OR JOINTS AT ALL.

- Before applying ice or a cold pack, mix 4 to 5 drops of peppermint or the Soothing blend in 1/3 cup of water and shake. Soak a gauze or small flannel cloth in it and apply it to the painful area. Secure it with a cling bandage. Cover it with a dry cloth and apply an ice or cold pack.

- After 24 hours and when or if it becomes appropriate to apply heat to the area to aid healing, use the Inflammation blend or the Soothing blend. The Inflammation blend has a deep action that lowers inflammation, but is a little less effective at helping with pain. Create a compress similar to the cold compress above, but this time apply a warm, damp cloth, a dry cloth, and a heat pack. But apply heat only when all signs of inflammation have ceased.

- To speed healing, lightly massage the area around the injury with 4 to 5 drops of the circulation blend in a teaspoon of a carrier oil.

Upper Body Joint & Muscle Conditions

(shoulders, bursitis, tennis elbow, wrists, tendonitis, carpal tunnel syndrome, etc.)

WHAT THEY ARE

Bursitis is inflammation, swelling, and irritation of a bursa, a fluid-filled sac that cushions movement of muscles, tendons, and joints of the shoulder, elbow, and knee. Tennis elbow is an inflammation of the tendons of the elbow from repetitive motions like tennis movements. The pain is on the outside of the upper arm near the elbow. Similarly, carpal tunnel syndrome comes from excessive pressure on the median nerve in the wrist that permits feeling and movement in parts of the hand. It is characterized by numbness, tingling, weakness, or muscle damage in hands and fingers.

RECOMMENDED OILS

Eucalyptus radiata		Helichrysum	
Wintergreen		Birch	
Marjoram			

RECOMMENDED BLENDS

Soothing blend

Massage blend

Inflammation blend

Comforting blend

Circulation blend

INSTRUCTION

If arthritis is ruled out, consult an authoritative self-help book or a health care professional for guidelines on evaluating your symptoms to make sure that you don't have something far more serious that should be treated at home.

- For tennis elbow Dr. Pénoël recommends using a drop of helichrysum on the small painful area. Do not massage the area.

- For tennis elbow Dr. Pénoël also recommends a blend of Eucalyptus radiata (90%) and wintergreen (10%) for an undiluted application to the elbow several times a day **+++P**.

- If there is both inflammation and pain, use either the Soothing blend or the Inflammation blend. If the area is small (wrist or finger), apply the oil undiluted. If the area is larger (shoulder), blend 4 to 5 drops in a teaspoon of carrier oil and apply several times daily.

- Use the Foot Massage blend with the Massage blend (a.m.) or the Comforting blend (p.m.) to release any energy blockage throughout your body. Focus on the areas that corresponding to the problem in the body.

- Use the circulation blend in dilution (4 to 5 drops per teaspoon of carrier oil) around affected areas to accelerate healing.

Pain in the Joints and Muscles of the Lower Body

(tendonitis, Plantar fasciitis, tendonitis, etc.)

WHAT IT IS

Painful joints, tendons, and muscles of the legs, feet, and hips that are not associated with arthritis will all respond to similar treatment. Plantar fasciitis is a common painful disorder on the heel and underside of the feet. All these conditions can be caused by overuse due to exercise, excess weight, being on the feet too long, weight, or age.

RECOMMENDED OILS

Wintergreen

Birch

Eucalyptus radiata

Balsam fir

Cypress

Peppermint

Marjoram

RECOMMENDED BLENDS

Soothing blend

Massage blend

Inflammation blend

Comforting blend

Circulation blend

INSTRUCTION

If arthritis is ruled out, consult an authoritative self-help book or a health care professional for guidelines on evaluating your symptoms to make sure that you don't have something far more serious that should be treated at home.

- Exercising on a slant board with feet elevated can help with all conditions related to the hips, knees, ankles, and feet.

- Use the Massage blend to warm up the joints before exercise of these joints.

- For tendonitis, use a blend of Eucalyptus radiata (90%) and wintergreen (10%) for undiluted application to the tendon several times a day.

- If there is both inflammation and pain, use either the Soothing blend or the Inflammation blend. If the area is small (feet, toes, or ankle), apply the oil undiluted. If the area is larger (hip or knee), blend 4 to 5 drops in a teaspoon of carrier oil and apply several times daily.

- Use the Foot Massage blend with the Massage blend (a.m.) or the Comforting blend (p.m.) to release any energy blockage throughout your body.

- Use the circulation blend in dilution (4 to 5 drops per teaspoon of carrier oil) around affected areas to accelerate healing.

Muscle Cramps

(Charley horse, menstrual cramps, spasms, etc.)

WHAT THEY ARE

Sudden, severe, involuntary muscle contractions causing mild to severe pain and immobility. They affect both smooth muscle (menstrual cramps) and skeletal muscle (charley horses).

RECOMMENDED OILS

Rosemary		Birch	
Wintergreen		Lavender	
Marjoram		Bergamot	
Roman chamomile		German chamomile	
Clary sage		Black pepper	

RECOMMENDED BLENDS

Soothing blend		Circulation blend	

INSTRUCTION

- Create a blend of rosemary 50:50 with a carrier oil and apply topically with a gentle massage increasing the pressure to loosen up the muscle 2 – 4 times a day ++++P.

- For spasms, massage into the muscle 4 to 5 drops of the Comforting blend diluted in a teaspoon of a carrier oil. Then wait a few minutes before you do another massage with a similar diluted blend using the Massage blend to warm muscles and tendons. Carefully stretch and move your muscles and joints if they remain pain-free. Rotate massages using these two blends to both calm and energize with increasing activity and range of movement.

- For menstrual cramps create a compress by applying 3 to 4 drops of sweet basil directly on the lower abdomen then applying a warm, damp cloth, a dry cloth, and a hot pad or hot water bottle. Add a carrier oil if the basil begins to feel uncomfortably hot. Gentle massage over the lower abdomen with a 50:50 blend of any of the recommended oils and a carrier oil may also be helpful.

Nausea/Vomiting

(See Vomiting)

WHAT THEY ARE

An unsettled stomach and throwing up are common symptoms with many causes. Morning sickness is one, and it is covered under pregnancy later in this chapter. The other most common causes are chemotherapy, poor functioning of stomach muscles, general anesthesia, migraines, motion sickness, overdose of alcohol or drugs, vertigo, a form of childhood diarrhea (rotavirus), and infection from contaminated food.

RECOMMENDED OILS

Spearmint		Peppermint
Lemon		Tangerine
Sweet basil		Tea tree

RECOMMENDED BLENDS

Respiratory blend		Digestion blend
Comforting blend		Protecting blend

INSTRUCTION

- For suggestions regarding vomiting in children less than four years old, see "Infant and Child Care" earlier in this chapter.

- Stop food intake for a few hours. Gradually add mild foods such as vegetable broth, stewed apples, steamed vegetables, or brown rice with a few drops of tropical basil, spearmint, or the respiratory or digestion blends.

- Dr. Pénoël suggests applying a few drops of undiluted tangerine just below the breast bone two to three times a day +++P.

- He also suggests creating a blend of peppermint (25%), lemon (25%), and carrier oil (50%), filling capsules with a dropper and taking one capsule 3 times a day +++P.

- Mix a drop or two of spearmint, lemon, the Respiratory blend, or the Digestion blend in a quart of drinking water. For smaller amounts, dip a toothpick in the oil and stir it into a glass of hot or cold water.

- Mix a drop of spearmint, lemon, tangerine, the respiratory blend or the digestion blend in a teaspoon of honey and dissolve it slowly in your mouth. Mix it in hot or cold water.

- For nausea due to motion sickness, put a trace of peppermint or spearmint on your hand, rub your hands together, cup them over your nose and mouth and inhale. Or you can put a drop in a tissue and inhale. Avoid getting peppermint into your eyes or the mucous membranes of your nose.

- Because nausea, especially from motion sickness, can cause such a strong emotional reaction, it can easily create a powerful aversion to certain oils. Make sure the amounts of oils used are not too strong in order to avoid creating this reaction. Rotate oils to find the best, most agreeable ones.

- If you suspect that contaminated food or drinking water might be the cause of the nausea or vomiting, take lick traces of tea tree off the back of your hand every few minutes for an hour. Also create a blend 50:50 with tea tree and a carrier oil, fill capsules and take a capsule 3 times a day with food. Use this for prevention when traveling in countries or areas where food or water may be contaminated.

- Refer to an authoritative medical guide, website, or health care professional for signs that vomiting may be more serious than you should try to treat with home remedies alone.

CLINICAL SUPPORT

Peppermint essential oils is safe and effective for preventing chemotherapy-induced nausea and vomiting in patients, as well as being cost-effective (Tayarani-Najaran Z, et al., 2013).

"The aim of the present study is to review the available literature to determine if there is evidence for effectiveness of aromatherapy in surgical patients to treat anxiety and insomnia, to control pain and nausea, and to dress wounds. Efficacy studies of lavender or orange and peppermint essential oils, to treat anxiety and nausea, respectively, have shown positive results. Finally, there are encouraging data for the treatment of infections, especially for tea tree oil..." (Stea S, Beraudi A, De Pasquale D., 2014).

Neck Pain

WHAT IT IS

A common complaint that is typically caused by poor posture or hunching over a workbench or computer terminal. Various forms of arthritis are also common causes. In rare cases it can be more serious. Seek a professional diagnosis if your neck pain comes with numbness or loss of strength in arms or hands or if you have shooting pain into your shoulder or down your arm.

RECOMMENDED OILS

Helichrysum		Balsam fir	
Lavender		Marjoram	
Rosemary		Peppermint	

RECOMMENDED BLENDS

Soothing blend		Circulation blend	
Massage blend		Balancing blend	
Inflammation blend			

INSTRUCTION

- Neck pain can be caused by many things—tense muscles, poor structural alignment, inadequate circulation, nerve damage, pain in the bones, or inflammation in tendons or cartilage. One way to identify the cause is to experiment on the neck of the big toe with different oils to see which ones reduce the pain most effectively.

- For tense muscles, test with the Comforting blend.

- For alignment, use the Soothing blend or the Inflammation blend. You can also try the alignment or the Foot Massage blend.

- For inadequate circulation, try the circulation blend.

- For nerve damage, try helichrysum.

- For bone pain, try balsam fir or peppermint.

- For inflammation in tendons or cartilage, test with the Massage blend.

- When you have discovered those that are most effective, use it (them) undiluted on your neck. Start right where your head meets your neck and massage down and out onto your shoulders. You could also dilute 4 to 5 drops of essential oil in a teaspoon of carrier oil if you want a more mild application.

Nephrotic Syndrome

WHAT IT IS

A kidney disorder with a number of signs: protein in the urine rather than where it should be in the blood, and swelling of the tissues from fluid retention. You could also see elevated cholesterol levels and a predisposition for blood clotting. It increases your chances of infections.

RECOMMENDED OILS

Lemon	💧	Lime	💧
Tangerine	💧	Orange	💧

RECOMMENDED BLENDS

Protecting blend	💧	Immune balancing blend	💧

INSTRUCTION

In-home suggestions as part of a plan involving your health care professional:

- Increase your water intake by adding a drop of the Protecting blend and a drop of the Immune Balancing blend to every quart of your drinking water. Consume at least 2 quarts of this blended water every day. Have a little more each day to the point where you may be able to drink as much as a gallon a day.

- You can also use a drop of each of these blends in a cup of herbal tea.

- Create a lemon juice drink each morning by mixing the juice of 1/2 lemon in a large glass of water with a drop or two of lemon essential oil to buffer the sour taste.

Nervous Tics

WHAT THEY ARE

An involuntary, compulsive, repetitive, movement or vocalization involving various muscle groups. They can be invisible to the observer, such as toe clenching or abdominal tensing. Blinking the eyes and clearing the throat are common tics.

RECOMMENDED OILS

Lavender	🌫️💧	Sweet basil	🌫️💧💧
Roman chamomile	🌫️💧💧	German chamomile	🌫️💧💧

RECOMMENDED BLENDS

Comforting blend	🌫️💧	Stress control blend	🌫️💧
Intimacy blend	🌫️💧		

INSTRUCTION

- Take a warm bath with 10 to 15 drops of lavender, the Comforting blend, the Stress control blend, or the Intimacy blend mixed with a cup of Epsom Salts.

- Diffuse 10 to 20 drops of lavender, the Intimacy blend, or the Comforting blend whenever you need a calming influence.

- Take a drop of chamomile or sweet basil in a cup of herbal tea or a quart of water.

Neuralgia

WHAT IT IS

Pain along the pathway of a nerve that may be caused by many different things, including damage to the nerve, nerve irritation, infection, etc. Some of the most common types of neuralgia include: severe facial nerve pain (trigeminal neuralgia), shingles (postherpetic neuralgia), postoperative nerve pain, pelvic nerve pain, wrist nerve pain (carpal tunnel syndrome), and nerve pain down the leg (sciatica).

RECOMMENDED OILS

Wintergreen	💧	Peppermint	💧
Birch	💧	Clove	💧
Lavender	💧	Rosemary	💧
Helichrysum	💧	Black pepper	💧

RECOMMENDED BLENDS

Soothing
blend

Comforting
blend

INSTRUCTION

Follow these suggestions as part of an overall plan with advice from your health care professional as needed:

- Apply a drop or two of the Soothing blend or the Comforting blend, undiluted, on a small, localized area; for a larger area, use 4 to 5 drops in a teaspoon of carrier oil and gently massage the area.

- Create a cooling compress by mixing 4 to 5 drops of lavender, the Soothing blend, or the Comforting blend in a tablespoon of water. Soak a piece of gauze or a cloth in the solution and put it on the painful area, keeping it in position with a cling film. Add a dry cloth and an ice pack to add to the cooling action. If you wish to try a stimulating, warming action, try replacing the cooling oils with two drops of a warming oil—black pepper or rosemary—blending it safely with a teaspoon of carrier oil.

- For treating shingles Dr. Pénoël recommends creating a 50:50 blend with peppermint and a carrier oil, filling capsules and taking 3 to 4 a day with food +++++P.

- Blend a drop or two of wintergreen and a drop or two of peppermint in a teaspoon of carrier oil and massage the painful nerve pathway ++++P. Add a drop of clove for additional pain relief.

- Dr. Pénoël suggests a 50:50 peppermint and carrier oil blend. Fill capsules and take a capsule 3 times a day with food ++++P.

- Take warm bath with 5 to 10 drops of the Comforting blend or lavender dispersed in a cup of Epsom Salts.

- Diffuse 10 to 20 drops of lavender, the Stress control blend, or the Comforting blend whenever you need a calming influence.

- Use a drop of bergamot or the Comforting blend in a cup of herbal tea or a quart of drinking water.

CLINICAL SUPPORT

"[Rosemary essential oil] is used for problems involved in central nervous system, cardiovascular system, genito-urinary conditions, liver treatments, the reproductive system and respiratory system. The volatile oil of the plant is used in oils and lotions for the treatment of various ailments like arthritis, gout, muscular pain, neuralgia, wounds and rubbed into hair for stimulating the hair bulbs to renewed activity, to prevent premature baldness" (Begum A, et al., 2013).

Nosebleed

WHAT IT IS

Epistaxis or bleeding from the nose usually comes from the area that separates the nostrils in the front of the nose where there are many blood vessels close to the surface. They may be caused by local infections like colds and sinus conditions, drying of the membranes of the nose during cold seasons, overuse of nasal sprays, foreign objects in the nose, fist fights, and bleeding disorders.

RECOMMENDED OILS

Lemon		Cypress	
Peppermint		Eucalyptus radiata	

INSTRUCTION

- Avoid applying essential oils directly on the fragile mucous membranes on the inside of the nose (especially if you have allergies).

- Try putting a trace of lemon on the surface of the nose without getting it on the mucous membranes inside the nose.

- Patricia Davis suggests soaking a gauze pad in a mixture of a drop or two of lemon oil, a 1/2 teaspoon of lemon juice and a 1/2 teaspoon of carrier oil. Put it up the nose (Davis, p. 55).

- Apply a cold, damp cloth or ice pack to the base of the neck (apply a few drops of undiluted peppermint first to enhance the cooling action). Do not put peppermint on the necks of children under 30 months.

Obesity & Weight Loss

WHAT IT IS

Traditionally 20% to 40% over ideal weight was considered mildly obese. Forty to 100% over ideal weight was obese, and over 100% was considered morbidly obese. Other guidelines use BMI (body mass index). It is your weight multiplied by 703 divided by twice your height in inches. BMI of 25.9 to 29 is considered overweight. Over 30 is obese.

RECOMMENDED OILS

Rosemary		Bergamot	
Black pepper		Grapefruit	
Lemon		Peppermint	
Orange		Tangerine	

RECOMMENDED BLEND

Weight loss blend

INSTRUCTION

- Create a 50:50 blend using the weight loss blend and a carrier oil. Create capsules using a dropper, and take 3 to 4 a day with food to decrease appetite and help with the product's natural thermogenic effect to burn calories.

- Dr. Pénoël suggests a capsule with lemon (25%), tangerine (25%), and carrier oil (50%). Use a dropper to create capsules and take 2 a day with food ++P.

- He also suggests a massage oil for obesity including Eucalyptus radiata 20%, sage, 20%, peppermint 10%, and 50% carrier oil ++P.

- Pamper yourself with a bath using 10 to 15 drops of any of these oils: birch, tangerine, lemon, or orange in a cup of Epsom Salts ++P.

CLINICAL SUPPORT

"Abdominal subcutaneous fat and waist circumference in the experimental group significantly decreased after aromatherapy massage compared to the control group. Body image in the experimental group was significantly better after aromatherapy massage than in the control group. These results suggest that aromatherapy massage could be utilized as an effective intervention to reduce abdominal subcutaneous fat, waist circumference, and to improve body image in post-menopausal women" (Kim HJ., 2007).

Osteoarthritis (See Arthritis)

Osteoporosis

WHAT IT IS

A medical condition in which your bones become fragile and brittle. The bone loses density, typically because of hormonal changes or insufficient available calcium or vitamin D.

RECOMMENDED OILS

Clary sage		Rosemary	
Eucalyptus radiate		Pine	

RECOMMENDED BLENDS

Massage blend		Circulation blend	
Soothing blend		Inflammation blend	

For the discomfort associated with osteoporosis and with the involvement of your health care professional as needed, use the following procedures:

- Massage the muscles and joints of the affected areas with a mixture of 4 to 5 drops of the Massage blend or the circulation blend in a teaspoon of carrier oil.

- For pain associated with osteoporosis, massage the painful areas with a diluted blend 50:50 of the Soothing blend with a carrier oil. Or you can massage on alternate days with a diluted blend (50:50) with the Inflammation blend. If you wish a single application, dilute 4 to 5 drops in a teaspoon of carrier oil.

- You can help prevent osteoporosis by following this book's dietary guidelines. It's important to understand how your bones become slowly dissolved by having too much acid in your body because of eating too

many proteins and other acid-forming foods. You'll want to enjoy a diet rich in green, leafy vegetables and sprouted grains to help you maintain healthy bones.

Paget's Disease

WHAT IT IS

A chronic disorder that involves abnormal bone deterioration and regrowth, resulting in deformity especially in the skill, pelvis, or spine. Typically a disease of the elderly that can sometimes cause significant pain.

RECOMMENDED OILS

Peppermint		Wintergreen	
Birch			

RECOMMENDED BLENDS

Soothing blend		Inflammation blend	

INSTRUCTION

With the involvement of a competent health care professional as needed, use the following suggestions:

- For relief of pain apply 4 to 5 drops of the Soothing blend undiluted on the area of greatest pain. If the area is a large one, mix the Soothing blend 50:50 with a carrier oil and massage the area twice a day.

- It may be important to alternate the Soothing blend with the inflammation blend. Use both blends the same but simply use the Soothing blend in the morning and the Inflammation blend in the evening.

Pancreatitis (Chronic)

WHAT IT IS

Chronic inflammation in the pancreas. The pancreas produces critical enzymes that help digestion as well as hormones that help regulate how the body processes sugar (glucose). Mild cases may go away without treatment, but severe ones can be life-threatening. Symptoms include unexpected weight loss without dieting, upper abdominal pain, and oily stools with a bad odor.

RECOMMENDED OILS

Peppermint   Orange

RECOMMENDED BLENDS

Liver blend   Digestion blend

Immune balancing blend

INSTRUCTION

Suggestions that are part of an overall health maintenance plan involving your health care professional as needed:

- Create a blend of equal quantities of the liver blend, the digestion blend, and the immune balancing blend and use it in the following four ways:

- Use 3 or 4 drops of the blend undiluted with a drop or two of the foot massage blend for a daily reflexology massage of the feet.

- Mix the blend 50:50 with a carrier oil for a massage over the area of the body where the pancreas is located.

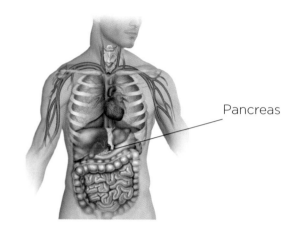

Pancreas

- Add a drop of the blend in a quart of your drinking water or a cup of herbal tea and drink it twice daily.

- Create a 50:50 mixture of the blend with a carrier oil. Fill capsules with a dropper and take capsule 3 times a day with food. Keep taking the capsules for an additional 3 or 4 months after you have seen an improvement.

- For a deep healing, do a Liver Cleanse according to the instructions on Cleansing earlier in this chapter. You'll want to do it for about a year to make sure there is a deep healing taking place.

Parasites (intestinal)

WHAT IT IS

A parasite is an opportunistic organism that lives on or in the body. An intestinal parasite typically populates the digestive tract, but it can also migrate and live throughout the body. Parasites enter the body from eating undercooked meat, drinking contaminated water, and through skin absorption. Giardia is an example. There are also worms: tapeworms, flatworms, roundworms, etc.

RECOMMENDED OILS

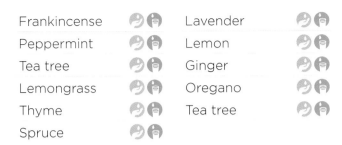

Frankincense		Lavender		
Peppermint		Lemon		
Tea tree		Ginger		
Lemongrass		Oregano		
Thyme		Tea tree		
Spruce				

RECOMMENDED BLENDS

Protecting blend		Liver blend	
Digestion blend			

INSTRUCTION

As a complement to the advice of your health care professional and with his/her approval, follow these suggestions:

- Take up to 16 drops daily of any of the recommended oils or blends. This can conveniently be done by mixing the oils into a blend then creating a 50:50 mixture with a carrier oil. Fill capsules with a dropper and take 3 capsules a day with food. An example of a strong blend would be tea tree (20%), cypress (20%), thyme (10%) and carrier oil (50%) +++P. A milder blend would be would be frankincense (20%), lavender (30%), and carrier oil (50%).

- Take 1 or 2 drops of the Liver blend, the Protecting blend, or the Digestion blend in an herbal tea with honey, a quart of drinking water, juice, or recipes (after taking the it off the stove).

- When traveling in locations where the water may be contaminated with parasites, use a drop of tea tree, lemon, or the Protecting blend to purify all drinking water. One drop per quart is sufficient. Also take one or two

of the capsules for prevention when traveling in these areas.

CLINICAL SUPPORT

Giardia is one of the most important worldwide causes of intestinal infections. Essential oils or some of their constituents may be useful in the clinical management of giardia infections (Machado M, et al, 2010).

There are many plant-derived agents that are more effective against human tropical diseases than the synthetic alternatives. Tropical diseases studied include: amebiasis, Chagas disease, cholera, cryptosporidiosis, dengue, epidemic typhus, filariasis (elephantiasis), giardia, human African trypanosomiasis (sleeping sickness), isosporiasis, leishmaniasis, Lyme disease, malaria, onchocerciasis, plague, recurrent fever, sarcocystosis, scabies, spotted fever, toxoplasmosis, West Nile fever, and yellow fever. Essential oils exhibiting noxious or toxic activity are comparable or superior to the synthetic control agents of choice for many tropical diseases (Pohlit AM, et al., 2011).

Phobias (See Aromatic Behavioral Conditioning under Addictions and Self-Defeating Behavior)

Pink Eye & Stye
(Conjunctivitis)

WHAT IT IS

Inflammation of the lining of the eyelids and the white part of the eye. Symptoms include a bloodshot look to the eye, itchiness, a gritty feeling, some discharge or a crust that forms overnight, and increased tearing. It is highly contagious for up to 2 weeks after symptoms begin. A stye is an inflamed oil gland on your eyelid. It looks like a pimple and is tender to the touch.

RECOMMENDED OILS

Tea tree

Roman chamomile

German chamomile

Eucalyptus radiata

Myrtle

Lavender

RECOMMENDED BLEND

Inflammation blend

INSTRUCTION

With the approval of your health care professional if needed, follow these simple suggestions:

- If you wear contacts, stop wearing them until your condition clears up.

- Never put even a trace of essential oils into your eyes.

- Soak a piece of sterile gauze in this solution and apply over closed eyes: 1 drop of tea tree, lavender, Eucalyptus radiata, Roman chamomile, or German chamomile oil in a cup of sterile tepid water mixed with 1/4 teaspoon of salt. Throw away the gauze after each treatment to avoid spreading the infection.

- For allergic conjunctivitis Dr. Pénoël recommends using myrtle for this treatment ++++P. For bacterial conjunctivitis he recommends an equal blend of Eucalyptus globulus and Roman chamomile ++++P. Use the saturated gauze treatment with water mentioned above.

- There is no harm in treating both eyes at the same time to avoid spreading the infection from one eye to the other.

CLINICAL SUPPORT

Tested a treatment of conjunctivitis with a lid scrub containing tea tree oil. Improvement in 10 out of 11 individuals tested (Gao YY, et al., 2007).

Pneumonia

WHAT IT IS

Pneumonia can apply to many types of lung inflammations, bacterial or viral. Symptoms include a cough that produces mucous, chest pain, sweating, faster breathing and pulse rates, and often a high fever. The tiny sacks of the lungs (alveoli) fill with pus and other liquid, making it hard to get oxygen to the red blood cells.

RECOMMENDED OILS

Eucalyptus radiata

Tea tree

Rosemary

Lavender

Pine

Cajeput

Frankincense

Peppermint

Lemon

RECOMMENDED BLENDS

Protecting blend

Respiratory blend

Massage blend

INSTRUCTION

Pneumonia can be life-threatening and requires the involvement of a health care professional. The following steps can be taken with his or her approval and to supplement his or her recommendations:

- Because essential oils are both antibacterial and antiviral, diffusing tea tree, Eucalyptus radiata, the Respiratory blend, and the Protecting blend will be helpful in the healing process. Alternating from one essential oil or blend to another every few hours can also be particularly effective at addressing all the possible bacteria or viruses that may be involved.

- To help prevent secondary infections coming from a cough, apply a trace of tea tree, frankincense, peppermint, the Respiratory blend, or the Protecting blend to the tongue and hold it there for a minute before swallowing. Do this often throughout the day.

- Steam inhalations using lemon, tea tree, Eucalyptus radiata, or the Respiratory blend will help loosen mucous and get life-giving essential oils to where they need to be in the respiratory system. Put 3 to 4 drops of one of the recommended oils in a bowl or pan of boiling water. Put a towel over your head and inhale deeply. Blowing into the water will disperse the aromatic molecules more quickly. Reheat the water and add more oils as needed.

- Lavender and balsam fir in this steam application will be especially beneficial for reducing coughing spasms.

- Warm compresses on both the back and the chest can be helpful. Mix 6 to 8 drops of the Respiratory blend or the Protecting blend in a cup of hot water. Soak a small towel in the mixture, wring it out slightly, and put it on the back or chest for 20 minutes. This can also be done by applying the oil undiluted to the body then putting a warm, damp towel over it. If the oil becomes at all uncomfortable, you may want to add a little carrier oil to calm it down.

- Use one of the recommended essential oils or blends 50:50 with carrier oil. Fill capsules with a dropper and take 3 to 6 capsules a day with food.

- Bacteria and viruses thrive on mucous-producing foods that contain dairy, white flour, and white sugar. Eliminate them as much as possible while you are trying to heal and for a few weeks afterwards.

- Drink more water than usual with a drop or trace of a respiratory oil in it. Add more fresh fruits and vegetables to your diet. Enjoy more foods than usual containing fresh garlic, cayenne pepper, and chili peppers. They can help alleviate pneumonia symptoms.

- To rapidly get a lot of essential oil molecules into your system, try Dr. Penoel's "Live Embalming" therapy found in Chapter 4. Use 5 to 10 drops at a time for a total of 20 or 30 drops of Eucalyptus radiata or ravintsara with a hair dryer to get a large amount of essential oils to penetrate the body in a short amount of time. Be sure to change locations on the body with each application. Be sure to read the instructions in Chapter 4 before trying this therapy.

Poisoning (see Detoxification after Poisoning or Addiction)

Pregnancy
(Using essential oils during and after)

Because your senses and emotions are more active than usual during and after pregnancy, essential oils can be amazingly helpful at helping you with some of the challenges of pregnancy. They will also help you enjoy many of the wonderful new feelings associated with pregnancy. The dietary guidelines in this book are important rules for a trouble-free pregnancy. Exercise, enough water, rest, and great relationships are also essential parts of a healthy pregnancy.

Avoid using these oils during pregnancy:

Peppermint, birch, sweet basil, camphor, clary sage, cypress, juniper, marjoram, oregano, rosemary, sage, thyme, wintergreen, the Massage blend, the Circulation blend, or the Soothing blend

These oils have some minor constituents that have been linked in some studies to inducing labor. It's wise to double dilute your oil during pregnancy because a little goes a long way when your whole system is involved in making a baby. So when the instructions say 50:50, dilute them 25:75.

With the blessing of your gynecologist or other health care professional, use the following essential oils for the conditions described:

Breast Tenderness

WHAT IT IS

Hormones are helping your breasts prepare for nursing a baby. They will be especially tender during the first trimester.

RECOMMENDED OILS

Lavender   Roman chamomile

German chamomile

RECOMMENDED BLEND

Inflammation blend

INSTRUCTION

- Use 2 to 3 drops of lavender, Roman chamomile, German chamomile, or the inflammation blend in a teaspoon of carrier oil. Massage gently on the tenderest areas.

Nausea/Morning Sickness

WHAT IT IS

This common condition can happen at any time of the day or night, not just in the morning. It's most common during the first trimester but can happen throughout your pregnancy. On rare occasions it can require hospitalization and IVs to avoid dehydration.

RECOMMENDED OILS

Lavender   Ginger

Roman chamomile   German chamomile

RECOMMENDED BLENDS

Digestion blend   Inflammation blend

INSTRUCTION

- Use a single drop of spearmint, lemon, tangerine, lime, or the digestion blend in each quart of your drinking water.

- A drop of any of these can also be used in a calming herbal tea. A trace of ginger in your tea may also be beneficial.

- Inhale your favourite of these oils from a tissue to help alleviate nausea.

Constipation

WHAT IT IS

A condition that often begins early in pregnancy due to hormones relaxing the smooth muscle of the body including digestive muscles. The problem can be even more severe late in pregnancy as the heavy baby presses on the digestive organs. Iron supplements may need to be adjusted because they can contribute to the problem.

RECOMMENDED OILS

Lavender		Roman chamomile	
German chamomile			

RECOMMENDED BLENDS

Digestion blend		Inflammation blend	

Instruction

Drink water containing a drop of the digestion blend or one of the other recommended oils. Massage your lower back in a counter-clockwise direction with 2 to 3 drops of the digestion blend or the other oils mixed in a teaspoon of carrier oil. Patricia Davis

recommends that you sit on a stool next to the massage couch. You are leaning on your forearms, which are folded on the couch (see illustration). The one giving the massage can kneel on the floor and use that leverage to give a comforting massage (Davis, p. 258). This may be more comfortable and allow a firmer, more comforting massage during the last trimester than lying on your back.

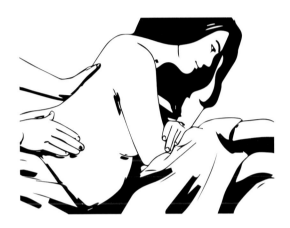

Massage the arch of your feet in a clockwise motion with 2 to 3 drops of one of the recommended oils and 2 to 3 drops of the foot massage blend.

Heartburn

WHAT IT IS

A condition that typically arrives in the second and third trimesters. It's a burning sensation of the esophagus caused by reflux of stomach contents (coming back up). Changing hormones may relax the smooth muscles and cause this condition.

Prevention and Treatment of Heartburn During Pregnancy

To reduce heartburn during pregnancy without hurting your baby, you should try the following:

RECOMMENDED OILS

Lavender		Lemon		
Tangerine		Ginger		
Roman chamomile		German chamomile		

RECOMMENDED BLENDS

Digestion blend		Inflammation blend	

INSTRUCTION

- Drink a glass of water with a trace of lemon or another citrus oil added with a toothpick.

- Use a drop or two of lemon oil or another citrus oil in each quart of your drinking water.

- Use a drop of lemon or another citrus oil in a cup of herbal tea.

- Massage two or three drops of lemon or another citrus oil and a little carrier oil on the balls of your feet.

- Eat more small meals each day, and eat slowly, enjoying your food.

- Avoid rich, fried, spicy foods.

- Don't drink as many liquids while eating

- Don't lie down right after eating.

- Sleep with your head higher than your feet

- Wear loose-fitting clothing.

Swollen Ankles

WHAT IT IS

A condition that often begins late in the pregnancy due to hormones relaxing the smooth muscle of the body including digestive muscles. The problem can be even more severe late in pregnancy as the heavy baby presses on the digestive organs. Iron supplements may need to be adjusted because they can contribute to the problem.

RECOMMENDED OILS

Lavender		Lemon	
Helichrysum		Balsam fir	
Roman chamomile		German chamomile	

RECOMMENDED BLENDS

Digestion blend		Inflammation blend	

INSTRUCTION

- Massage your ankles and legs in a direction leading toward the heart with a mixture of 3 to 4 of any of the recommended oils or blends in a teaspoon of carrier oil. It's best to have someone else give you this massage while your legs are slightly elevated, but rather than not doing it, do it for yourself. Do this massage twice daily if possible.

- Avoid adding extra salt or drinking coffee and strong tea

Stretch marks

WHAT IT IS

When the skin is constantly stretched, it can break down, leaving a form of scarring behind.

Initially is can be reddish or purplish, but then it becomes glossy, making the skin look streaked in silver or white.

RECOMMENDED OILS

Tangerine   Neroli

Lavender

RECOMMENDED BLENDS

Comforting blend

INSTRUCTION

- Prevention is the key with stretch marks. They're difficult to get rid of once they have formed. From the 4th month, you will want to massage your abdomen daily to increase the elasticity of the skin. A carrier oil like rose hip or jojoba alone will work, but 3 or 4 drops of a pleasant essential oil like tangerine or neroli will help even more. You can also add these oils to non-toxic lotions, but oils will likely be more effective overall.

- If you already have stretch marks, apply 2 to 3 drops of lavender undiluted on the marks. You can mix them with jojoba oil for a more moisturizing effect.

Backache (Possible sciatica)

WHAT IT IS

Your enlarged uterus will shift your center of gravity while it stretches and weakens your abdominal muscles, putting a strain on your back. Hormonal changes also loosen your joints and ligaments, making you feel less stable and causing pain when you do almost anything from turning over in bed to walking. Most pregnancy-related back pain is in the lower back, but you can also experience posterior pelvic pain in the back of your pelvis. Some women have pain that radiates to their legs and even their feet. If you feel serious sciatic pain or numbness, be sure to contact your health care professional or gynecologist right away.

RECOMMENDED OILS

Lavender   Roman chamomile

German chamomile

RECOMMENDED BLENDS

Inflammation blend   Foot massage blend

INSTRUCTION

- Patricia Davis recommends that early in your pregnancy your massage your back and abdomen very lightly, but as the back pain comes on, a more aggressive massage can be most helpful. For the best position she recommends that you sit on a stool next to the massage couch. You are leaning on your forearms, which are folded on the couch (see illustration). The one giving the massage can kneel on the floor and use that leverage to give a comforting massage (Davis, p. 258). This may be more comfortable and allow a firmer, more beneficial massage during the last trimester than lying on your back.

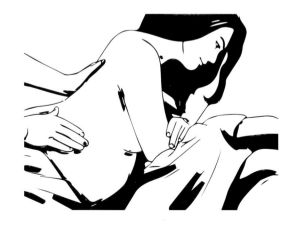

- Davis further cites research suggesting that mothers who are massaged regularly throughout their pregnancy, especially near the end of pregnancy, have calmer babies. The baby inside seems to settle down with frequent calming massage as well, and the calming oils and movements seem to settle any anxieties.

- Use 3 or 4 drops of lavender and the inflammation blend with the foot massage blend for a thorough massage along the inside bottoms of the feet.

- Use 3 to 4 drops of the Comforting blend in a teaspoon of carrier oil for a calming lower back massage.

- Use a drop of the Inflammation blend or the Comforting blend on the abdominal area of the ears as well.

- Ask for specific directions on how to guard your posture and exercise throughout your pregnancy to help strengthen the muscles that keep your back pain from becoming debilitating. Careful, pregnancy-adjusted yoga may prove helpful.

Shortness of Breath

WHAT IT IS

Women need more oxygen during pregnancy, and the amount of air you inhale and exhale with each breath increases significantly because you're breathing for two. Later, as the uterus presses on your diaphragm, your breathing might feel more difficult. You want to decrease the risk of any respiratory infection during pregnancy, so essential oils can help substantially with that.

RECOMMENDED OILS

Lavender		Eucalyptus radiata	
Roman chamomile		German chamomile	

RECOMMENDED BLENDS

Respiratory blend		Comforting blend	

INSTRUCTION

- Diffuse a few drops of the respiratory blend or Eucalyptus radiata whenever you feel short of breath.

- Apply a trace of any of the recommended blends on each side of your nostrils. Avoid putting it inside the nose near the mucous membranes.

Insomnia

WHAT IT IS

It's hard to sleep because it's hard to get comfortable. You may need to get up multiple times in the night to go to the bathroom. You may have leg cramps. You may be both excited and anxious about the baby's arrival.

RECOMMENDED OILS

Lavender		Tangerine	
Roman chamomile		German chamomile	
Balsam fir			

RECOMMENDED BLENDS

Comforting blend		Foot massage blend	
Inflammation blend			

INSTRUCTION

- Enjoy evening foot reflexology massages with 2 to 3 drops of lavender, the Comforting blend, and the Foot Massage blend undiluted or diluted in a teaspoon of carrier oil.

- Diffuse 5 to 10 drops of the Comforting blend or lavender for a few minutes every evening.

- Take warm (not hot) baths with 5 to 10 drops of one of the recommended oils dispersed with a cup of Epsom Salts.

Postpartum Depression After Childbirth

WHAT IT IS

The "baby blues" affects up to 80 percent of new mothers. It typically lasts two weeks. If it lasts longer, it could be clinical postpartum depression with anxiety, obsessive-compulsive disorder, irritability, hypersensitivity, difficulty concentrating, excessive crying, anger, hopelessness, difficulty sleeping, exhaustion, changes in appetite, headaches, dizziness, trembling, hot or cold flashes, fear of losing control, and fear of harming your baby or others. Seek professional help if your conditions become debilitating or if you fear you might act out on something harmful. There can be multiple causes—hormonal, biochemical, environmental, psychological, and genetic— that contribute to postpartum depression. Fortunately essential oils can help.

RECOMMENDED OILS

Lavender		Frankincense	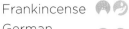
Roman chamomile		German chamomile	
Tangerine		Balsam fir	

RECOMMENDED BLENDS

Comforting blend		Foot massage blend	
Intimacy blend		Inflammation blend	

INSTRUCTION

- Enjoy evening foot reflexology massages with 2 to 3 drops of any of the recommended oils with the foot massage blend undiluted or diluted in a teaspoon of carrier oil.

- Take warm (not hot) baths with 5 to 10 drops of any of the recommended oils dispersed with a cup of Epsom Salts.

- Diffuse 5 to 10 drops the Comforting blend, lavender, lemon, the Intimacy blend, or frankincense. Alternate oils.

- Enjoy back massages using the Layer Therapy technique found in chapter 4. Layer only the calming oils recommended here, not the strong oils recommended elsewhere for this technique. Start and end with 3 to 4 drops of balsam fir applied undiluted up your back then, kneading the oils in with your knuckles on each side of the spine. Then feather the oil out with your fingernails on the sides of the back to wake up your nerves. Do each action 3 times. Finish by massaging with 2 to 3 drops of balsam fir mixed with a teaspoon of carrier oil down the back. Apply a drop of balsam fir on the sternum area and relax for 20 minutes.

CLINICAL SUPPORT

This study examined the benefits of aromatherapy-massage in postpartum mothers. Thirty-six first-time mothers participated. Scores significantly improved for those experiencing aromatherapy massage (Imura M, Misao H, Ushijima H., 2006).

"The pilot study indicates positive findings with minimal risk for the use of aromatherapy as a complementary therapy in both anxiety and depression scales with the postpartum woman" (Conrad P, Adams C., 2012).

Difficulty Nursing

WHAT IT IS

Breastfeeding can take time and practice. The following can present challenges: sore nipples (pinching, itching, or burning), breast fullness, not enough milk, plugged ducts, breast infections, and thrush are among the most common problems. There are many experts available to help with overcoming all these difficulties.

RECOMMENDED OILS

Lavender		Lemon	
Roman chamomile		German chamomile	
Tea tree		Frankincense	

RECOMMENDED BLENDS

Comforting blend		Foot massage blend	
Intimacy blend		Protecting blend	
Inflammation blend			

INSTRUCTION

Problems with breastfeeding are common and can be easily treated or solved with the help of a lactation consultant. With that professional assistance, try these suggestions:

- To help you relax, enjoy evening foot reflexology massages with 2 to 3 drops of any of the recommended oils with the Foot Massage blend undiluted or diluted in a teaspoon of carrier oil.

- Take warm (not hot) baths with 5 to 10 drops of any of the recommended oils dispersed with a cup of Epsom Salts.

- Diffuse 5 to 10 drops the Comforting blend, the Intimacy blend, lavender, lemon, or frankincense.

- Create a mixture with a teaspoon of carrier oil and a drop each of lavender and the inflammation blend. Gently massage breasts and upper back with this mixture.

- If breasts become infected (mastitis), add a drop of tea tree and a drop of the Protecting blend to the mixture.

- You can create alternating warm and cold compresses with cloths soaked in a drop or two of lavender mixed in a cup of water. Cover the cloth with a thin plastic film to help penetration and alternate applying cool then warm towels at 5-minute intervals.

Toxemia (Pre-eclampsia)

WHAT IT IS

A condition in pregnancy characterized by a sharp rise in blood pressure, a large amount of protein in the urine, blurry vision, and swelling in the hands, feet and face. It typically occurs in the third trimester. It is common in women with diabetes or who carry twins. It is a sign of serious problems: the detachment of the placenta, coma, or seizures. It is treated by bed rest and sometimes medication. It is resolved after the baby is born.

RECOMMENDED OILS

Lavender		Lemon	
Roman chamomile		German chamomile	
Frankincense			

RECOMMENDED BLENDS

Comforting blend		Intimacy blend	

INSTRUCTION

- Because this is such a serious condition, it is imperative that a health care professional become involved. The following suggestions may help.

- Massage ankles daily with 3 to 4 drops of the Comforting blend, the inflammation blend, and lavender. The massage should be in an upward direction toward the heart.

- Diffuse 10 to 15 drops of any of the oils listed.

Premenstrual Syndrome (PMS)

WHAT IT IS

A condition that happens a week to 10 days before menstruation. Symptoms include fluid retention, breast tenderness, swollen abdomen, headaches, nausea, high emotions, depression, and personality changes.

RECOMMENDED OILS

Rosemary		Peppermint	
Roman chamomile		German chamomile	
Sweet basil		Bergamot	
Frankincense			

RECOMMENDED BLENDS

Comforting blend		Intimacy blend	

INSTRUCTION

With the approval of your health care professional if needed, try the following in-home procedures:

- Patricia Davis recommends a lymphatic drainage massage done monthly 2 to 3 days before the anticipated onset of the PMS symptoms. It will help ease fluid retention, but it can mitigate many of the other effects of PMS (Davis, p. 260).

- Use a natural progesterone cream following careful instructions from a health care professional or an authoritative book on the subject.

- For breast tenderness, use a few drops of either lavender or the inflammation blend in a teaspoon of carrier oil. Gently massage the tender areas.

- For insomnia, have a foot massage every evening with 2 to 3 drops of lavender, the Comforting blend, and the Foot Massage blend undiluted.

- For insomnia you can also diffuse 5 to 10 drops of lavender or the Comforting blend for 5 minutes every evening. And take warm baths using 5 to 10 drops of lavender or the Comforting blend dispersed into a cup of Epsom Salts.

- For headaches, use a drop of peppermint or frankincense in a cup of herbal tea or a quart of drinking water. Also apply a trace of either of these oils on your temples, forehead, and back of the neck.

- Use a drop of sweet basil in herbal teas and many recipes as well (after taking the food off the stove). Use sweet basil in dips, salad dressings, and any recipe you can find to serve during the PMS days of the month.

- For emotional challenges, do frequent reflexology foot massages with 2 to 3 drops of peppermint, 2 to 3 drops of frankincense, and the foot massage blend. Concentrate under the anklebones the heel of the foot.

- For menstrual cramps massage the ankles and heel with 3 or 4 drops of sweet basil.

- Also for cramps do a massage of the lower abdomen using 3 to 4 drops of sweet basil in a teaspoon of carrier oil. Massage in a clockwise direction on the lower abdomen but use a counter-clockwise direction on the lower back.

- For fluid retention, gently massage the swollen areas toward the heart with a blend of 3 to 5 drops of the circulation blend or lavender in a teaspoon of carrier oil.

Prostate (Inflammation, enlargement, infection, and cancer)

WHAT IT IS

A gland unique to men that surrounds the neck of the bladder. It can become swollen (benign prostatic hyperplasia or BPH), inflamed, infected (prostatitis), and develop cancer, causing serious problems with urinary retention, especially among older men.

RECOMMENDED OILS

Tea tree		Spearmint	
Cypress		Myrtle	
Sweet basil		Peppermint	
Lavender		Frankincense	

RECOMMENDED BLEND

Foot massage blend

INSTRUCTION

Here are in-home procedures suggested as part of an overall plan involving your health care professional as needed.

- A thorough digestive cleanse will help clear up deep-seated infections and help balance all the organs and glands of the body. A balanced diet that is rich in fruits and vegetables, sufficient exercise, and good relationships all contribute to a healthy prostate and cancer prevention. Because hormones are a factor, you can try using a natural progesterone cream according to instructions for men.

- Create a blend of frankincense (25%), tea tree (25%), lavender (20%), peppermint (15%), and spearmint (15%). Ask for supplies for a fleet enema at your pharmacy. Mix 6 drops of this blend in a tablespoon of carrier oil to be used as a retention enema through the night each night for 7 days. Then take four days off, and repeat. Disinfect all supplies with soap and water after each application.

- Use the same blend of oils undiluted on your feet and ears on the areas corresponding to the prostate. Massage the points just below the ankle bones on the feet. Use with a few drops of the foot massage blend if desired.

- L'aromatherapie exactement, by Dr. Pénoël suggests the following oils as a prostate decongestant: cypress ++P, myrtle++P and sweet basil++P.

- For its anti-inflammatory effect, he also suggests spruce. Create a 50:50 blend with spruce and a carrier oil, then massage the area just above the pubic bone on the lower abdomen ++P.

Rabies

WHAT IT IS

An infection that affects the nervous system. It is transmitted in the saliva from a bite by an infected animal.

RECOMMENDED OILS

Tea tree		Thyme	
Spruce		Vetiver	
Orange		Eucalyptus globulus	
Frankincense			

RECOMMENDED BLEND

Protecting blend	

INSTRUCTION

Use the following in-home procedures with the approval of your health care professional:

- Create a blend of tea tree (40%), thyme (10%) and a carrier oil (50%). Or you can create a 50:50 mixture with the Protecting blend and a carrier oil. Fill capsules with a dropper and take three capsules daily with food.

- Take one or two drops of either the Protecting blend or tea tree in an herbal tea with honey, a quart of drinking water, juice, or recipes (after taking them off the stove).

- Children will typically prefer taking the oils in water, juice, or mild foods like applesauce.

- You can also massage the feet of children and even babies with 1 or 2 drops of Protecting blend, tea tree, or frankincense diluted in a teaspoon of carrier oil.

Rashes (See Hives & Rashes)

Raynaud's Syndrome

WHAT IT IS

A condition that causes some areas of your body (fingers, toes, nose, and ears) to feel numb and cool in cold temperatures or stress. Small arteries narrow, limiting circulation. It can be severe and lead to gangrene, but for most people, it is more of a nuisance than a disability. However, it is not just having cold hands and feet, nor is it the same as frostbite. During an attack the skin turns white then blue. It feels cold and numb. As circulation returns, the skin may turn red, sting, throb, tingle or swell.

RECOMMENDED OILS

Lavender		Orange	
Roman chamomile		German chamomile	
Tangerine		Lime	
Grapefruit		Neroli	
Lemon		Cinnamon	
Clove		Frankincense	

RECOMMENDED BLEND

Comforting blend		Foot massage blend	
Massage blend			

INSTRUCTION

Contact your health care professional if the condition is severe and you develop an ulcer or infection in one of your affected areas. Otherwise use these suggestions:

• Incorporate lavender and the Comforting blend in a diluted massage (2 to 3 drops of each oil in a teaspoon of carrier oil). Massage your neck and shoulders for calming the upper body.

• Use the Massage blend 50:50 with a carrier oil for gently massaging muscles to energize and restore feeling. You can also use the circulation blend this way.

• Use any of these blends undiluted with a few drops of the Foot Massage blend for calming reflexology massage.

• Create an energizing spice blend using 90% orange (or a mixture of various citrus oils),

5% cinnamon, and 5% clove. Ingest one or two drops of this delicious, energizing blend in your water or herbal tea. You can also use a toothpick to adjust the flavour in a glass of water or a cup of hot water.

• Diffuse 5 to 10 drops of the calming blend or lavender for 5 minutes for its restorative affect.

• Take a warm bath frequently with 5 to 10 drops of the Comforting blend or lavender dispersed in a cup of Epsom Salts.

Rheumatism (see Arthritis)

Ringworm

WHAT IT IS

A contagious skin infection usually on the scalp, appearing as small round circles that may or may not itch. It is not a worm but a fungus. It is similar to athlete's foot. There can be several patches on the scalp at once.

RECOMMENDED OILS

Lavender		Tea tree	
Peppermint		Spearmint	

RECOMMENDED BLEND

Protecting blend	

INSTRUCTION

• Use any of the recommended oils to create a 50:50 blend with a carrier oil and apply it to the affected area.

- You can also mix a few drops of any of the recommended oils in a few drops of water and apply it to the infection several times a day for a more drying action.

- Add 3 – 4 drops of any of the recommended oils to each application of your hair care products and massage them into your scalp as you apply them.

CLINICAL SUPPORT

"This study highlights the broad spectrum antifungal activity of essential oils against drug-resistant fungi" (Khan MS, Ahmad I., 2011).

Rubella (German measles)

WHAT IT IS

This condition usually causes little more than a mild rash. Though it is usually mild, it can severely damage a developing fetus.

Use the following in-home procedures with the agreement of your health care professional:

- Take up to 16 drops of a blend of equal parts of the following oils: Rosemary, tea tree, the Inflammation blend, and the Protecting blend. This can conveniently be done by taking 3 capsules a day with food as follows: mix 4 drops of the blend in a vegetable capsule and fill the capsule with carrier oil.

- Take 1 or 2 drops of the above blends or single oils in an herbal tea with honey, a quart of water, juice, or recipes (after taking the recipe off the heat).

- Small children will do better taking the oils in water, juice, or food.

- You can also rub the feet of children and even babies with 1 or 2 drops of the recommended oils diluted in a teaspoon of carrier oil. Do this several times a day.

- If there is a high fever or mild rash associated with rubella, mix a drop of the Inflammation blend in a cup of tepid water. Soak a cloth in it and wipe the child's back or effected area with it. This will cool the child safely and quickly and will sooth the rash.

Scabies (Itch mite)

WHAT IT IS

Scabies is a skin disease that is easily spread. It is caused by a very small mite that burrows in the skin and creates small, raised red spots. The itching is usually worst at night. Though any part of the body may be infected, it is most often found in folds between fingers, in armpits, around the waist, on the inner elbow, etc. Because it is so infectious, a whole family should be treated at the same time.

RECOMMENDED OILS

Bergamot		Lavender	
Lemongrass		Peppermint	
Spearmint		Pine	
Rosemary			

RECOMMENDED BLENDS

Protecting blend		Purifying blend	

INSTRUCTION

- Use any of the recommended oils to create a 50:50 blend with a carrier oil and apply it to the affected area.

- You can also mix a few drops of any of the recommended oils in a few drops of water and apply it to the infection several times a day for a more drying action.

- If the infection is in your scalp, add 3 – 4 drops of any of the recommended oils to each application of your hair care products and massage them into your scalp as you apply them.

CLINICAL SUPPORT

Resistance against other agents that treat scabies is mounting, so this test confirmed the recommendation of tea tree oil as an effective alternative (Walton SF, et al., 2004).

Scars & Stretch Marks

WHAT IT IS

When the skin is constantly stretched, as in pregnancy, scars can develop called stretch marks. A scar is a mark left on the skin where a wound, burn, or infection has not healed completely and a fibrous connective tissue has developed.

RECOMMENDED OILS

Tangerine		Neroli	
Patchouli		Rosewood	
Sandalwood		Lavender	
Frankincense			

RECOMMENDED BLENDS

Comforting blend

INSTRUCTION

- Prevention is the best way to avoid scars and stretch marks. They're difficult to get rid of once they have formed.

- For preventing stretch marks, from the 4th month, you will want to massage your abdomen daily to increase the elasticity of the skin. A carrier oil like rose hips or jojoba alone will work, but 3 or 4 drops of a pleasant essential oil like the Comforting blend, tangerine, or neroli will help even more. You can also add these oils to non-toxic lotions, but oils will likely be more effective overall.

- In the healing process of burns, wounds, or infections that could scar, with the advisement of an attending health care professional, we suggest applying a moisturizing carrier oils frequently with 2 to 3 drops of the Comforting blend, neroli, or tangerine in each application.

- If you already have stretch marks or scars, apply 2 to 3 drops of lavender undiluted on the scars. You can mix them with jojoba oil for a more moisturizing effect. Depending on the size and severity of the scar or stretch mark, it may take many months of daily applications to see improvement.

Scoliosis

WHAT IT IS

An abnormal curving of the spine in a "C" curve or an "S" curve. It can be mild or severe, affecting the functioning of internal organs and the body's balance. Everyone's spine curves a little. But people with scoliosis have a back bone that curves too much.

RECOMMENDED OILS

Sweet basil   Balsam fir

Spearmint

RECOMMENDED BLENDS

Comforting blend   Balancing blend

Massage blend   Foot massage blend

INSTRUCTION

With the approval of any needed health care professional, use the following suggestions to help straighten the back as a part of a complete program of exercise to strengthen the muscles that hold the spine in place. It is futile to straighten the back without also using therapeutic muscle strengthening. Yoga exercises help you become aware of your posture, your balance, and the complete, controlled stretch of the musculoskeletal systems of your body.

• For relaxing tensions in the back, massage the back with 3 to 5 drops of the Comforting blend neat, dripped down the spine and feathered out and upward with the fingertips then massaged in with the knuckles on both sides of the spine.

• Do the same massage procedure using the Massage blend for toning and energizing the muscles of the back before you doing any exercising like yoga or weight lifting.

• For assisting in the straightening and straightening process, follow these steps once a week. More detailed instructions are given in Chapter 4, "How to Use Essential Oils" under "Layer Therapy."

1. Begin by applying a few drops of the Balancing blend to the collar bone areas of your chest for calming your entire body.

2. Do a complete foot reflexology massage using 3 to 5 drops of the Balancing blend and 3 to 5 drops of the foot massage blend with a teaspoon of carrier oil. Massage each foot for at least five minutes. Concentrate with your knuckles on the spinal reflex points that extend along the inside edges of the soles of your feet.

3. Use 4 to 5 drops of each of the following oils undiluted, one after the other: the Balancing blend, sweet basil, balsam fir, the Massage blend, and spearmint. Drop 4 to 5 drops of each oil down the spine, massage the oils in with rocking motions using your knuckles alone both sides of the spine. Then feather the oils with your fingernails up and out onto the back. Then massage down the sides of the spine with your fingertips in small circular movements. Do each movement 3 times with each oil.

4. After each oil has been massaged in, place a warm towel on the back for 10 to 20 minutes to enhance the penetration of the oils.

5. End the therapy by lying on your back and holding your knees to your chest for a stretch and alignment of the back for about 3 minutes.

• Do back strengthening, posture positioning, and stretching exercises at least every other day. When sitting at a computer or in one place for many hours, be sure to stand and walk around at least every half hour to readjust your posture.

Sexual Dysfunction & Healthy Sexual Relationships

The role of aroma is a powerful yet often ignored element of our sexual reactions. Like beautiful music, texture and touch, and romantic visual images; the high emotional element of aroma can bring an intensely pleasurable sexual response that defies the ability of language to explain. Aromas can relax the adverse hyperactive "neurochatter" that could be going on in our head and getting in the way of our focused experience. We can learn to use the power of aroma to train or re-train our senses and their emotional and physical responses. This is, of course, a personal journey for companions who love one another. Because they go directly to the brain, aromas can easily and instantly retrieve from our library of emotions those memories that are mostly unconscious.

RECOMMENDED OILS

Bergamot		Neroli	
Tangerine		Ylang ylang	
Grapefruit		Patchouli	
Vanilla		Balsam fir	
Juniper		Spruce	
Frankincense			

RECOMMENDED BLENDS

Comforting blend		Balancing blend	
Focusing blend		Stress control blend	
Intimacy blend		Foot massage blend	

INSTRUCTION

- When a couple has a happy and healthy sexual life together, it is wonderful to use aromatic massage as part of their preparation for love making. Agree with one another which of the oils are most pleasurable and appealing to both of you. Then create a blend in a bowl you can easily reach.

- Ten drops of your favorite intimacy blend in a tablespoon of carrier oil will create a wonderful emotional memory for both partners. This will place into the unconscious library of the mind feelings and emotions that can then be retrieved throughout life whenever those aromas are revisited.

- Then, for anyone with some sexual dysfunction, a few drops of the blend you used in the best of times can be used for light massage either for sexual pleasure or simply for "sensate focus"— non-sexual massage.

- It is important to have used the oil when all was going well so the wonderful aromas will be become associated both in the subconscious and conscious mind with the best of sexual memories. Then, if a time comes when it is more difficult to trigger desire, the same oils can be used for massage, and the desire and sexual energy may return more easily. An intense and pleasurable aroma helps direct the senses away from distracting messages the brain may be sending.

- Where serious sexual problems exist, a couple who is fundamentally in opposition with one another may be unable to use aroma to perform the miracles they need. The first steps may need to be psychological, spiritual, or even marriage counseling. While a happy sexual relationship can help to reinforce a strong relationship, if there is little unity and too much unkindness, the sexual relationship alone will not be enough to make the union a lasting one.

- On the other hand, when both partners are united in all the most important ways, and when it is only the sexual issues that are dysfunctional, it would be sad to tear the relationship apart without trying to improve the sexual issues. You may need to consult a professional in this area as well. The use of aroma may play an important complementary role, especially as you relax and retrain your senses through "sensate focus" exercises.

- An unsatisfactory sexual life can create not only hidden resentments but also physical blockages in the energy flow inside the body. This can then contribute to many different pathological issues both physical and psychological. This is as true for men as it is for women. The relationship must be based on true, unselfish, compassionate love. We cannot escape that fact no matter how hard we try.

Sexually Transmitted Infections

(STIs, STDs, chlamydia, herpes, gonorrhea, syphilis or HIV)

WHAT ARE THEY

Infections usually acquired by sexual contact, though some can also be transmitted nonsexually, like from a mother to her baby during pregnancy or childbirth, or through blood transfusions or shared needles.
It is possible to contract STIs from people who seem perfectly healthy and aren't even aware that they are infected. Many have no symptoms. That's why experts prefer the term "sexually transmitted infections" (STIs) to "sexually transmitted diseases" (STDs). Left untreated STIs can cause infertility in both men

and women and even be fatal to all involved, including babies. Symptoms can include poor muscle coordination, paralysis, numbness, blindness, and dementia (mental disorder).

RECOMMENDED OILS

Tea tree		Eucalyptus radiata	
Lemon		Sweet basil	

RECOMMENDED BLENDS

Protecting blend	

INSTRUCTION

Suggestions as part of an overall plan involving your health care professional:

- You may be able to minimize the negative impact of using the significant load of antibiotics you may need by following an Immune Strengthening Cleanse discussed under "Cleansing" in this chapter.

- Whenever you are using antibiotics for any reason, you should use more anti-infectious essential oils at the same time in the water you drink, the food you eat, and even in capsules. Put a drop per quart in all your drinking water, put a drop in your herbal tea, and add oils like sweet basil and lemon to as many recipes as you can (after you take them off the heat).

- For chlamydia, Dr. Pénoël recommends creating a 25:75 blend of thyme and a carrier oil, filling capsules with a dropper, and taking 3 a day with food ++++P.

- Diffuse 20 drops of an essential oil or blend at least twice a day to get antimicrobial molecules in your bloodstream. Use any of your favorite diffusing oils for this—

Comforting blend, intimacy blend, Focusing blend, Stress control blend, tangerine, neroli, spearmint, lemon, etc.

- The best oils to use for STIs are Rosemary, tea tree, and the Protecting blend. If you are on a heavy dose of antibiotics, it may be well to create a blend of one of these three oils 50:50 with a carrier oil, fill capsules with a dropper, and take a capsule 3 times a day with food.

Shin Splints & Leg Cramps

WHAT THEY ARE

The term "shin splints" refers to pain along the shinbone (tibia), a common complaint in runners and dancers. They happen from overworking muscles, tendons and bones.

Leg cramps (charley horses) are involuntary spasms of the muscles and can happen any time during the day or even in the middle of the night. They are caused by many things: medication, too much exercise, pregnancy, etc. Children and pre-teens can get "growing pains" that wake them in the night. They don't appear to be linked to growth spurts, however.

RECOMMENDED OILS

Peppermint		Black Pepper	
Marjoram		Lavender	
Birch		Wintergreen	
Rosemary			

RECOMMENDED BLENDS

Soothing blend

INSTRUCTION

In-home procedures:

- Mix 4 to 5 drops of the Soothing blend or any of the other recommended oils in a teaspoon of carrier oil and massage. Use hot oils like black pepper and marjoram if you are applying heat and cooling oils like peppermint if you prefer using an ice pack because of hot inflammation.

- Use the foods you eat to add more calcium to your diet— low-fat dairy products and green, leafy vegetables. Avoid acid-forming foods such as sugary foods, refined flours, and soft drinks.

- Patricia Davis suggests that for spasms you use any of the oils recommended above for deep muscle massage. Start with a lighter "warm up" massage and gradually go deeper (Davis, p. 300).

Shingles (Herpes zoster)

WHAT IT IS

A painful inflammation of nerve tissues with blistering skin eruptions often forming a circle around the midsection of the body. Its cause is the same virus as chickenpox.

RECOMMENDED OILS

Tea tree		Ravitsara	
Eucalyptus radiata		Lemon	
Lavender			

RECOMMENDED BLENDS

Protecting blend

INSTRUCTION

In-home procedures:

- Use the following in-home procedures with the approval of your health care professional:

- At the first sign of the infection, apply a trace of the Protecting blend undiluted only on the area of the blisters. If the skin is highly sensitive, use a tiny brush to apply the oil only on each blister. It is better to not use a carrier oil in this case because it will slow the penetration speed.

- Dr. Pénoël recommends a 50:50 blend of peppermint and a carrier oil. Fill capsules with a dropper and take 3 to 4 capsules a day with food +++++P

- Do not eat meat or meals with heavy protein while you have the disease.

- If you prefer using single oils, create a blend of equal amounts of tea tree, lavender, and possibly lemon.

- Depending on how severe your pain is, try a back massage with the Protecting blend according to the instruction on Layer Therapy in Chapter 4: How to Use Essential Oils. Apply 3 to 4 drops of the blend undiluted along the spine. Work the oil in by rocking and massaging with your knuckles along each side of the spine. Then use your fingernails to gently feather the oil upward and outward on the back.

Shock (Psychological)

WHAT IT IS

Acute shock can be a medical emergency that can result in serious damage or death. It can be caused by sudden loss of blood flow because the heart stops pumping adequately, circulation is interrupted due to blood loss or dehydration, or a serious infection leads to toxic buildup, blood clots, and uncontrollable bleeding (sceptic shock). Immediate first-aid measures must be used during the first two stages of shock to stop bleeding, restart the heart, and control the infection. This can prevent escalation and death. Essential oils are not a relevant treatment for acute shock.

Psychological shock can occur when a traumatic event so overwhelms the psyche that one can no longer integrate ideas and emotions. It can manifest in both physical and psychological symptoms. Both types of shock can occur simultaneously.

RECOMMENDED OILS

Peppermint		Roman chamomile	
Lavender		Lemon	
Tangerine		Marjoram	

RECOMMENDED BLENDS

Comforting blend

INSTRUCTION

- To help with psychological shock, use peppermint on a tissue or inhaled directly from the bottle. An undiluted drop on the sternum and a drop massaged into the center of the balls of the feet may be helpful.

- In keeping the patient relaxed, apply the "M" technique massaging the hands with the a few drops of the Comforting blend or lavender in a teaspoon of carrier oil.

- Administer a gentle reflexology foot massage using 2 to 3 drops of the Foot Massage blend and a drop or two of lavender or the Comforting blend mixed into a teaspoon of carrier oil.

- Simply smelling lavender or the Comforting blend directly from the bottle or in a tissue will help prevent shock from progressing and aid recovery.

- Dr. Pénoël suggests a blend of lemon, tangerine, and neroli mixed 50:50 with a carrier oil to calm agitation +++P.

Sinusitis

WHAT IT IS

An inflammation of the sinus cavities that sometimes accompanies upper respiratory infections but can be chronic allergic conditions as well. Symptoms can include severe headache, earache, toothache, facial pain, cranial pressure, loss of a sense of smell, fever, a stuffy nose, and mucous drainage. Chronic sinus infections over many months, whether through infections or allergies, can lead to significant and serious health issues elsewhere in the body.

RECOMMENDED OILS

Peppermint	🔵🔵	Lavender	🔵🔵
Lemon	🔵🔵	Eucalyptus radiata	🔵🔵
Pine	🔵🔵	Thyme	🔵🔵
Frankincense	🔵🔵	Tea tree	🔵

RECOMMENDED BLENDS

Respiratory blend	🔵🔵	Antimicrobial blend	🔵🔵
Comforting blend	🔵🔵		🔵🔵

INSTRUCTION

With the possible involvement of your health care professional as needed, use these procedures:

- Give yourself steam inhalations of 4 or 5 drops of Eucalyptus radiata, tea tree, lavender, lemon, the respiratory blend, or the Protecting blend in a pan or bowl of hot water breathed deeply through the nose. Cover your head with a cloth to contain the steam. If started early enough this therapy alone can sometimes prevent a respiratory infection from spreading into the sinuses.

- Put a drop or two of one of the recommended oils in a tissue and breathe through it or put a drop on your hand, rub your palms together, cup your hands over your mouth and nose, and breathe deeply several times.

- To help relieve the pain of a sinus headache, apply 1 or 2 drops of frankincense or peppermint on each temple.

- To help relieve plugged sinuses, mix 2 drops of peppermint in a teaspoon of honey and hold the mixture in the back of your mouth long enough for the aromatic molecules to begin to penetrate your nasal cavities from the back of your throat. You can clear your sinuses quickly using this therapy.

- Breathe slow-diffusing essential oils through the night while sleeping, especially Eucalyptus radiata or the respiratory blend.

- Increase the amount of aromatic drinking water you consume to at least 1/2 gallon every day. Put a drop of oil in every quart of drinking water.

- While you are trying to recover, avoid mucous-producing food products containing dairy, white flour, and white sugar.

- Patricia Davis suggests aromatic facial massage including a diluted respiratory blend and light drumming (tappotement) on the sinus areas of the face to help with drainage. This cannot be used when the facial pain is at its most severe, but will help in complete recovery if it is used as sinuses begin to clear (Davis p. 293).

- In many people just lightly massaging the sinus areas of the face with well-diluted (5:95) blends of essential oils will be effective.

- When diffusing an essential oil, however, it is important to get the aromatic molecules into the sinuses instead of simply breathing them deeply into the lungs. Here's a breathing technique that will help. First take a deep breath and hold it. Then place a nostril right next to the diffuser opening and turn it on to its lowest setting. When you need to exhale, turn the diffuser off. Take another deep breath and turn the diffuser on again. Repeat 5 to 7 times with each nostril. Use 20 drops of tea tree at a time. Tea tree is antimicrobial and doesn't burn the sinuses when diffused. Learn more details about this special procedure in Chapter 4.

- For acute sinusitis, try Dr. Penoel's "Live Embalming" therapy found in Chapter 4. Use 5 to 10 drops at a time for a total of 20 or 30 drops of Eucalyptus radiata or ravintsara with a hair dryer to get a large amount of essential oils to penetrate the body in a short amount of time. Be sure to change locations on the body with each application. Be sure to read the instructions in Chapter 4 before trying this therapy.

CLINICAL SUPPORT

These tests of essential oils in chronic bronchitis, sinusitis and COPD confirmed that orange oil, Eucalyptus oil and a standardized extract called Myrtol had antioxidative properties and potent anti-inflammatory activity (Rantzsch U, et al., 2009).

Frankincense takes away sinus congestion

If I get a little sinus congestion, I apply a drop of frankincense on the sides of my nose and around my sinus area. The congestion seems to always go away and doesn't come back.

Skin Conditions

General guidelines

Skin conditions ranging from acne to eczema are often symptoms of a deep-seated, sometimes hidden infection, inflammation, or autoimmune condition that must be treated holistically to prevent what Dr. Pénoël calls "morbid transfer" or the transfer of a symptom or condition from one area or system of the body to another. As disease moves and transfers in this way, it usually becomes even more serious and much more difficult to heal. This is where essential oils excel—at safely, gently, and thoroughly going to the root of all these conditions and correcting them. No synthetic substance has the power to do this deep work.

RECOMMENDED OILS

Peppermint	🔵🟢	Lavender	🔵🟢
Lemon	🔵🟢	Eucalyptus radiata	🔵🟢
Pine	🔵🟢	Thyme	🔵🟢
Frankincense	🔵🟢	Tea tree	🟢

RECOMMENDED BLENDS

Respiratory blend	🔵🟡		Protecting blend	🔵🟡
Focusing blend	🔵🟡		Stress control blend	🔵🟡
Mental focus blend	🔵🟡		Intimacy blend	🔵🟡
Balancing blend	🔵🟡		Comforting blend	🔵🟡

INSTRUCTION

• Most of the symptoms and conditions that of the skin relate to skin conditions are important signals that you need to significantly reduce the toxic buildup in your body, especially in your digestive system and your organs of metabolism like the pancreas and liver. They are also a sign that you must add critical whole-food nutrients and unblock healing energy pathways in your body through essential oil massage.

• Always begin with your dietary habits. The simple rules are clearly defined in this book. Skin problems will often reoccur unless dietary laws are obeyed on a consistent basis.

• You may need to drink more water (1/2 gallon a day) and exercise (the equivalent of a 2-mile walk every day) to improve your circulation and continually flush toxins out of your body through movement, perspiration, and deep breathing.

• You need to examine your emotional life as well and reduce toxic buildup of unresolved conflicts, resentments, unfounded fears, selfishness, self-pity, criticism, etc. Diffusing oils to help release these emotions and calming massage can help significantly, but skin problems will recur if emotional issues are not addressed and resolved.

• Incorporate stress-reducing activities into your day. Take time for meditation while diffusing balsam fir, lemon, the Comforting blend, the Stress control blend, or an intimacy blend.

• Take spare moments to treat yourself to relaxing massages of your feet, hands, abdomen, neck, shoulders, ears, or joints with 3 to 4 drops of lavender, neroli, lemon, the Comforting blend, the Focusing blend, the Stress control blend, the Mental Focus blend, the Intimacy blend, or the Balancing blend diluted in a small amount of carrier oil. Premix your favorites and use them at work from time to time to help with your concentration or relaxation.

• Eliminate any unsafe, self-defeating addictions you use to escape your problems, such as overeating, overworking, smoking, drugs, or alcoholism.

• For persistent skin conditions, it may be vital to spend a year and complete one or more of the cleanses described earlier in this chapter. There are four of them: The Liver, Digestion, Immune Strengthening, or Mind/Body Cleanse.

Smoking Cessation

WHAT IT IS
Attempting to stop smoking is challenging both physiologically and psychologically because smoking is an addiction. Both sides of the addiction need to be addressed, and essential oils can be particularly helpful.

RECOMMENDED OILS

Peppermint	🔵🟡		Lavender	🔵🟡
Lemon	🔵🟡		Neroli	🔵🟡
Eucalyptus globulus	🔵🟡🔴		Eucalyptus radiata	🔵🟡
Pine	🔵🟡		Frankincense	🔵🟡
Tea tree	🟡			

RECOMMENDED BLENDS

Respiratory blend		Protecting blend	
Focusing blend		Stress control blend	
Mental focus blend		Intimacy blend	
Balancing blend		Comforting blend	

INSTRUCTION

• Apply the steps of Aromatic Behavioral Conditioning described in the section on "Addictions" in this chapter.

• Choose from among these five oils the one that is most pleasing to you—the Protecting blend, the respiratory blend, Eucalyptus radiata, peppermint, and balsam fir. These blends will be most effective at helping to restore the complete functionality of your respiratory system. For Behavioral Conditioning try the Comforting blend, the intimacy blend, or any of the other blends listed above.

• Dr. Pénoël suggests that Eucalyptus globulus is particularly effective at helping his patients overcome smoking addictions. "They take the oil internally with a toothpick or 'lick trick' (a trace on the tongue) whenever they are tempted to smoke. The taste of eucalyptus appears to make the taste of smoking more repulsive to them" (Pénoël Guide, p. 172).

Sore Throat & Strep Throat

WHAT IT IS

Pain, scratchiness or irritation in the throat that feels worse when you swallow. The most common cause of sore throat (pharyngitis) is a viral infection from a cold or flu. Strep throat (streptococcal infection) is caused by bacteria and can be more serious.

RECOMMENDED OILS

Peppermint		Lavender	
Lemon		Neroli	
Eucalyptus radiata		Pine	
Frankincense		Tea tree	

RECOMMENDED BLENDS

Respiratory blend		Protecting blend	
Focusing blend		Stress control blend	
Mental focus blend		Intimacy blend	
Balancing blend		Comforting blend	

INSTRUCTION

With the approval of your health care professional, use the following in-home procedures:

• Dr. Pénoël suggests creating this blend of thyme (20%), tea tree (60%), and peppermint (20%). Blend this mixture 50:50 with a carrier oil, use a dropper to fill capsules, and take 3 to 6 capsules a day with food +++++P.

• Here's another blend he recommends: cinnamon (30%), tea tree (33%), and thyme (30%). Blend this mixture 50:50 with a carrier oil, use a dropper to fill capsules, and take 3 to 6 capsules a day with food +++++P.

• Mix a drop of the Protecting blend into a teaspoon of honey. Hold this mixture in the back of your throat as it mixes with saliva and coats the membranes of your throat. Swallow the mixture after a minute or two, and as it passes through your digestive system, it will continue its healing.

- Complement the ingestion with an external application of 2 to 3 drops of tea tree undiluted along the sides of the throat and chest where there are the most lymph nodes. That would be from the mastoid bone behind the ear to the collar bone (clavicle). Also apply 2 or 3 drops of tea tree mixed in an equal amount of carrier oil down the back of the neck. If your neck feels stiff, add 2 or 3 drops of lavender.

- Use a toothpick to add a trace of the respiratory blend to a cup of warm water. This is like an antimicrobial "aromatic tea" that you can drink between meals on an empty stomach for maximum antimicrobial action. Sip it slowly, allowing the molecules to coat your throat as you swallow.

- Lick a trace of tea tree, frankincense, the respiratory blend, or the Protecting blend off the back of your hand and take it to the back of your throat. You can use a toothpick if you wish to adjust the amount. Hold it in your mouth for at least a minute, mixing it with your saliva. Repeat this important action once a minute for the first 15 minutes, then do it about every 5 minutes for the next couple of hours. Gradually decrease the frequency as the soreness goes away.

- Put a drop of the Respiratory blend or the Protecting blend in every quart of drinking water you consume. Enjoy this aromatic water for several months after all your symptoms have gone away.

- Try Dr. Pénoël's "Live Embalming" therapy found in Chapter 4. Use 5 to 10 drops at a time for a total of 20 or 30 drops of Eucalyptus radiata or ravintsara with a hair dryer to get a large amount of essential oils to penetrate

the body in a short amount of time. Be sure to change locations on the body with each application. Be sure to read the instructions in Chapter 4 before trying this therapy.

> ### Slow-healing sprained ankle heals quickly with a pain blend
>
> Whenever I've sprained my ankle, it's taken a long time to heal, so when it happened again (I'm in my 60s) I was convinced I was in for a long healing time. I used a pain blend on my ankle for a couple of days, and it was fine.

Sprains

WHAT THEY ARE

A sprain is a damaged ligament that is inflamed and swollen.

RECOMMENDED OILS

Lavender	🌀	Helichrysum	🌀
German chamomile	🌀	Roman chamomile	🌀
Peppermint	🌀	Spearmint	🌀
Birch	🌀	Wintergreen	🌀

RECOMMENDED BLENDS

Soothing blend	🌀	Circulation blend	🌀

INSTRUCTION

Follow first aid instructions and cautions found in an authoritative health care guide or website or consult a health care professional for advice. If home care is indicated, follow these suggestions:

- Immediately control pain by applying either peppermint or the Soothing blend. If the area is small (finger, wrist, etc.) put a drop of oil on your little finger and dab the area. For a bit larger area (ankle, elbow, or shoulder), use a pipette and apply a few drops undiluted and spread it gently with your little finger. For a larger area (hip, leg, back), dilute the oil, 4 to 5 drops in a teaspoon of carrier oil, and spread it on the area. Do not massage the area.

- Before applying ice or a cold pack, mix 4 to 5 drops of peppermint or the Soothing blend in 1/3 cup of water and shake. Soak a gauze or small flannel cloth in it and apply it to the painful area. Secure it with a cling bandage. Cover it with a dry cloth and apply an ice or cold pack.

- After 24 hours and when the swelling has gone down and it becomes appropriate to try heat on the sprained area to aid healing, use the inflammation blend or the Soothing blend. The Inflammation blend has a deep action that lowers Inflammation, but is a little less effective at helping with pain. Create a compress similar to the cold compress above, but this time apply a warm, damp cloth, a dry cloth, and a heat pack. But apply heat only when all signs of inflammation have ceased.

- To speed healing, lightly massage the area around the injury with 4 to 5 drops of the circulation blend in a teaspoon of a carrier oil.

- IMPORTANT NOTE: as long the area shows signs of inflammation—hot, red, swollen, and with acute pain—do not use a hot compress because it will add more heat and make the situation worse. Listen to what your body is telling you, not what is written in a book or on a website. If you feel more relief with a cold compress, use cold. If you feel better with a warm one, that is what you need.

Stomach Flu

WHAT IT IS

A gastrointestinal illness that is caused by a microorganism. It usually comes from something you ate. It is not related to the flu virus.

RECOMMENDED OILS

Lavender		Peppermint	
Roman chamomile		German chamomile	
Spearmint		Tea tree	
Sweet basil			

RECOMMENDED BLENDS

Protecting blend		circulation blend	

INSTRUCTION

- Add a drop of the Protecting blend in every quart of drinking water you have. Or you can put a trace of the blend on a toothpick and stir it into a cup of hot or cold drinking water.

- Also use a drop or two of lemon or sweet basil in mild steamed vegetable recipes or vegetable bouillon recipes after they are taken off the stove.

- To dispel nausea, take a drop each of sweet basil and peppermint in an herbal tea or warm water. Adjust the quantity with a toothpick so you get the flavor right.

- Massage 2 to 3 drops each of tea tree and Eucalyptus radiata undiluted on the lower back. Massage it into both sides of the spine using downward motions. To massage larger areas, add these oils to a tablespoon of carrier oil and massage the entire back or chest.

- Use this blend for an abdominal massage. Start just below the navel and lightly massage the area in a clockwise spiral moving gradually outward to the edges of the rib cage and pelvis.

- Massage the bottoms of your feet (the arch area), the palms of your hands, and the upper part of your ears (inside and out) with any of the following oils undiluted: tea tree, Eucalyptus radiata, sweet basil, peppermint, or the Protecting blend.

- Refer to an authoritative medical guide, website, or medical professional to learn whether your symptoms are more serious than should be treated only at home.

Stye (see Pink Eye & Stye)

Sunburn

WHAT IT IS

Painful skin that is red and feels hot to the touch appearing after too much sun or UV exposure. It increases your risk of other skin diseases as serious as skin cancer (melanoma). It will also accelerate the aging process with accompanying wrinkles, dark spots, and rough spots.

RECOMMENDED OILS

Lavender		Peppermint	
German chamomile		Roman chamomile	
Spearmint		Tea tree	

RECOMMENDED BLENDS

Protecting blend	

INSTRUCTION

Suggestions as part of an overall plan involving your health care professional as needed for serious, infected burns.

- Act quickly to run tepid water over a sunburn for 10 minutes. This will help reduce the swelling and inflammation.

- For small areas of sunburn, put a drop or two of lavender in your palm along with a few drops of water and apply the mixture on a small area. Lavender takes the pain away quickly and speeds healing.

- For a serious second-degree sunburn with blistering and possibly cracked and infected skin, follow the direction of your health care professional, but suggest using lavender in a sterile solution sprayed on the burn. It can be sprayed on frequently to cool the burn, help take away some of the pain, and speed up the healing process. Mix 4 to 5 drops of lavender in 1/2 cup of sterile water. You may want to add a drop of peppermint for its cooling action, a drop of helichrysum for its restorative action, and a drop of tea tree for its antimicrobial action. Shake the bottle to mix the oils before each application. Spray the sunburn every 15 or 20 minutes for your first 3 or 4 hours whenever you feel the heat. Spray it again daily after your shower until it heals.

- For a smaller area with a major sunburn, you can use a sterile gauze dipped in a 1/2 cup of water with 5 drops of lavender added. Place the damp gauze on the minor burn. If you cover it with a cling film, or a piece of clear plastic wrap to aid the penetration, keep it cool by spraying it with cold water or a lavender and water solution. You can also apply cold cloths and ice packs.

TMJ Syndrome

(temporomandibular joint disorder)

What It Is

Pain or tenderness in your jaw and the muscles that move it. It may come from arthritis, a jaw injury, or grinding your teeth. You may also experience pain in your face and around your ear, headaches, difficulty chewing or swallowing, aching facial pain, and in the most severe cases, a locking of the joint, making it difficult to open or close the mouth. It can also create clicking sounds when you chew.

RECOMMENDED OILS

Lavender   Peppermint

RECOMMENDED BLENDS

Comforting blend   Balancing blend

Massage blend   Foot massage blend

INSTRUCTION

With the approval of your health care professional, try the following in-home procedures:

- Massage 1 or 2 drops of the Comforting blend, the Stress control blend, or the Balancing blend around the joint of the jaw to relax the area. Manipulate the jaw until it is not hurting, then apply a drop of the Massage blend to stimulate the muscles of the jaw to position it so that it is not painful. Your goal is to re-train the joints and ligaments so they automatically move into a position that is not painful.

- Emotional stress may aggravate your condition so calming reflexology massage using the foot massage blend on the feet with various calming oils before bed will be excellent for helping you unwind and reduce stress.

Tetanus (Lockjaw)

WHAT IT IS

A serious bacterial disease that affects the nervous system, leading to painful muscle contractions, especially of the jaw and neck. It can interfere with swallowing, breathing, and even threaten your life. The infection typically comes from a deep puncture wound or scratch where bacteria from dust, dirt, or animal feces may be present.

RECOMMENDED OILS

Tea tree   Eucalyptus radiata

RECOMMENDED BLENDS

Protecting blend

INSTRUCTION

In addition to immunizations and tetanus booster shot that may be needed, the following in-home procedures may be helpful along with advice as needed from your health care professional.

- To prevent tetanus from taking hold, after washing and disinfecting any wound, especially those involving dirt, dust, or possibly animal feces; use 3 or 4 drops of tea tree, Eucalyptus radiata, and/or the Protecting blend undiluted for additional disinfecting. Place a few drops of any of these oils on an adhesive bandage or gauze pad to cover the wound and protect it.

- Because this infection is potentially so serious, it's important to disinfect the body on a deep level. Create a blend of any of the recommended oils 50:50 with a carrier oil and use your dropper to fill capsules. Take 3 capsules a day with food.

- Take a drop or two of any recommended oil in hot water or an herbal tea with a little honey. You can also have a drop in each quart of drinking water, in a glass of juice, or in recipes (after taking it off the stove).

Thyroiditis

(Hashimoto's disease, hypothyroidism)

WHAT IT IS

An autoimmune condition in which your immune system attacks your thyroid, a gland at the base of your neck beneath your Adam's apple. This often leads to an underactive thyroid (hypothyroidism). You may may notice a swelling at your throat (goiter). The disease progresses slowly, causing chronic thyroid damage, leading to a drop in thyroid hormone. Symptoms include fatigue; sensitivity to cold; constipation; pale, dry skin; a puffy face; a hoarse voice; unexplained weight gain, most of which is fluid; muscle aches; stiffness in shoulders and hips; swelling and pain in hands and feet; muscle weakness; excessive menstrual bleeding; and depression.

RECOMMENDED BLEND

Immune balancing blend

INSTRUCTION

In-home procedures suggested as part of an overall plan involving your health care professional:

- Allergies are often a part of autoimmune conditions. So, if you have allergies, avoid applying essential oils topically to any part of the body but the feet. You may be able to ingest them, however.

- In times of severe symptoms use 2 – 3 drops of the immune balancing blend, undiluted, on the thyroid area of the feet.

- If you have tested a drop of the immune balancing blend on the inside of your arm for an allergic reaction and it seems to be okay to use it topically, dilute 2 – 3 drops of the blend and apply over the thyroid area at the base of the neck and upper chest over the thyroid.

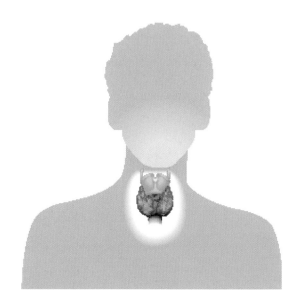

- Add a drop of the immune balancing blend in a cup of hot water or herbal tea.

- Take the time to enjoy benefits of the Immune Strengthening Cleanse for at least one year to help your body do all it can to recover from autoimmune issues.

Ticks (see Lyme disease and Insect Repellent)

Tinnitis (Ringing in the ears)

WHAT IT IS

Noises in the ears when there is no actual source for the sounds. They can be soft or loud and seem like ringing, blowing, roaring, buzzing, hissing, humming, whistling, or sizzling.

RECOMMENDED OILS

Cypress

Helichrysum

Sweet basil

INSTRUCTION

With the advice of your health care professional as needed, try the following suggestions:

• Apply a few drops of helichrysum to the outer ear as well as around the ear. Pull the ear in various directions to help the oil penetrate. This may take frequent applications over an extended period of time because damage may be a long time in healing.

• Dr. Pénoël recommends an equal blend of sweet basil and cypress applied around the ear twice daily +++P.

Tonsillitis

WHAT IT IS

An inflammation of the tonsils, the two glands made of lymph tissue located on either side of the back of the throat. Symptoms include redness, pain, swelling, inflammation of the tonsils, difficulty swallowing, hoarseness, and coughing. The inflammation may be caused by a virus or bacteria.

RECOMMENDED OILS

Tea tree

Lemon

Eucalyptus radiata

RECOMMENDED BLENDS

Respiratory blend

Antimicrobial blend

INSTRUCTION

With the advice of your health care professional as needed, try the following suggestions:

• Lick a trace of tea tree or the Protecting blend off the back of your hand and distribute it to the back of your throat to help soothe inflamed tonsils and fight infection. Do this every minute for 15 minutes when you feel the very first sign of a sore throat. Then do it every five minutes for two or 3 hours as the pain eases. Continue doing it several times a day for several days even after the pain is gone.

• Use steam inhalations often to help control the infection and relieve pain. Use 2 to 3 drops of lemon, tea tree, Eucalyptus radiata, the Respiratory blend, or the Protecting blend in a bowl or pan of hot, steaming water. Put a towel over your head to contain the vapors and inhale deeply. Reheat the water, add more oil, and repeat the treatment as long as you wish to break up any mucous and treat the infection.

• If the condition becomes severe, create a blend of one of the four oils 50:50 with a carrier oil. Fill capsules using a dropper and take 3 to 6 capsules a day with food.

Toothache

WHAT IT IS

The mouth is the most fertile area of the body for the growth and proliferation of microbes. Therefore, keeping your teeth clean, your breath fresh, and your mouth free of all infection are important goals for the health of your whole body. A toothache is a sign that bacteria has eaten through the enamel and made its way into a tooth. There is a cavity or an infection forming in or around the tooth. Decay is the main cause of most toothaches. The first symptom may be a sensation of pain when you eat something sweet, cold, or hot. An infection may grow into an abscess.

RECOMMENDED OILS

Clove	🌀🔵	Peppermint	🌀🔵
Roman chamomile	🌀🔵	German chamomile	🌀🔵
Spearmint	🌀🔵		🌀🔵

RECOMMENDED BLENDS

Soothing blend	🌀🔵	Protecting blend	🌀🔵

INSTRUCTION

Call your dentist and make an appointment at the first sign of a toothache. Infection can become more severe quickly; the sooner the toothache gets taken care of, the better your overall health will be.

- To help limit infection and control the pain while you are waiting for your dental appointment, put a few drops of tea tree undiluted on a cotton ball or gauze pad and place it between your cheek and the infected tooth or gum.

- If pain is acute, a tract of clove or peppermint can be added to the cotton ball or gauze pad.

Put a drop of clove on a cotton swab and dab the gum area to deaden the pain.

- To fight infection, in addition to whatever antibiotics the dentist may suggest, mix a blend of tea tree or the Protecting blend 50:50 with a carrier oil. Fill capsules and take one capsule three times a day with food.

- Brush teeth twice daily with a tooth powder mixed with a drop of tea tree, peppermint, clove, or the Protecting blend. Create your own tooth powder by mixing 2 parts baking soda to 1 part fine-ground, natural salt. Thoroughly mix in drops of peppermint or clove oil to taste. Sprinkle some in your hand, add a drop of tea tree or the Protecting blend, wet your toothbrush, and enjoy brushing your teeth without the toxic chemicals.

Tuberculosis (TB)

WHAT IT IS

A highly contagious bacterial disease of the lungs that is easily transmitted through coughing and sneezing. The cough can bring up blood and pus-filled phlegm. Other symptoms include low fever, weakness, weight loss, chills, and night sweats. This is a serious disease that is reappearing more a more often, due to drug-resistant strains of the bacteria.

RECOMMENDED OILS

Lemon	🌀🌀🔵	Tea tree	🌀🌀🔵
Balsam fir	🌀🌀🔵	Eucalylptus radiata	🌀🌀
Roman chamomile	🌀🔵	German chamomile	🌀🔵

RECOMMENDED BLENDS

Respiratory blend		Antimicrobial blend	

INSTRUCTION

This is a serious disease that requires the intervention of a health care professional. The following procedures may be helpful.

- To reduce exposure to all other potential infections during recovery and to maximize the antimicrobial properties of essential oils throughout the respiratory system and the circulatory system, diffuse 20 drops at a time of any of the following: tea tree, Eucalyptus radiata, lemon, balsam fir, the Respiratory blend, or the Protecting blend. Do this two or three times a day.

- To improve breathing and to soothe the severe cough, try steam inhalations using Eucalyptus radiata or the Respiratory blend. Add 3 to 6 drops of either of the oils to a steaming bowl or pan of water. Place a cloth over the head, blow into the water to disperse the aromatic molecules, and breathe deeply. Reheat the water, add more oils and repeat as often as needed.

- TB can remain dormant in someone who has been infected but who has a strong immune system.

- To strengthen and stimulate your immune system use lemon essential oil. It seems to stimulate white-blood-cell production in the bones. Massage lemon essential oil into the lung reflex points on the balls of the feet. Also drink an aromatic lemon tea by placing one drop of lemon essential oil in a cup of warm water. Add the juice of real lemons for a healthy immune-boosting drink.

- To rapidly get a lot of essential oil molecules into your system, try Dr. Penoel's "Live Embalming" therapy found in Chapter 4. Use 5 to 10 drops at a time for a total of 20 or 30 drops of Eucalyptus radiata or ravintsara

with a hair dryer to get a large amount of essential oils to penetrate the body in a short amount of time. Be sure to change locations on the body with each application. Be sure to read the instructions in Chapter 4 before trying this therapy.

Ulcers

WHAT THEY ARE

Open sores that form on the lining of the esophagus, stomach and upper portion of the small intestine. Abdominal pain is the most common symptom. A bacterial infection (Helicobacter pylori) is the main cause, but too many pain medications and other drugs may contribute or cause ulcers. Symptoms are at their worst when the stomach is empty and can be temporarily relived by eating buffering foods or taking something to reduce stomach acid. More severe signs including nausea, vomiting, unexplained weight loss, dark blood in stools, and appetite changes. Left untreated, ulcers can lead to severe bleeding, serious infections, and scar tissue that can severely inhibit healthy digestion.

RECOMMENDED OILS

Lemon		Tea tree	
Lavender		Sweet basil	

RECOMMENDED BLENDS

Digestion blend		Antimicrobial blend	

INSTRUCTION

In-home suggestion that can be part of an overall plan with the approval of your health care professional:

- Mix a drop of tea tree, lemon, lavender, sweet basil, Protecting blend or digestion blend in a quart of water or a trace on a toothpick stirred into a cup of hot or cold water. Drink 1/2 gallon per day.

- Use a drop or two of either of the Antimicrobial or the Digestion blend in mild steamed vegetable recipes or vegetable bouillon (after they are taken off the stove).

- Refer to a medical diagnostic guide, authoritative website, or health care professional for signs that your symptoms may be more serious than home remedies alone should treat.

- Blend 2 to 3 drops of both neroli and tangerine in a teaspoon of carrier oil and massage on the upper abdomen 3 or 4 times a day +++P.

Urinary Tract Disorders

(Kidney, bladder, & prostate infections; see also Kidney Stones)

WHAT THEY ARE

Serious urinary tract disorders can be the result of many damaging habits and lifestyle choices that involve improper diet, lack of exercise, lack of sufficient liquids (especially water), toxic emotional habits, and unhealthy relationships. A person who wishes to clear up these conditions must be willing to drink at least 1/2 gallon of water every day, exercise the equivalent of walking two miles daily, and follow the dietary guidelines in this book. To merely control a symptom is not true healing. The involvement of family members can be extremely important to your success. Your health care professional is also an important

advisor in all serious conditions of the urinary tract, especially the infections, inflammations, and pre-cancerous and cancerous conditions. Symptoms include: burning urine, severe back pain, nausea, too-frequent trips to the bathroom especially at night, cloudy urine, strong-smelling urine, blood in urine, inability to urinate, pelvic pain (women), or rectal pain (men).

RECOMMENDED OILS

Bergamot		German chamomile	
Roman chamomile		Eucalyptus radiatai	
Tea tree		Lavender	
Sweet basil		Sandalwood	
Lemon		Juniper	

RECOMMENDED BLEND

Protecting blend		Soothing blend	

INSTRUCTION

If a urinary tract infection (UTI) doesn't resolve itself in a day or two, seek professional help. A UTI can quickly spread to the kidneys, causing serious problems. Kidney infections will almost certainly require you to resort to professional help and antibiotics. Here are suggestions as part of an overall plan involving your health care professional:

- Act quickly at your first sign of an infection. Begin by taking a 50:50 blend of the Protecting blend with a carrier oil in capsules. Fill capsules with a dropper. Take 6 capsules with food within the first hour. Take two immediately, two on the half hour, and two on the hour. After that adapt other capsules to your symptoms, 6 capsules a day. One of the biggest problems Dr. Pénoël sees with infections is not getting enough strong essential oils often enough to take out the infection quickly. If you are not aggressive enough in the first hours of the infection, it will grow and take over. So you want to get a lot of essential oils in your body for a couple of hours at the first hint of an infection.

- Prompt treatment can sometimes keep a urinary tract infection from spreading, especially if it is accompanied by drinking a large amount of aromatic water with a drop of essential oils (especially lemon) in each quart and a drop in each hot drink (herbal tea).

- Drink large amounts of chamomile tea (made with either the tea bags or a trace of one of the chamomile essential oils in an herbal tea or hot water).

- Take aromatic baths using 10 to 15 drops of any of the recommended oils mixed in a cup of Epsom Salts.

- Massage using a 50:50 blend with carrier oil and one of the recommended oils to relieve the depression often associated with UTIs.

- If you are taking antibiotics, be sure to supplement with probiotic foods or supplements so you don't destroy all your healthy bacteria that keep future UTIs under control and prevent the constant cycling of UTIs and antibiotics that so many people dread.

- Switch oils frequently so your body is experiencing different sensations and receiving different antimicrobial profiles. Replace bergamot with sandalwood, and tea tree with sweet basil occasionally.

FOR MEN

- For prostatitis, after notifying your urologist for direction, create compresses with 50:50 blends with a carrier oil and one of these essential oils: Roman chamomile, juniper, or pine. Apply the oil over the lower abdomen and cover it with a hot, damp towel, a dry towel, and a heating pad or hot water bottle. Use the same compress on the lower back and again over the kidneys to relieve pain and help clear the infection.

- To help with kidney or prostate pain, massage the lower abdomen, lower back, and kidney area with 3 – 4 drops of the Soothing blend, undiluted. Add a carrier oil as needed.

FOR WOMEN

- Use 5 to 10 drops of one of the chamomile oils diluted in water to wash all infected areas daily

- Take an aromatic bath using 10 to 15 drops of any of the recommended oils dispersed in a cup of Epsom Salts.

- Massage the lower abdomen with bergamot or lavender frequently.

- If there is a lot of pain, create a compress using one of the chamomiles undiluted and covered with a hot, damp towel, a dry towel, and a heating pad or hot water bottle.

- Take a lemon oil and carrier oil blend (50:50) in a capsule 3 times a day +++P.

Urinary Incontinence

WHAT IT IS

This embarrassing condition can have many causes, some of which may be psychological in origin. It can limit your social interaction and severely limit how you conduct your life. Its causes can come from weak muscles, pregnancy, childbirth, prostate enlargement, prostate cancer, hysterectomy, a tumor, etc.

RECOMMENDED OILS

Balsam fir

Lavender

Bergamot

Lemon

RECOMMENDED BLENDS

Comforting blend

Intimacy blend

Use these suggestions and always involve your health care professional as needed. There are multiple interventions, exercises, and treatments that can be successfully implemented.

- For calming the psychological issues, mix 3 to 4 drops of any of the following essential oils in a teaspoon of mixing oil for a regular back massage: balsam fir, lavender, the Comforting blend, or the Intimacy blend.

- Use 5 to 10 drops of any of the recommended oils with a cup of Epsom Salts in an aromatic bath at least 3 times a week.

- Massage the feet after each bath with 3 drops of any of the recommended oils mixed with the foot massage blend neat.

- Diffuse 5 to 10 drops of any of these oils for 5 minutes before retiring.

Vaginitis

WHAT IT IS

An inflammation of the vagina that can result in discharge, itching, and pain that is usually caused by a disruption of the normal balance of vaginal bacteria or a bacterial or yeast infection. It can also come from reduced estrogen levels after menopause.

RECOMMENDED OILS

Tea tree

Lavender

RECOMMENDED BLENDS

Protecting blend

INSTRUCTION

With the approval of your health care professional as needed, try the following in-home procedures:

- Mix 20 drops of tea tree or 10 drops of tea tree and 10 drops of lavender in a pint of water. Flush using a vagina irrigation system available at your pharmacy. This kind of cleansing douche is the most important treatment at the earliest sign of the infection. Douche twice daily.

- Mix tea tree (5%) and lavender (5%) in a carrier oil (90%). Stir or shake the mixture. Dip a tampon into the blend. Insert it into the vagina overnight.

- Do an immune-strengthening cleanse to stop the cycle of infection and inflammation that may have developed, especially if have used antibiotics frequently.

- To help clear up deep-seated infections, prepare a 50:50 blend of the Protecting blend and a carrier oil, fill capsules, and take a capsule daily with food.

- Consume plenty of probiotic foods or supplements to replenish beneficial bacteria that keep pathogens under control.

Varicose Veins & Spider Veins

WHAT THEY ARE

Gnarled, enlarged veins, usually in the legs and feet. Standing, walking upright, and sitting improperly can increase pressure on the veins of the lower body. They can ache and be very uncomfortable. They may alert you to an increased risk of other circulatory problems. Spider veins are a mild variation of varicose veins – a cosmetic concern.

RECOMMENDED OILS

Lavender		Cypress	
Helichrysum		Juniper	
Rosemary		Balsam fir	

RECOMMENDED BLENDS

Circulation blend		Inflammation blend	

INSTRUCTION

• Apply a highly diluted a blend of cypress (25%) with a carrier oil (75%) and lightly massage your veins in a direction leading toward the heart. You can also create a mixture of 3 to 4 of any of the recommended oils or blends in a teaspoon of carrier oil. It's best to have someone else give you this massage while your legs are slightly elevated, but rather than not doing it, do it for yourself. Do this massage twice daily if possible. It may take many months of this daily treatment to see improvements.

• Massage varicose veins with the circulation or inflammation blends diluted 75:25 with a carrier oil, very lightly in the direction of the heart.

• Vary the essential oils you are using from time to time.

Vascular Disorders

(Critical arteries)

WHAT IT IS

Various diseases of the arteries—coronary, kidney, arteries to the brain, the lungs, etc. These are serious conditions requiring the involvement of health care professionals and quick response. There can be ballooning of the arteries (aneurysm), hardening and possible blockage of the arteries from arteriosclerosis, and many variations on these. Clotting or thrombosis can also result in loss of life or limb.

RECOMMENDED OILS

Lavender		Bergamot	
Roman chamomile		German chamomile	

RECOMMENDED BLENDS

Circulation blend	

INSTRUCTION

In-home procedures suggested as part of an overall plan under the direction of your health care professional:

• All conditions involving thrombosis (blood clotting) may be helped by applying lavender either undiluted or in dilution (3 to 4 drops per teaspoon of carrier oil) for a reflexology foot massage.

• Gently apply this same massage blend to affected areas or generally all over the body for its calming effects.

- Use the "M" technique described in Chapter 4 for calming stress.

- Diffuse 5 to 15 drops of lavender at any time of the day for its calming, restorative action.

Vertigo/Dizziness
(vestibular infection of the ear)

WHAT IT IS

A sensation of whirling and loss of balance. It can be caused by a disease of the inner ear or the vestibular nerve. Dizziness is more associated with being lightheaded.

RECOMMENDED OILS

Ginger			Sweet basil		
Peppermint			Frankincense		
Cypress			Lavender		
Roman chamomile			German chamomile		
Helichrysum			Bergamot		

RECOMMENDED BLEND

Protecting blend

INSTRUCTION

With the involvement of your health care professional as needed, use the following suggestions:

- The oils that may be most effective at overcoming conditions of the inner ear are the Protecting blend and sweet basil. Create a 50:50 blend with either of these oils and a carrier oil, fill capsules with a dropper, and take 3 capsules a day with food.

- Take one or two drops of the Protecting blend or sweet basil in an herbal tea with honey. Put a drop in each a quart of drinking water you consume. Use a drop in tomato juice or recipes (after taking the recipe off the stove).

- For dizziness or lightheadedness, try aromatic use of frankincense, peppermint, cypress, ginger, lavender, Roman chamomile, or German chamomile. Diffuse 10 to 15 drops of any of these oils or inhale them from a few drops on a tissue or cotton ball.

- Vertigo associated with the nerves of the inner ear may be benefitted by putting 2 drops of helichrysum on a small cotton ball and inserting it into the ear. You must never drop oils, even diluted into the ear canal. On a cotton ball the molecules are absorbed safely into the areas of infection. Massage a few drops around the ear as well.

Viral Hepatitis
(See Hepatitis, Viral)

Vomiting (See Nausea/Vomiting)

WHAT IT IS

Throwing up or involuntarily forcing the contents of the stomach up through the esophagus and out of the mouth.

RECOMMENDED OILS

Spearmint				Peppermint			
Lemon				Tangerine			
Sweet basil				Tea tree			

RECOMMENDED BLENDS

Respiratory blend		Digestion blend	
Comforting blend		Protecting blend	

INSTRUCTION

- Stop all food intake for a few hours and then gradually add mild foods such as clear vegetable broth, stewed apples, steamed vegetables, or brown rice with a few drops of sweet basil, spearmint, or the digestion blend.

- Add a drop or two of spearmint, lemon, or the digestion blend to each quart of your drinking water. For smaller amounts, dip a toothpick into the oil and stir it in a glass of cold water or mug of hot water. Add honey if needed.

- Mix a drop of spearmint, lemon, or the digestion blend in a teaspoon of honey and suck on it slowly.

- If vomiting is happening because of motion sickness, prevent it by using a trace of peppermint on your hand or a tissue and inhaling. Be sure to avoid getting peppermint into your eyes or into the mucous membranes of your nose.

- If you suspect contaminated food or drinking water may be the cause of vomiting, take traces of tea tree oil on your tongue every few minutes for an hour. Also prepare a 50:50 blend of tea tree or the Protecting blend. Fill capsules and take one 3 times a day with food. This may also prevent nausea and vomiting from contaminated food or water.

- Refer to a medical guide, website, or medical professional for signs that your vomiting is more serious than you should treat with home remedies.

Warts & Corns

WHAT THEY ARE

Warts are small growths on the skin, usually painless and harmless. They are caused by the human papillomavirus (HPV). Some warts are spread through sex. They can be embarrassing. They may itch or hurt, especially if they're on your feet. A corn is a small callus on the skin, often caused by local pressure that irritates tissues over a bone. Although the surface area may be small, the hardened area can extend through deep layers of the skin and flesh.

RECOMMENDED OILS

Cinnamon		Lemongrass	
Eucalyptus globulus		Eucalyptus radiata	
Lemon		Lime	
Tea tree		Helichrysum	
Oregano		Thyme	

RECOMMENDED BLEND

Protecting blend	

INSTRUCTION

- Do a Liver Cleanse and an Immune Strengthening Cleanse of at least a year to clear viral infections out of your body.

- Apply tea tree, eucalyptus, lemon, or the Protecting blend undiluted on each individual affected area two or three times daily.

- Take a drop of lemongrass on a cotton swab and apply it on a wart. Put a piece of plastic over it. Then cover that with a little gauze and a bandage to hold it in place. Replace daily and be patient until the wart disappears. It can be a long process.

Weight Management

WHAT IT IS

Your ideal weight is the weight at which you will have the least risk of health problems. Although a healthy body mass index (BMI) and a waist size that is within an acceptable range are easy measurements to monitor, it is your healthy eating and exercise habits that are more important. When you're exercising regularly and eating well, your body will settle into the weight that is most healthy for you. If your goal is to be at your best weight, the way to get there is to establish optimally healthy lifestyle habits.

RECOMMENDED OILS

Rosemary		Bergamot		
Black pepper		Grapefruit		
Sweet basil		Lemon		
Peppermint		Orange		
Tangerine				

RECOMMENDED BLEND

Weight loss blend

INSTRUCTION

- Create a 50:50 blend using the weight loss blend and a carrier oil. Create capsules using a dropper, and take 3 to 4 a day with food to decrease appetite and help with the product's natural thermogenic effect to burn calories.

- Dr. Pénoël suggests a capsule with lemon (25%), tangerine (25%), and carrier oil (50%). Use a dropper to create capsules and take 2 a day with food ++P.

- He also suggests a massage oil for obesity including Eucalyptus radiata 20%, sage, 20%, peppermint 10%, and 50% carrier oil ++P.

- Pamper yourself with a bath using 10 to 15 drops of any of these oils: birch, tangerine, lemon, or orange in a cup of Epsom Salts ++P.

- A citrus blend, the Comforting blend, or various other food associated oils such as sweet basil or the Digestion blend can be used with Aromatic Behavior Conditioning described above in the section on Addictions. Find the aroma that is most pleasurable for you and use it to anchor positive healthy weight messages for yourself.

- To break any nervous habit associated with bingeing, put a trace of sweet basil on the back of your hand before each meal and enjoy the aroma. Rehearse in your mind how good you will feel when you have reached your ideal weight. Imagine the most pleasurable ways you will use to get there.

- Also lean forward. Put your elbows on the table and massage your neck with a few drops of sweet basil.

- Brush your teeth immediately after each meals and use a trace of tea tree or another breath-freshening oil to break the digestive response that could lead to bingeing.

- Massage the lower parts of your ears, both on the front and back, with a drop of sweet basil.

- Create a new tradition of enjoying an "aperitif drink" before each meal. Add one drop of your favorite flavoring oil (possibly two if you wish a stronger action) to a teaspoon of honey. Stir them together and then stir them into a small glass of water. This will significantly improve your healthy digestion and assimilation.

- Even if you have weight concerns, do not try to "kill" your appetite. The battle over becoming thin can create a dangerous love/hate relationship, even with healthy food. You need to retrain your unconscious mind that you must nourish your cells to the depth of their requirements by choosing the best-tasting and finest whole, natural foods that you can find and afford so that they will satisfy your body, your mind, and your emotions.

- Also establish a new tradition of enjoying an aromatic warm drink at the end of each meal to stop the snacking and signal the end of the meal. Many people use coffee for this, but you can use a healthier herbal tea with many essential oil options. Be sure to make them as delicious as possible and create a wide variety of choices your family and your guests can enjoy.

Habits that will help you eat in a relaxed way and fully enjoy your healthy meals or snacks

- Prior to eating, develop habits and routines that will help you unwind and relax for a few minutes.

- Develop the habit of expressing gratitude to God and those who prepared your meal before beginning to eat.

- Reprogram your brain to become more aware of the smells and tastes of your food by chewing your foods more slowly. Attempt to describe to others the nuances in flavors you are experiencing so everyone can become more conscious of the pleasures associated with healthy food.

- Make it a rule to avoid all arguments and conflicts while eating.

- Avoid eating in distracting, noisy places. Never watch TV or work on your computer or laptop while eating.

- Stop eating before you are completely full, even if you need another meal a short time later.

- Have a little rest after the meal if possible. Even a short, relaxing conversation will help.

CLINICAL SUPPORT

"Abdominal subcutaneous fat and waist circumference in the experimental group significantly decreased after aromatherapy massage compared to the control group. Body image in the experimental group was significantly better after aromatherapy massage than in the control group. These results suggest that aromatherapy massage could be utilized as an effective intervention to reduce abdominal subcutaneous fat, waist circumference, and to improve body image in post-menopausal women" (Kim HJ., 2007).

Wrinkles & Mature Skin

WHAT IT IS

Mature and wrinkled skin are a natural part of aging. They are most prominent on sun-exposed skin: the face, neck, hands, feet, and forearms. Although genetics may play a part, sun exposure is also a major cause of wrinkles, especially in those who are fair-skinned. Pollutants, dry climates, and smoking, also contribute to wrinkling.

RECOMMENDED OILS

Frankincense		Lavender	
Tangerine		Neroli	
Patchouli		Rosewood	
Clary sage		Sandalwood	
Ylang ylang			

RECOMMENDED BLENDS

Circulation blend

INSTRUCTION

Massage wrinkled areas of the face with a drop of undiluted frankincense. Do not get too close to the eyes, but do gently apply the oil to wrinkles and puffy areas near the eyes. This oil can work as well as the most expensive night serum.

Create 50:50 blends with the finest carrier oils and any of the essential oils listed. Rotate the oils to maximize the therapeutic benefits of a variety of oils. Massage your face, hands, neck, and feet with these oils.

Take a therapeutic bath using 10 to 15 drops of essential oils in a cup of Epsom Salts. Add a few teaspoons of carrier oil to the water for a moisturizing effect.

Add 2 to 3 drops of your favorite skin-care essential oils to each application of lotions or creams. Blend them into your lotions or creams by adding 10 to 20 drops to each 8 ounce jar or bottle.

Yellow Fever

WHAT IT IS

A tropical disease transmitted by mosquitos that affects the liver and kidneys, causing jaundice and fever. It is often fatal.

RECOMMENDED OILS

Tea tree		Peppermint	
Lemon		Thyme	

RECOMMENDED BLENDS

Protecting blend

INSTRUCTION

Use the following in-home procedures with the approval of your health care professional:

- The most effective oils for yellow fever are a blend of peppermint (25%), lemon (15%), thyme (10%), and a carrier oil (50%). This combination is then blended 50:50 with a carrier oil +++P.

- You can then use a dropper to fill capsules and take 4 a day for 20 to 30 days. After having been in a country where you may have been infected, continue taking the capsules for 14 days+++P.

- You can also apply this blend two or three times a day to the area of the chest directly over the liver. Do this for 20 or 30 days+++P.

- Try taking 1 or 2 drops of any of the recommended oils in an herbal tea with honey. Adjust the flavor by adjusting the quantity of oil used from a couple of drops down to a trace. Do the same in a quart of drinking water, juice, or recipes (after taking the recipe off the stove).

- Small children will typically do better taking essential oils in water, juice, or food rather than in a capsule. If you are treating small children, dilute these oils down to 10% or even less. A little of the strongest oils goes a long way with children. They also respond to a lot less essential oil in their drinking water or foods than adults, so involve them in deciding the flavors they enjoy.

- You can also massage the feet of children and even babies with 1 or 2 drops of tea tree or the antimicrobial diluted in a teaspoon of carrier oil. Do this several times daily to help with this and similar stubborn infections.

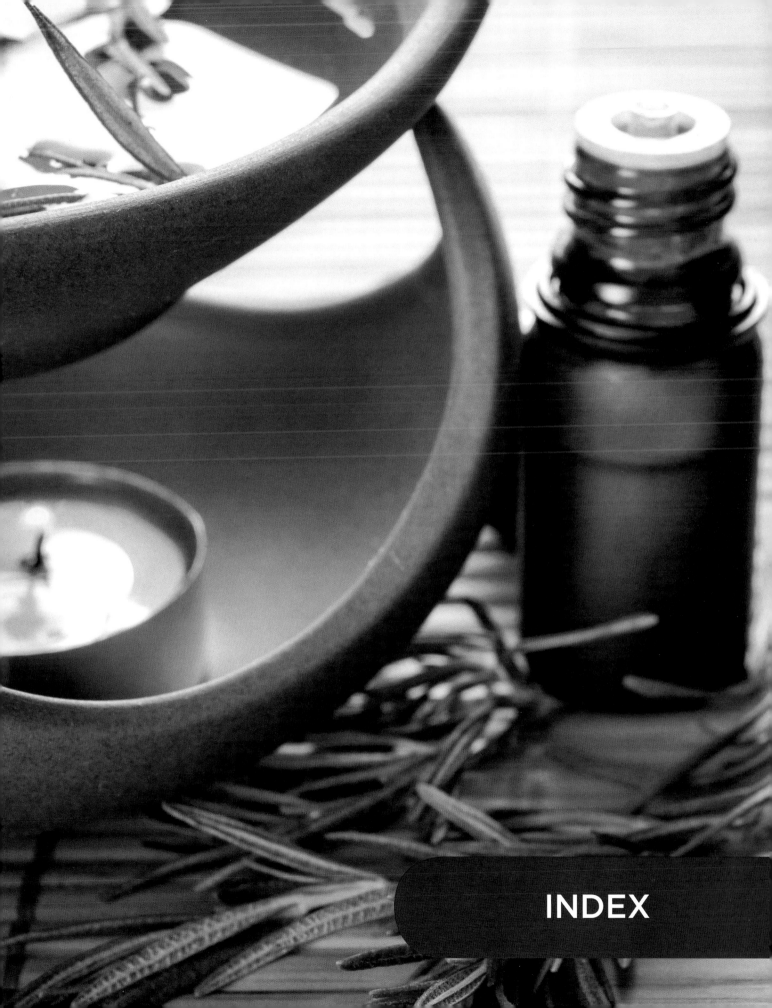

INDEX

Bibliography

Here is only a small sample of the vast number of published studies and research from all over the world on the clinical uses of essential oils. For a quick look at the most recent research or to focus on a particular use or function of an essential oil, go to www.pubmed.gov and search for the oil and the medical condition you wish to research. As of August 2014, there were...

- 4,132 studies on using essential oils for the skin
- 4,024 studies on using essential oils in cancer treatment
- 3,591 studies on using essential oils on children
- 2,490 studies on using essential oils for diabetes
- 1,761 studies on uses of essential oils for depression
- 1,707 studies on using essential oils for cardiovascular conditions
- 1,598 studies on using essential oils during pregnancy
- 1,543 studies on using essential oils and hormones
- 1,491 studies on using essential oils for antibiotic-resistant bacteria
- 1,118 studies on uses of essential oils for anxiety
- 821 studies on anti-inflammatory uses of essential oils
- 765 studies on antimicrobial uses of essential oils
- 662 studies on using essential oils for pain relief
- 633 studies on antibacterial uses of essential oils
- 445 studies on antifungal uses of essential oils
- 278 studies on dental applications for essential oils

Now ask yourself, "is the clinical use of essential oils considered a serious focus of attention by the scientific community?" Glance through the following studies if you are still uncertain.

Aazza S. et al. "Anti-oxidant, anti-inflammatory and anti-proliferative activities of Moroccan commercial essential oils." Nat Prod Commun. 2014 Apr;9(4):587-94.

Abraham C, Amoros M, Girre L. 1983. Etude de l'activité antifongique des plantes supérierures: action de 39 plantes indigènes sur 4 champignons phytopathogènes. Ann. Pharm. franç.

Abu-Al-Basal MA. Healing potential of Rosmarinus officinalis L. on full-thickness excision cutaneous wounds in alloxan-induced-diabetic BALB/c mice. J Ethnopharmacol. 2010 Sep 15;131(2):443-50.

Abu-Darwish, M. S. , C. Cabral, I. V. Ferreira, M. J. Gonçalves, C. Cavaleiro, M. T. Cruz, T. H. Al-bdour, and L. Salgueiro. "Essential Oil of Common Sage (Salvia officinalis L.) from Jordan: Assessment of Safety in Mammalian Cells and Its Antifungal and Anti-Inflammatory Potential." Biomed Res Int. 2013; 2013: 538940.

Ackerman, Diane. Natural History of the Senses. Random House, 2011.

Adorjan, B and Buchbauer, G (2010). "Biological properties of essential oils: an updated review." Flavour and Fragrance Journal 25, 407-426

Al-Bayati FA. 2008. Synergistic antibacterial activity between Thymus vulgaris and Pimpinella anisum essential oils and methanol extracts. J Ethnopharmacol;116(3):403-6. Epub.

Al-Hader A, Hasan Z. 1994. Hyperglycemic and insulin release inhibitory erects of Rosmarinus officinalis. Journal of Ethnopharmacology. 43(3) 217-211.

Allegrini J, Simeon de Buochberg M. 1972. Une technique d'étude du pouvoir antibactérien des huiles essentielles. Labotatoire de microbiologe. Faculté de Montpellier.

Ammar AH et al. "Chemical composition and in vitro antimicrobial and antioxidant activities of Citrus aurantium l. flowers essential oil (Neroli oil). Pak J Biol Sci. 2012 Nov 1;15(21):1034-40).

Anderson C, Lis-Balchin M, Kirk-Smith M. 2000. Evaluation of massage with essential oils on childhood atopic eczema. Phytotherapy Research. 14(6) 452-456.

Ansari M, Razdan R. 1995. Relative efficacy of various oils in repelling mosquitos. Indian Journal of Malariology. 32:104-111.

Armaka M, Papanikolaou E, Sivropoulou A, et al. 1999. Antiviral properties of volatile oils. Journal of Applied Microbiology. 88(2) 308-316.

Arnal-Schnebelen B, 1998. Fighting Gynecological Infection with Aromatherapy. Int. Symp. Integrated Arom. Med. Franchomme P, ed. 7-12.

Arnal-Schnebelen B, 2000. Statistical Analysis of Essential Oils in Gynecological Infectious Treatments: Using Aromatograms. Int. Symp. Integrated Arom. Med. Franchomme P, ed. 27-36.

Arrien, Winter, 1958. The significance of volatile oils for the treatment of urinary passage infections. Planta médica G.B.

Arzi A, et al. 2010. The influence of odorants on respiratory patterns in sleep. Chem Senses. 35(1):31-40.

Asgary S. et al. "Chemical analysis and biological activities of Cupressus sempervirens var. horizontalis essential oils." Pharm Biol. 2013 Feb;51(2):137-44.

Asnaashari S, Delazar A, Habibi B, Vasfi R, Nahara L, Hamedeyazdan S, Sarker SD. "Essential oil from Citrus aurantifolia prevents ketotifen-induced weight-gain in mice." Phytother Res. 2010 Dec;24(12):1893-7.

Bhalla Y, Gupta VK, Jaitak V. Anticancer activity of essential oils: a review. J Sci Food Agric. 2013 Dec;93(15):3643-53.

Balacs T, 1993. Antimicrobial Lamiaceae. In Research Reports, International Journal of Aromatherapy. 5(4) 34.

Bardeau F, 1976. The use of essential oils to purify and deodorize the air. Chirugien-Dentiste de France (Paris). 46(319) 53.

Bassett IB, et al. 1990. A comparative study of tea-tree oil versus benzoyl peroxide in the treatment of acne. Med J Aust. 153(8) 455-8.

Baser, K. Husnu Can, Buchbauer, Gerhard. (2009) Handbook of Essential Oils: Science, Technology, and Applications. CRC Press.

Bassolé IH, Juliani HR. 2012. Essential oils in combination and their antimicrobial properties. Molecules. 17(4):3989-4006. Review.

Bath-Hextall FJ, et al. 2012. Dietary supplements for established atopic eczema. Cochrane Database Syst Rev.;2:CD005205.

Begum A, Sandhya S, Shaffath Ali S, Vinod KR, Reddy S, Banji D. An in-depth review on the medicinal flora Rosmarinus officinalis (Lamiaceae). Acta Sci Pol Technol Aliment. 2013 Jan-Mar;12(1):61-73.

Belaiche P, 1976. Bronchites chroniques. Compte rendu du 1er Congrès International de Phytothérapie et d'Aromathérapie, Paris.

Belaiche P, 1976. Infections de la sphère genitor-urinaire, in Compte rendu du 1er Congrès International de Phytothérapie et d'Aromathérapie, Paris.

Belaiche P, 1977. Bronchites chroniques. Compte rendu du 2e Congrès International de Phytothérapie et d'Aromathérapie, Monaco.

Belaiche P, 1985a. Treatment of skin infections with essential oils of Melaleuca alternifolia. Phytotherapy. 15:15-17.

Benencia F, Courreges M, 2000. In vitro and in vivo activity of eugenol on human herpes virus. Phytotherapy Research. 14:495-500.

Benko S, Macher A, Effect of essential oils on atherosclerosis of cholesterol-fed rabbits. Nature, G. B.

Benouda A, Hassar M, Benjilali B, 1988. Antimicrobial activity of clove oil. Journal of Applied Bacteriology. 66(1) 69-75.

Bentley R, 1874. Rôle de l'eucalyptus dans la bronchite et l'asthme. Yearbook Pharm., 24, 19.

Bezanger-Beauquesne L, Andrieu S, Zad B, 1977. Sensibilté des champignons pathogènes aux antifongiques d'origine végétale. Les huiles essentielles. Bulletin de société de pharmacie de Lille.

Bonnaure F, 1919. Essai sur les propriétés bactericides de quelques huiles essentielles. Thèse Lyon.

Boonchird D, Flegel T, 1982. In vitro activity of eugenol and vanillin against Candida albicans and Cryptococcus neoformans. Canadian Journal of Microbiology. 28(11) 1235-1241.

Boonyuan Wasana et al. "Excito-Repellency of Essential Oils against an Aedes aegypti (L.) Field Population in Thailand." Journal of Vector Ecology 39(1):112-122. 2014.

Boses SM, Bhima Rac. Cn, Subramanyan V, 1949. Relation between chemical constitution and constituents of certain essential oils and their bactericidal properties. J. Sci. Ind. Research (India) 8B, 157-162.

Botelho MA, et al. 2007/ Antimicrobial activity of the essential oil from Lippia sidoides, carvacrol and thymol against oral pathogens. Braz J Med Biol Res; 40(3):349-56.

Bouchra C, et al. "Chemical composition and antifungal activity of essential oils of seven Moroccan Labiatae against Botrytis cinerea Pers: Fr." J Ethnopharmacol. 2003 Nov;89(1):165-9.

Boyd E, Sheppard E, 1968. The effect of steam inhalation of volatile oils on the output and composition of respiratory tract fluid. Journal of Pharmacology and Expermental Therapeutics. 163(4) 250-256.

Braden R, Reichow S, Halm MA. "The use of the essential oil lavandin to reduce preoperative anxiety in surgical patients." J Perianesth Nurs. 2009 Dec;24(6):348-55.

Bradshaw R, Marchant J, Meredith M, et al. 1998. Effects of lavender straw on stress and travel sickness in pigs. Journal of Alternative & Complementary Medicine. 4(3) 271-275.

Brun G, 1952. Les huiles essentielles en tant qu'agent de pénétration tissulaire. Thèse Pharmacie Strasbourg.

Buchbauer G, Jirovetz L, Jager W, 1991. Aromatherapy: Evidence for sedative effects of the essential oil of lavender after inhalation. Zeitschrift fur Naturforschung 46(11-12) 1067-1072.

Buck D, Nidorf D, Addino J, 1994. Comparison of two topical preparations for the treatment of onychomycosis: Melaleuca alternifolia (teatree) oil and clotrimazole. Journal of Family Practice. 38(6) 601-605.

Buckle J, 1999. Use of aromatherapy as a complementary therapy of chronic pain. Alternative Therapies in Health & Medicine. 5(5) 42-51.

Buckle, Jane. (2003) Clinical Aromatherapy: Essential Oils in Practice, Churchill Livingstone.

Budhiraja SS, Cullum ME, Sioutis SS, Evangelista L, Habanova ST. Biological activity of Melaleuca alternifola (Tea Tree) oil component, terpinen-4-ol, in human myelocytic cell line HL-60. J Manipulative Physiol Ther. 1999 Sep;22(7):447-53.

Budzyńska A, et al. "Enzymatic profile, adhesive and invasive properties of Candida albicans under the influence of selected plant essential oils." Acta Biochim Pol. 2014;61(1):115-21.

Bowles, E. Joy. (2004) The Chemistry of Aromatherapy. Allen & Unwin Academic. 34th Ed.

Burfield T, 2000. Safety of essential oils. International Journal of Aromatherapy. 10(1/2) 16-29.

Butt MS et al. "Black pepper and health claims: a comprehensive treatise." Crit Rev Food Sci Nutr. 2013;53(9):875-86.

Cabo J, Crespo M, Jimenez J, et al. 1986. The spasmolytic activity of various aromatic plants from the province of Grananda. The activity of major components of their essential oils. Plantes Medicinales et Phytotherapie. 20(3) 213-218.

Cade AR, 1957. Essential oils, antiseptics, disinfectants, fungicides, and chemical and physical sterilization, Reddish C.F. éd. Philadelphia.

Caelli M, Porteous J, Carson C, et al. 2001. Tea tree oil as an alternative topical decolonization for methicillin-resistant Staphylococcus aureus. Journal of Hospital Infection. 46(3) 236-237.

Caldwell N. "The effects of ylang ylang on craving of women with substance abuse." Hunter, N.Y.: R J Buckle Associates.

Camarda L, et al. 2007. Chemical composition and antimicrobial activity of some oleogum resin essential oils from Boswellia spp. (Burseraceae). Ann Chim.;97(9):837-44.

Cannas S et al. "Antifungal, anti-biofilm and adhesion activity of the essential oil of Myrtus communisL. against Candida species." Nat Prod Res. 2014 Jun 24:1-5.

Capua M, 1974. Consideration on the phototoxicity of bergamot oil. Essenze derive, agrum. Ital.

Carson C, Cookson B, Farrelly H, et al. 1995. Susceptibility of methicillin-resistant Staphylococcus aureus to the essential oil of Melaleuca alternifolia. Journal of Antimicrobial Chemotherapy. 35(3) 421-424.

Carson C, Riley T, 1993. Antimicrobial activity of essential oil of Melaleuca alternifolia. Letters in Applied Microbiology. 16:49-55.

Carson CF, et al. 1995. Antimicrobial activity of the major components of the essential oil of Melaleuca alternifolia. J Appl Bacteriol. 78(3) 264-269.

Casey M, 2002. Aromatherapy: Pain management. Aromatherapy Today. 21:26-29.

Caujolle F, 1942. Hysope: vasolilatation accélération du rythme repiatore, lavande, lavandin: hypotension, diminution de l'amplitude. Soc. Med. Chirurgie Pharm., Toulouse.

Cecchini C, et al. 2012. Antimicrobial efficacy of Achillea ligustica All. (Asteraceae) essential oils against reference and isolated oral microorganisms. Chem Biodivers; 9(1):12-24. doi: 10.1002/cbdv.201100249.

Ceschin C, 1985. Composés perfluorés. Microémulsification. Utilisation pour la croissance des bactéries anaérobies. Thése de doctorat nouveau régime, UPSP Toulouse.

Chalcat J, 1998. Antimicrobial activity of softwood essential oils. Int. Symp. Integrated Arom. Med. Franchomme P, ed. 23-26.

Chan C, Loudon K, 1998. Activity of tea tree oil on methicillin-resistant Staphylococcus aureus (MRSA). Journal of Hospital Infection. 39(3) 244-245.

Chanus H, 2000. Essential Oils and Hospital Germs. Proceedings from the International Symposium of Integrated Aromatic Medicine. Franchomme P, ed. 5-7.

Charabot. Les huiles essentielles. Encyclopédie scientifique éd.

Charron J, 1997. Use of Lavandula latifolia as an expectorant. Journal of Alternative & Complementary Medicine. 3(3) 211.

Chaudhari, et al. "Antimicrobial activity of commercially available essential oils against Streptococcus mutans." J Contemp Dent Pract. 2012 Jan 1;13(1):71-4

Chaumont J-P, 2000. Inventory of Fungi Colonizing Humans: Treatment Options. Int. Symp. Integrated Arom. Med. Franchomme P, ed. 17-19.

Chaumont JP, Jolivet J, 1978. Recherche de substances antifongiques d'origine végétale: action de 100 extraits de plantes des Alpes françaises sur sept champignons phytopathogénes. Phytiatrie-Phytopharmacie.

Chaumont JP, 1985. Plantes antifongiques. Phytothérapy.

Chen W. et al. "Camphor—a fumigant during the Black Death and a coveted fragrant wood in ancient Egypt and Babylon—a review." Molecules. 2013 May 10;18(5):5434-54.

Chesne C, 2001. Antineo-angiogenesis and terpenoids, a path of research in the treatment of rheumatoid arthritis and psoriasis. Int. Symp. Integrated Arom. Med. Franchomme P, ed. 151-152.

Chesne C, Amoros M, Girre L, 1984. Etude de l'activité antifongique de plantes supérieures. Action de 49 plantes indigenes sur 11 champignons phytopathogénes. Ann. Pharm. franç.

Chung MJ, et al. 2010. Anti-diabetic effects of lemon balm (Melissa officinalis) essential oil on glucose- and lipid-regulating enzymes in type 2 diabetic mice. Br J Nutr. 104(2):180-8.

Clark, Sue. (2005) Essential Chemistry for Aromatherapy. 2nd Ed. Churchill Livingstone, Edinburgh.

Concha JM, et al. 1998. William J. Stickel Bronze Award. Antifungal activity of Melaleuca alternifolia (tea-tree oil) against various pathogenic organisms. J Am Podiatr Med Assoc. 88(10) 489-492.

Cornillot P, 2000. The Place of Aromatherapy in Today's Therapeutic Arsenal. Int. Symp. Integrated Arom. Med. Franchomme P, ed. 21-26.

Conrad P, Adams C. "The effects of clinical aromatherapy for anxiety and depression in the high risk postpartum woman - a pilot study." Complement Ther Clin Pract. 2012 Aug;18(3):164-8.

Cornwell S, et al. 1995. Lavender oil and perineal repair. Mod Midwife 5(3) 31-33.

Cox et al. 2000 Jan. The mode of antimicrobial action of the essential oil of Melaleuca alternifolia (tea tree oil). J Appl Microbiol. 88(1) 170-175.

Cwikla C. et al. "Investigations into the antibacterial activities of phytotherapeutics against Helicobacter pylori and Campylobacter jejuni." Phytother Res. 2010 May;24(5):649-56

Dakhil MA, Morsy TA, 1999. The larvicidal activities of the peel oils of three citrus fruits against Culex pipiens. J Egypt Soc Parasitol. 29(2) 347-352.

Dalvi et al. 1991 Jul. Effect of peppermint oil on gastric emptying in man: a preliminary study using a radiolagelled solid test meal. Indian J Physiol Pharmacol. 35(3) 212-214.

Daudet-Vedis J, 2000. Candidiases in Women. Int. Symp. Integrated Arom. Med. Franchomme P, ed. 37-40.

Davenne D, 2001. Study of the photoprotective activity of essential oils on human keratinocytes. Int. Symp. Integrated Arom. Med. Franchomme P, ed. 163-165.

Davis, Patricia. (1995) An A – Z Aromatherapy. Barnes & Noble Books, New York.

Dean S, Ritchie G, 1987. Antibacterial properties of plant essential oils. International Journal of Food Microbiology. 5:165-180.

Debelmas A, 1953. Contribution à l'étude du pouvoir anthelmintique des huiles essentielles et de certains de leurs constituents. Thèse Pharm. Paris.
Dehaut, 1945. Pouvoir antibactérien du thymol, du carvacrol et de quelques derives. Thèse Pharmacie, Toulouse.
Delaveau P, et al. 1989. Neuro-depressive properties of essential oil of lavender. C R Seances Soc Biol Fil. 183(4) 342-348.

Delioux de Savignac, 1988. L'essence dementhe et ses proptiétés analgésiantes. Bull. Mem. Soc. Ther., 1875, 1er s., 4, 41-57.
De Martino L, De Feo V, Nazzaro F. 2009. Chemical composition and in vitro antimicrobial and mutagenic activities of seven Lamiaceae essential oils. Molecules. 2009 Oct 20;14(10):4213-30.
Diego MA, et al. 1998. Dec. Aromatherapy positively affects mood, EEG patterns of alertness and math computations. Int J Neurosci. 96(3-4) 217-224.
Dikshit A, Husain A, 1984. Antifungal Action of Some Essential Oils Against Animal Pathogens. Fitoterapia.
Dobetsberger, C. and Buchbauer, G. (2011) "Actions of essential oils on the central nervous system: an updated review." Flavour and Fragrance Journal 26, 5, 300-316.
Dolara P, Corte B, Ghelardini C, et al. 2000. Local anesthetic, antibacterial and antifungal properties of sesquiterpenes from myrrh. Planta Medica. 66(4) 356-358.
Dolara P, et al. 1996 Jan 4. Analgesic effects of myrrh. Nature. 379(6560) 29.
Dorman H, Dean S, 2000. Antimicrobial agents from plants: Antibacterial of plant isoborneol, a potent inhibitor of herpes simplex virus type 1. Antiviral Research. 43(2) 79-92.
Dube S, Upadihay P, Tripathi S, 1989. Antifungal, physiochemical and insect-repelling activity of the essential oil of Ocimum basilicum. Canadian Journal of Botany. 67(7) 2085-2087.
Dutta BK, Karmakar S, Naglot A, Aich JC, Begam M. "Anticandidial activity of some essential oils of a mega biodiversity hotspot in India." Mycoses. 2007 Mar;50(2):121-4.
Duwenuis P, 1968. Utilization des huiles essentielles en pharmacie, leur normalization et l'europe du medicament. Parfums, cosmet. savons.
Duwiejua M, Zeitlin I, Waterman P, et al. 1992. Anti-inflammatory activity of resins from some species of the plant family Burseraceae. Planta Medica. 59(1) 12-16.
El Keltawi NEM, Megalla SE, Ross SA, 1980. Antimicrobial Activity of Some Egyptian Aromatic Plants. Herba polonica.
Elisabetsky E, de Souza G, Dos Santos M, et al. 1995. Sedative properties of linalool. Fitoterapia. 66(5) 407-415.
Elisabetsky E, Marschner J, Souza D, 1995a. Effects of linalool on glutamatergic system in the rat cerebral cortex. Neurochem Res. 20(4) 461-465.
Elsethager T, 2000. The use of lemongrass and tea tree for fungal infections of feet and nails. Unpublished dissertation. Hunter, NY:R J Buckle Associates.
Enshaieh S et al. "The efficacy of 5% topical tea tree oil gel in mild to moderate acne vulgaris: a randomized, double-blind placebo-controlled study. Indian J Dermatol Venereol Leprol. 2007 Jan-Feb;73(1):22-5.
Erler F, Ulug I, Yalcinkaya B. Fitoterapia. "Repellent activity of five essential oils against Culex pipiens." 2006 Dec;77(7-8):491-4.
Fakim G, Sewaj M, 1992. Studies on the antisickling properties of extracts of Sideroxylon puberulum, Faujariopsis flexuosa, Cardispermum halicacabum and Pelargonium graveoleus. Planta Medica. 58 (Suppl.) A648-A649.
Falsetto, Sharon, Authentic Aromatherapy, 2014.
Faoagali JL, et al. 1998. Antimicrobial effects of melaleuca oil. Burns. 24(4) 383.
Faouzia H, Fkih-Tetouani S, Tantaoui-Elaraki A, 1993. Antimicrobial activity of twenty-one Eucalyptus Essential oils. Fitoterapia. 64:1.
Fauron R, 1998. Using EOs in treating specific pathologies: intestinal, bronchopulmonary, and dermatological. Int. Symp. Integrated Arom. Med. Franchomme P, ed. 37-42.
Feneyriu, 1951. Contribution à l'étude du pouvoir antiseptique de certains dérivés sulfurés du phenol, du thymol et du carvacrol. Thèse Pharmacie. Toulouse.
Ferley J, Poutignat N, Mirou D, 1989. Prophylactic aromatherapy for supervening infections in patients with chronic bronchitis. Statistical evaluation conducted in clinics against a placebo. Phytotherapy Research. 3(3) 97-100.
Figuenick R, 1998. Essential oil of peppermint: A 3-part audit on nausea. Unpublished dissertation. R J Buckle Associates, Hunter, NY.
Fine et al. "An investigation of the effect of an essential oil mouthrinse on induced bacteraemia: a pilot study." J Clin Periodontol. 2010 Sep;37(9):840-7
Franchomme P, 2000. Intestinal Parasitoses and Malnutrition and a Catalog of Antimicrobial Aromatics. Int. Symp. Integrated Arom. Med. Franchomme P, ed. 9-15.
Franchomme, Pierre and Pénoël, Daniel. (2001) L'Aromathérapie Exactement: Encyclopédie de l'utilisation therapeutique des huiles essentielles. Roger Jollois.
Franchomme P, Les chlamydioses, nº 2 février 1987. La grippe et Ravensara aromatica, nº 3 juin 1987. L'aromathérapie à vise anti-infectieuse, nº 4 septembre 1987 revue Epidaure.
Franchomme P, 1998. Using eubiotic and antibiotic EOs in resetting aerobic and anaerobic intestinal flora. Int. Symp. Integrated Arom. Med. Franchomme P, ed. 51-56.
Fu Y, et al. 2007. Antimicrobial activity of clove and rosemary essential oils alone and in combination. Phytother Res. 2007 Oct;21(10):989-94.
Galal E, Adel M, El-Sherif S, 1973. Evaluation of certain volatile oils for their antifungal properties. Journal of Drug Research. 5(2) 235-245.
Garg S, Dengre S, 1988. Antifungal activity of some essential oils. Pharmacie. 43(2) 141-142.
Garg SC, 1974. Antifungical activity of some essential oils. Indian J. Pharm. India.
Garozzo A, Timpanaro R, Stivala A, Bisignano G, Castro A. "Activity of Melaleuca alternifolia (tea tree) oil on Influenza virus A/PR/8: study on the mechanism of action." Antiviral Res. 2011 Jan;89(1):83-8.
Gao YY, Di Pascuale MA, Elizondo A, Tseng SC. "Clinical treatment of ocular demodecosis by lid scrub with tea tree oil." Cornea. 2007 Feb;26(2):136-43.
Gershbein LE, 1977. Regeneration of rat liver in the presence of essential oil. Food Cosmet. Toxicol.
Ghelardini C, Galeotti N, Salvatore G, et al. 1999. Local anesthetic activity of essential oil of Lavandula angustifolia. Planta Medica. 65(8) 700-703.
Girault M, Traité de phytothérapie et d'aromathérapie (P. Belaiche), tome III. Gynécologie, Maloine éd.
Gobel H, Schmidt G, Soyka, D. 1991. Effect of peppermint and eucalyptus oil preparations on neurophysiological and experimental algesimetric headache parameters. Cephalalgia. 14:228-234.
Goetz P, 2000. Acne Treatment Options. Int. Symp. Integrated Arom. Med. Franchomme P, ed. 53-56.
Goldway G, Teff D, Schmidt R, et al. 1995. Multidrug resistance in Candida albicans: Disruption of the BEN gene. Antimicrobial Agents and Chemotherapy. 39(2) 422-426.
Guba R, 2002. Beyond Aromatherapy. Center for Aromatic Medicine. NSW, Australia. Notes published by Center for Aromatic Medicine.
Guba R., "Toxicity Myths: The actual risks of essential oil use." International Journal of Aromatherapy. 10(1/2), 37-49.
Guerin JC, Reveillere HP, 1984. Activité antifongique d'extraits végétaux à usage thérapeutique. II. Etude de 41 extraits sur 9 sources fongiques. Ann. Pharm. franç.
Guerin JC, Reveillere HP, 1985. Activité antifongique d'extraits végétaux à usage thérapeutique. II. Etude de 27 extraits sur 9 sources fongiques. Ann. Pharm. franç.
Guerra et al. "Increasing antibiotic activity against a multidrug-resistant Acinetobacter spp byessential oils of Citrus limon and Cinnamomum zeylanicum." Nat Prod Res. 2012;26(23):2235-8
Guilhon CC, et al. 2011. Characterisation of the anti-inflammatory and antinociceptive activities and the mechanism of the action of Lippia gracilis essential oil. .J Ethnopharmacol. 135(2):406-13.
Guillemain J, et al. 1989. Neurodepressive effects of the essential oil of Lavandula angustifolia Mill. Ann Pharm Fr. 47(6) 337-343.
Gutierrez, L, et al. "Effect of mixed antimicrobial agents and flavors in active packaging films." J Agric Food Chem. 2009 Sep 23;57(18):8564-71.
Hadji-Minaglou F, 1998. ADHD in children: phytoaromatherapy—an alternative to Ritalin. Int. Symp. Integrated Arom. Med. Franchomme P, ed. 57-60.
Hadji-Minaglou F, 2000. Computer-assisted Infectiology Prescriptions. Int. Symp. Integrated Arom. Med. Franchomme P, ed. 41-44.
Hamidpour M, Rafie Hamidpour, Soheila Hamidpour, and Mina Shahlari. "Chemistry, Pharmacology, and Medicinal Property of Sage (Salvia) to Prevent and Cure Illnesses such as Obesity, Diabetes, Depression, Dementia, Lupus, Autism, Heart Disease, and Cancer." J Tradit Complement Med. 2014 Apr-Jun; 4(2): 82–88.
Han S, Hur M, Buckle J, 2003. A randomized trial effect of aromatherapy on the menstrual cramps in college students. In press.
Hancianu M, Cioanca O, Mihasan M, Hritcu L. "Neuroprotective effects of inhaled lavender oil on scopolamine-induced dementia via anti-oxidative activities in rats." Phytomedicine. 2013 Mar 15;20(5):446-52.
Harris B, Harris R, 1995. Essential oils as antifungal agents. Aromatherapy Quarterly. 44:25-27.
Haze et al. "Grapefruit oil attenuates adipogenesis in cultured subcutaneous adipocytes." Planta Med. 2010 Jul;76(10):950-5.
Hermann EC Jr, Kucera LS, 1967. Antiviral Substances in Plants of the Mint Family (Labiatae). Proc. Soc. Exp. Biol. Med. I + II 124, 369-374, 865-869.
Herriset A, Jolivet J, Rey P, 1971. Essences de lavande officinale, de lavande aspic, de lavandins Pl. Méd. Et Phyt. 5, 1305-1314.
Herriset A, Jolivet J, Rey P, 1971. Essences de menthe poivrée. Pl. Méd. Et Phyt. 5, 188-198.
Herriset A, Jolivet J, Rey P, 1973. Essences de citron, d'orange douce, d'orange amère, de bergamote. Pl. Méd. Et Phyt. 7.
Hervieus L, 1998. Aromatherapy for HIV-positive patients. Int. Symp. Integrated Arom. Med. Franchomme P, ed. 61-62.
Holmes P, 1995. Aromatherapy: applications for clinical practice. Alternative Medicine. 1(3) 177-182.
Hudson R, 1996. The value of lavender for rest and activity in the elderly patient. Complementary Therapies in Medicine. 4(1) 52-57.
Imanishi J, Hiroko Kuriyama, Ichiro Shigemori, Satoko Watanabe, Yuka Aihara, Masakazu Kita, Kiyoshi Sawai, Hiroo Nakajima, Noriko Yoshida, Masahiro Kunisawa, Masanori Kawase, and Kenji Fukui. "Anxiolytic Effect of Aromatherapy Massage in Patients with Breast Cancer." Evid Based Complement Alternat Med. Mar 2009; 6(1): 123–128.
Imura M, Misao H, Ushijima H. The psychological effects of aromatherapy-massage in healthy postpartum mothers. J Midwifery Women's Health. 2006 Mar-Apr;51(2):e21-7.
Inouye S, Takizawa T, Yamaguchi H, 2001 May. Antibacterial activity of essential oils and their major constituents against respiratory tract pathogens by gaseous contact. J Antimicrob Chemother. 47(5) 565-573.
Inouye S, Uchida K, Nishiyama Y, Hasumi Y, Yamaguchi H, Abe S. "Combined effect of heat, essential oils and salt on fungicidal activity against Trichophyton mentagrophytes in a foot bath." Nihon Ishinkin Gakkai Zasshi. 2007;48(1):27-36.
Jacquemin M, 1998. Can chemotyped EOs relieve Benzodiazepene withdrawal? Int. Symp. Integrated Arom. Med. Franchomme P, ed. 63-76.
Jandera V, Hudson S, de West P, 2000. Cooling the burn wound: evaluation of different modalities. Burns. 26(3) 265-270.
Janssen AM, Scheffer JJ, Baerheim Svendsen A. 1987. Antimicrobial activities of essential oils. A 1976-1986 literature review on possible applications. Pharm Weekbl Sci. 21;9(4):193-7.
Jedlickova Z et al, "Antibacterial properties of the Vietnamese cajeput oil and ocimum oil in combination with antibacterial agents." J Hyg Epidemiol Microbiol Immunol. 1992;36(3):303-9
Jeong JB, et al. "Patchouli alcohol, an essential oil of Pogostemon cablin, exhibits anti-tumorigenic activity in human colorectal cancer cells." Int Immunopharmacol. 2013 Jun;16(2):184-90.
Johnson, Scott A. (2014) Surviving When Modern Medicine Fails: A Definitive Guide to Essential Oils That Could Save Your Life During a Crisis, CreateSpace.
Joksimovic N, Spasovski G, Joksimovic V, Andreevski V, Zuccari C, Omini CF. "Efficacy and tolerability of hyaluronic acid, tea tree oil and methyl-sulfonyl-methane in a new gel medical device for treatment of haemorrhoids in a double-blind, placebo-controlled clinical trial." Updates Surg. 2012 Sep;64(3):195-201.
Ju MS, Lee S, Bae I, Hur MH, Seong K, Lee MS. "Effects of aroma massage on home blood pressure, ambulatory blood pressure, and sleep quality in middle-aged women with hypertension." Evid Based Complement Alternat Med. 2013;2013:403251.
Juergens UR, et al. 1998. The anti-inflammatory activity of L-menthol compared to mint oil in human monocytes in vitro: a novel perspective for its therapeutic use in inflammatory diseases. Eur J Med Res. 3(12) 539-545.
Junor GO, et al. "Investigation of essential oil extracts from four native Jamaican species of Bursera for antibacterial activity." West Indian Med J. 2007 Jan;56(1):22-5.
Kačániová M, Vukovič N, Horská E, Salamon I, Bobková A, Hleba L, Fiskelová M, Vatľák A, Petrová J, Bobko M. "Antibacterial activity against Clostridium genus and antiradical activity of the essential oils from different origin." J Environ Sci Health B. 2014;49(7):505-12.
Kalemba D, Kunicka A.2003. Antibacterial and antifungal properties of essential oils. Curr Med Chem. 2003 May;10(10):813-29. Review.
Kapoor IP et al. "Chemistry and in vitro antioxidant activity of volatile oil and oleoresins of black pepper (Piper nigrum)." J Agric Food Chem. 2009 Jun 24;57(12):5358-64.
Kemper F, 2001. Pharmacological and toxicological aspects of essential oils. Int. Symp. Integrated Arom. Med. Franchomme P, ed. 107-112.
Kennedy DO, et al. 2011. Monoterpenoid extract of sage (Salvia lavandulaefolia) with cholinesterase inhibiting properties improves cognitive performance and mood in healthy adults. J Psychopharmacol. 2025(8):1088-100.
Khan MS, Ahmad I. "Antifungal activity of essential oils and their synergy with fluconazole against drug-resistant strains of Aspergillus fumigatus and Trichophyton rubrum." Appl Microbiol Biotechnol. 2011 May;90(3):1083-94.
Khoury M, El Beyrouthy M, Ouaini N, Iriti M, Eparvier V, Stien D. "Chemical composition and antimicrobial activity of the essential oil of Juniperusexcelsa M.Bieb. growing wild in Lebanon." Chem Biodivers. 2014 May;11(5):825-30.
Kim HJ. "Effect of aromatherapy massage on abdominal fat and body image in post-menopausal women." Taehan Kanho Hakhoe Chi. 2007 Jun;37(4):603-12.
Kim HM, et al. 1999. Lavender oil inhibits immediate-type allergic reaction in mice and rats. J Pharm Pharmacol. 51(2) 221-226.
Kim IH, et al. "Essential oil inhalation on blood pressure and salivary cortisol levels in prehypertensive and hypertensive subjects." Evid Based Complement Alternat Med. 2012;2012:984203.
Kline R, Kline J, Di Palma J, et al. 2001. Enteric coated pH dependent peppermint oil capsules for the treatment of irritable bowel syndrome in children. Journal of Pediatrics. 138:125-128.
Koch C, Reichling J, Schneele J, Schnitzler P. "Inhibitory effect of essential oils against herpes simplex virus type 2." Phytomedicine. 2008 Jan;15(1-2):71-8.
Koh KJ, Pearce AL, Marshman G, Finlay-Jones JJ, Hart PH. "Tea tree oil reduces histamine-induced skin inflammation." Br J Dermatol. 2002 Dec;147(6):1212-7.
Kozlowski G, 2000. Use of clary sage and geranium on menopausal symptoms. Hunter, NY: R J Buckle Associates.
Kristinsson KG, Magnusdottir AB, Petersen H, Hermansson A. Effective treatment of experimental acute otitis media by application of volatile fluids into the ear canal. J Infect Dis. 2005 Jun 1;191(11):1876-80.

Kucera L, Herrmann E, 1967. Antiviral substances in plants of the mint family. (Labiatae) Tannin of Melissa officinalis. Proceedings from the Society for Experimental Biology and Medicine. 124(3) 865-869.

Lachowicz KJ, et al. 1998. The synergistic preservative effects of the essential oils of sweet basil (Ocimum basilicum L.) against acid-tolerant food microflora. Lett Appl Microbiol. 26(3) 209-214.

Lahlou M, Berrada R, Agoumi A, et al. 2000. The potential effectiveness of essential oils in the control of human head lice in Morocco. International Journal of Aromatherapy. 10(3/4) 108-123.

Larrondo J, Agut M, Calvo-Torres M, 1995. Antimicrobial ativity of essences from labiates. Microbios. 82:171-172.

Larrondo J, Calvo M, 1991. Effecto of essential oils on Candida albicans: A scanning electron microscope study. Biomedical Letters. 46(184) 269-272.

Lavabre, Marcel. (1990) Aromatherapy Workbook. Healing Arts Press, Rochester, VT.

Lawless, Julia. (2013) The Encyclopedia of Essential Oils: The Complete Guide to the Use of Aromatic Oils in Aromatherapy, Herbalism, Health & Well-Being. Conari Press, San Francisco.

Legault J et al. "Antitumor activity of balsam fir oil: production of reactive oxygen species induced by alpha-humulene as possible mechanism of action." Planta Med. 2003 May;69(5):402-7.

Leicester R, Hunt R, 1982. Peppermint oil to reduce colonic spasm during endoscopy. Lancet. 2(8305) 989-990.

Lin RF, et al. "Prevention of UV radiation-induced cutaneous photoaging in mice by topical administration of patchouli oil." J Ethnopharmacol. 2014 Jun 11;154(2):408-18.

Liju VB, Jeena K, Kuttan R. "Gastroprotective activity of essential oils from turmeric and ginger." J Basic Clin Physiol Pharmacol. 2014 Apr 21.

Liu et al. "Metabolomics of ginger essential oil against alcoholic fatty liver in mice." J Agric Food Chem. 2013 Nov 20;61(46):11231-40.

Lima DK et al. 2012. Evaluation of the antinociceptive, anti-inflammatory and gastric antiulcer activities of the essential oil from Piper aleyreanum C.DC in rodents. J Ethnopharmacol.142(1):274-82.

Lis-Balchin M, 1997. A preliminary study of the effect of essential oils on skeletal and smooth muscle in vitro. Journal of Ethnopharmacology. 58(3) 183-187.

Lockhart N, 2000. Inhalation of frankincense and its effect on asthmatics. Unpublished dissertation. Hunter, NY: R J Buckle Associates.

L M Lopes C, et al. 2011. Sedative, anxiolytic and antidepressant activities of Citrus limon (Burn) essential oil in mice. Pharmazie; 66(8):623-7.

Loizzo MR. et al. Antiproliferative effects of essential oils and their major constituents in human renal adenocarcinoma and amelanotic melanoma cells. Cell Prolif. 2008 Dec;41(6):1002-12.

Lorenzi et al. "Geraniol restores antibiotic activities against multidrug-resistant isolates from gram-negative species." Antimicrob Agents Chemother. 2009 May;53(5):2209-11).

Machado M, Sousa Mdo C, Salgueiro L, Cavaleiro C. Effects of essential oils on the growth of Giardia lamblia trophozoites. Nat Prod Commun. 2010 Jan;5(1):137-41.

Manivannan R et al, "A comparative antimicrobial study on the essential oil of the leaves of various species of cupressus." Anc Sci Life. 2005 Jan;24(3):131-3.

Maruzella J, Percival H, 1958. Antimicrobial activity of perfume oils. Journal of the American Pharmaceutical Association. XLVII, 471-476.

Maruzella J, Sicurella N, 1960. Antibacterial activity of essential oil vapors. Journal of the American Pharmaceutical Association (Scientific Edition). 49(11) 693-695.

Marzouk TM et al. The effect of aromatherapy abdominal massage on alleviating menstrual pain in nursing students: a prospective randomized cross-over study. Evidence Based Complementary Alternative Medicine. 2013;2013:742421.

Matiz G, Osorio MR, Camacho F, Atencia M, Herazo J. [Effectiveness of antimicrobial formulations for acne based on orange (Citrus sinensis) and sweet basil (Ocimum basilicum L) essential oils]. Biomedica. 2012 Jan-Mar;32(1):125-33 [Article in Spanish].

Matsubara E., et al. "Volatiles emitted from the roots of Vetiveria zizanioides suppress the decline in attention during a visual display terminal task." Biomed Res. 2012;33(5):299-308.

Maxia A, et al. "Essential oil of Myrtus communis inhibits inflammation in rats by reducing serum IL-6 and TNF-alpha." Nat Prod Commun. 2011 Oct;6(10):1545-8.

Mayaud L, et al "Comparison of bacteriostatic and bactericidal activity of 13 essential oils against strains with varying sensitivity to antibiotics." Lett Appl Microbiol. 2008 Sep;47(3):167-73.

Meneses R, Ocazionez RE, Martinez JR, Stashenko EE. "Inhibitory effect of essential oils obtained from plants grown in Colombia on yellow fever virus replication in vitro." Ann Clin Microbiol Antimicrob. 2009 Mar 6;8:8.

Michie, C A, et al. 1991. Frankincense and myrrh as remedies in children. J R Soc Med. 84(10) 602-605.

Mi-Yeon Cho, Eun Sil Min, Myung-Haeng Hur, and Myeong Soo Lee "Effects of Aromatherapy on the Anxiety, Vital Signs, and Sleep Quality of Percutaneous Coronary Intervention Patients in Intensive Care Units." Evid Based Complement Alternat Med. 2013; 2013: 381381.

Montrain B, 1998. Aromatherapy in the treatment of tinnitus. Int. Symp. Integrated Arom. Med. Franchomme P, ed. 85-87.

Moss M, et al. "Modulation of cognitive performance and mood by aromas of peppermint and ylang-ylang." Int J Neurosci. 2008 Jan;118(1):59-77.

Motiejūnaite O, Peciulyte D. "Fungicidal properties of Pinus sylvestris L. for improvement of air quality." Medicina (Kaunas). 2004;40(8):787-94.

Mustian, KM, Katie Devine, Julie L Ryan, Michelle C Janelsins, Lisa K Sprod, Luke J Peppone, Grace D Candelario, Supriya G Mohile, Gary R Morrow. "Treatment of Nausea and Vomiting During Chemotherapy." US Oncol Hematol. 2011; 7(2): 91–97.

Myers H, 1927. An unappreciated fungicidal action of certain volatile oils. Journal of the American Medical Association. 1834-1836.

Nascimento SS, Camargo EA, DeSantana JM, Araújo AA, Menezes PP, Lucca-Júnior W, Albuquerque-Júnior RL,Bonjardim LR, Quintans-Júnior LJ. "Linalool and linalool complexed in β-cyclodextrin produce anti-hyperalgesic activity and increase Fos protein expression in animal model for fibromyalgia." Naunyn Schmiedebergs Arch Pharmacol. 2014 Jun 24.

Nenoff P, Haustein U, Brndt W, 1996. Antifungal activity of Melaleuca alternifolia (tea tree oil) against pathogenic fungi in vitro. Skin Pharmacology and Applied Skin Physiology. 9:388-394.

Nicole M, 1998. Fibromyalgia and CFS: a real hope for a cure. Int. Symp. Integrated Arom. Med. Franchomme P, ed. 89-100.

Obistioiu D, Cristina RT, Schmerold I, Chizzola R, Stolze K, Nichita I, Chiurciu V. "Chemical characterization by GC-MS and in vitro activity against Candida albicans ofvolatile fractions prepared from Artemisia dracunculus, Artemisia abrotanum, Artemisia absinthium and Artemisia vulgaris." Chem Cent J. 2014 Jan 29;8(1):6.

Oboh G, Ademosun AO, Odubanjo OV, Akinbola IA. "Antioxidative properties and inhibition of key enzymes relevant to type-2 diabetesand hypertension by essential oils from black pepper." Adv Pharmacol Sci. 2013;2013:926047.

Ohno T, Kita M, Yamaoka Y, Imamura S, Yamamoto T, Mitsufuji S, Kodama T, Kashima K, Imanishi J."Antimicrobial activity of essential oils against Helicobacter pylori." Helicobacter. 2003 Jun;8(3):207-15).

Panizzi L, et al. 1993. Composition and antimicrobial properties of essential oils of four Mediterranean Lamiaceae. J Ethnopharmacol. 39(3) 167-170.

Pattnaik S, Subramanyam V, Bapaji M, et al. 1997. Antibacterial and antifungal activity of aromatic constituents of essential oils. Microbios. 89(358) 39-46.

Pattnaik S, Subramanyam V, Kole C, 1996. Anitbacterial and antifungal activity of essential oils in vitro. Microbios. 86(349) 237-246.

Pauli A, 2001. Specific selection of components of essential oils for the treatment of infectious diseases in children. Int. Symp. Integrated Arom. Med. Franchomme P, ed. 51-71.

Peace-Rhind, Jennifer (2012) Essential Oils: A Handbook for Aromatherapy Practice. Singing Dragon, London.

Peana A, Moretti M, Juliano C, 1999. Chemical compostition and antimicrobial action of the essential oils of Salvia desoliana and Salvia sclarea. Planta Medica. 65(8) 752-754.

Pellecuer J, 1998. Anti-infectious properties of essential oils. Int. Symp. Integrated Arom. Med. Franchomme P, ed. 101-107.

Pellecuer, J and Allegrini, J. "Place de l'essence de Satureia Montana L. dans l'arsenal therapeutique, » Plantes Medicinales et Phytotherapie 9, no. 2 (1975) : 99-106.

Pemberton E, Turpin PG. "The effect of essential oils on work-related stress in intensive care unit nurses." Holist Nurs Pract. 2008 Mar-Apr;22(2):97-102.

Pénoël D, 2000. A Severe Case of Acne: Methodology and Findings. Int. Symp. Integrated Arom. Med. Franchomme P, ed. 57-64.

Pénoël, Daniel and Rose-Marie. (2002) Guide to Home Use of Essential Oils, 2nd Ed. Essentia Publishing, Provo, Utah.

Pénoël, Daniel and Rose-Marie. (2000) Life Helping Life: Unleash Your Mind/Body Potential with Essential Oils. Essentia Publishing, Provo, Utah.

Pénoël, Daniel and Rose-Marie. (1998) Natural Home Health Care Using Essential Oils, Essential Science Publishing, Hurricane, Utah.

Phasomkusolsil S, Soonwera M."Insect repellent activity of medicinal plant oils against Aedes aegypti (Linn.), Anopheles minimus (Theobald) and Culex quinquefasciatus Say based on protection time and biting rate." Southeast Asian J Trop Med Public Health. 2010 Jul;41(4):831-40.).

Pichette A et al "Composition and antibacterial activity of Abies balsamea essential oil." Phytother Res. 2006 May;20(5):371-3.

Pitcher L., 2001. The Effects of Mentha piperita on chronic upper respiratory symptoms in adults. Unpublished dissertation. Hunter, N.Y: R J Buckle Associates.

Pohlit AM et al. "Plant extracts, isolated phytochemicals, and plant-derived agents which are lethal to arthropod vectors of human tropical diseases--a review." Planta Med. 2011 Apr;77(6):618-30.

Pohlit AM, Rezende AR, Lopes Baldin EL, Lopes NP, Neto VF. Plant extracts, isolated phytochemicals, and plant-derived agents which are lethal to arthropod vectors of human tropical diseases--a review. Planta Med. 2011 Apr;77(6):618-30).

Prasad CS, Shukla R, Kumar A, Dubey NK.2010. In vitro and in vivo antifungal activity of essential oils of Cymbopogon martini and Chenopodium ambrosioides and their synergism against dermatophytes. Mycoses; 1;53(2):123-9.

Price, Shirley and Len. (1996) Aromatherapy for Health Professionals. Churchill Livingstone, Edinburgh.

Ramadan W, et al. 1996 Jun. Oil of bitter orange: a new topical antifungal agent. Int J Dermatol. 35(6) 448-449.

Rantzsch U, Vacca G, Dück R, Gillissen A. "Anti-inflammatory effects of Myrtol standardized and other essential oils on alveolar macrophages from patients with chronic obstructive pulmonary disease." Eur J Med Res. 2009 Dec 7;14 Suppl 4:205-9.

Rasooli I, et al. "The effect of Mentha spicata and Eucalyptus camaldulensis essential oils on dental biofilm." Int J Dent Hyg. 2009 Aug;7(3):196-203.

Reddy AC, et al. 1994. Studies on anti-inflammatory activity of spice principles and dietary n-3 polyunsaturated fatty acids on carrageenan-induced inflammation in rats. Ann Nutr Metab. 38(6) 349-358.

Rojas J, Palacios O, Ronceros S. "[The effect of the essential oil from Aloysia triphylla britton (lemon verbena) on Trypanosoma cruzi in mice]." Rev Peru Med Exp Salud Publica. 2012 Mar;29(1):61-8 [Article in Spanish]

Rosato A, et al. 2009. In vitro synergic efficacy of the combination of Nystatin with the essential oils of Origanum vulgare and Pelargonium graveolens against some Candida species. Phytomedicine. (10):972-5. Epub 2009 Jul 18.

Rossi T, Melegari M, Bianchi A, et al. 1988. Sedative, anti-inflammatory and anti-diuretic effects induced in rats by essential oils of varieties of Anthemisnobilis: a comparative study. Pharmacological Research Communications. 20(Suppl.) 71-74.

Rusu A, 2000. Initial Results of a Brief Clinical Study of Acne and the Treatment of Athlete's Food with Essential Oils. Int. Symp. Integrated Arom. Med. Franchomme P, ed. 65-66.

Saad A, et al. 2010. Anticandidal activity of the essential oils of Thymus maroccanus and Thymus broussonetii and their synergism with amphotericin B and fluconazol. Phytomedicine;17(13):1057-60.

Sadlon AE, Lamson DW. 2010. Immune-modifying and antimicrobial effects of Eucalyptus oil and simple inhalation devices. Altern Med Rev. 15(1):33-47.

Saeed SA, et al. 1994. Antithrombotic activity of clove oil. JMPA J Pak Med Assoc. 44(5) 112-115.

Sah SP, Mathela CS, Chopra K. 2010. Elucidation of possible mechanism of analgesic action of Valeriana wallichii DC chemotype (patchouli alcohol) in experimental animal models. Indian J Exp Biol.48(3):289-93.

Sahi S, Shukla A, Bajaj A, et al. 1999. Broad spectrum antimycotic drug for the control of fungal infections in human beings. Cuttent Science. 76(6) 836-939.

Saiyudthong, S.; Ausavarungnirun, R.; Jiwajinda, S.; Turakitwanakan, W. "Effects of aromatherapy massage with lime essential oil on stress. International Journal of Essential Oil Therapeutics 2009 Vol. 3 No. 2/3 pp. 76-80.

Santos R.C. et al. "Antimicrobial activity of Amazonian oils against Paenibacillus species." J Invertebr Pathol. 2012 Mar;109(3):265-8.

Sasannejad P, Saeedi M, Shoeibi A, Gorji A, Abbasi M, Foroughipour M. "Lavender essential oil in the treatment of migraine headache: a placebo-controlled clinical trial." Eur Neurol. 2012;67(5):288-91.

Schafer D, Schafer W, 1981. Pharmacological studies with an ointment containing menthol, camphene and essential oils for broncholytic and secretolytic effects. Arzneimittelforschung. 31(1) 82-86.

Schnaubelt K, 1993. Aromatherapy Practitioner Reference Manual, Vol. 11. Tampa, FL: Atlantic Institute of Aromatherapy.

Schnaubelt K, 1999. Medical Aromatherapy. Berkley, CA: Frog Ltd., 179. Shapiro S, et al. 1994. The antimicrobial activity of essential oils and essential oil components towards oral bacteria. Oral Microbiol Immunol. 9(4) 202-208.

Schnaubelt, Kurt. (2011) The Healing Intelligence of Essential Oils: The Science of Advanced Aromatherapy. Healing Arts Press, Rochester, VT.

Schnitzler et al. "Antiviral activity of Australian tea tree oil and eucalyptus oil against herpes simplex cultures in cell culture." Pharmazie. 56(4).343-7.

Schnitzler P, Koch C, Reichling J. "Susceptibility of Drug-Resistant Clinical Herpes Simplex Virus Type 1 Strains to Essential Oils of Ginger, Thyme, Hyssop, and Sandalwood." Antimicrob Agents Chemother. May 2007; 51(5): 1859-1862.

Schröder C, 2000. The Use of Essential Oils in Gingivodental Treatments. Int. Symp. Integrated Arom. Med. Franchomme P, ed. 67-72.

Seol GH, Shim HS, Kim PJ, Moon HK, Lee KH, Shim I, Suh SH, Min SS. "Antidepressant-like effect of Salvia sclarea is explained by modulation of dopamine activities in rats." J Ethnopharmacol. 2010 Jul 6;130(1):187-90.

Shahat AA, et al. 2011. Chemical composition, antimicrobial and antioxidant activities of essential oils from organically cultivated fennel cultivars. Molecules;16(2):1366-77.

Shavakhi A, Ardestani SK, Taki M, Goli M, Keshteli AH. Premedication with peppermint oil capsules in colonoscopy: a double blind placebo-controlled randomized trial study. Acta Gastroenterol Belg. 2012 Sep;75(3):349-53.

Shemesh A, 1991. Australian tea-tree: A natural antiseptic and fungicidal agent. Australian Journal of Pharmacy. 12:802-803.

Shipradeep, 2012. Development of probiotic candidate in combination with essential oils from medicinal plant and their effect on enteric pathogens: a review. Gastroenterol Res Pract.;2012:457150.

Sienkiewicz M, et al 2012. The antimicrobial activity of thyme essential oil against multidrug resistant clinical bacterial strains. Microb Drug Resist. 18(2):137-48.

Siurein S A, 1997. Effects of essential oil on lipid peroxidation and lipid metabolism in patients with chronic bronchitis. Klin Med (Mosk). 75(10) 43-45.

Spadaro F, Costa R, Circosta C, Occhiuto F. "Volatile composition and biological activity of key lime Citrus aurantifolia essential oil." Nat Prod Commun. 2012 Nov;7(11):1523-6.

Spear B, 1999. Essential oils and their effectiveness in the relief of symptoms of asthma. Unpublished dissertation. Hunter, N.Y.: R J Buckle Associates.

Srivastava KC, 1993. Antiplatelet principles from a food spice clove. Prostaglandins Leukot Essent Fatty Acids. 48(5) 363-372.

Stea S, Beraudi A, De Pasquale D. "Essential oils for complementary treatment of surgical patients: state of the art." Evid Based Complement Alternat Med. 2014;2014:726341.

Steflitsch W. 2009. [Wound care with essential oils after enucleation of a chronic abscess]. Forsch Komplementmed.16(6):400-3. German.

Syed T, Qureshi Z, Ali S, et al. 1999. Treatment if toenail onychomycosis with 2% butenafine and 5% Melaleuca alternifoila (tea tree in cream). Tropical Medicine & International Health. 4(4) 284-287.

Sysoev NP, 1991. The effect of waxes from essential-oil plants on the dehydrogenase activity of the blood neutrophils in mucosal trauma of the mouth. Stomatologiia. 70(1) 12-13.

Tantaoui-Elaraki A, et al. 1994. Inhibition of growth and aflatoxin production in Aspergillus parasiticus by essential oils of selected plant materials. J Environ Pathol Toxicol Oncol. 13(1) 67-72.

Tao N, Jia L, Zhou H "Anti-fungal activity of Citrus reticulata Blanco essential oil against Penicillium italicum and Penicillium digitatum." Food Chem. 2014 Jun 15;153:265-71.

Tate S, 1997. Peppermint oil: A treatment for postoperative nausea. Journal of Advanced Nursing. 26(3) 543-549.

Tayarani-Najaran Z, et al. "Antiemetic activity of volatile oil from Mentha spicata and Mentha × piperita in chemotherapy-induced nausea and vomiting." Ecancermedicalscience. 2013;7:290.

Taylor, Pamela L., Simple Ways of Healing (Moline ILL.: Mid West Botanicals, 2007).

Thompson A et al. "Comparison of the antibacterial activity of essential oils and extracts of medicinal and culinary herbs to investigate potential new treatments for irritable bowel syndrome." BMC Complement Altern Med. 2013 Nov 28;13:338.

Tisserand R, 1988. Lavender beats benzodiazepines. International Journal of Aromatherapy. 1(1) 1-2.

Tisserand, Robert and Young, Rodney. (2013) Essential Oil Safety: A Guide for Health Care Professionals. Churchill Livingstone.

Tiwari BK, et al. 1966. Evaluation of insecticidal, fumigant and repellant properties of lemongrass oil. Indian J Exp Biol. 4(2) 128-129.

Tomić M. et al. "Antihyperalgesic and antiedematous activities of bisabolol-oxides-rich matricaria oilin a rat model of inflammation." Phytother Res. 2014 May;28(5):759-66).

Tong M, Altman P, Barnetson R. 1992. Tea tree oil in the treatment of Tinea pedis. Australasian Journal of Dermatology. 33(3) 145-149.

Tovey ER, et al. 1997. A simple washing procedure with eucalyptus oil for controlling house dust mites and their allergens in clothing and bedding. J Allergy Clin Immunol. 100(4) 464-466.

Tubéry P, 1998. Allergies and auto-immune diseases: treatment using plant products. Int. Symp. Integrated Arom. Med. Franchomme P, ed. 133-137.

Tumen I et al. "Topical wound-healing effects and phytochemical composition of heartwood essential oils of Juniperus virginiana L., Juniperus occidentalis Hook., and Juniperusashei J. Buchholz." J Med Food. 2013 Jan;16(1):48-55.

Valnet, Jean. (1980) The Practice of Aromatherapy: Holistic Health and the Essential Oils of Flowers and Herbs. Destiny Books, New York.

Van Leeuwen M, Slot D, Van der Weijden G. The effect of an essential-oils mouthrinse as compared to a vehicle solution on plaque and gingival inflammation: a systematic review and meta-analysis. Int J Dent Hyg. 2014 Aug;12(3):160-167.

Van Vuuren SF, Suliman S, Viljoen AM 2009. The antimicrobial activity of four commercial essential oils in combination with conventional antimicrobials. Lett Appl Microbiol. 2009 Apr;48(4):440-6.

Varney E, Buckle J. "Effect of inhaled essential oils on mental exhaustion and moderate burnout: a small pilot study." J Altern Complement Med. 2013 Jan;19(1):69-71.

Vericel M, 2001. Clinical results in ENT and respiratory pathology in children under aromatherapy. Int. Symp. Integrated Arom. Med. Franchomme P, ed. 73-79.

Vilaseca A, 2000. Natural Insect Repellants and Insecticides from the Aromatic Plant Species of Bolivian Flora. Int. Symp. Integrated Arom. Med. Franchomme P, ed. 83-88.

Viollon C, Chaumont J. 1994. Antifungal properties of essential oil components against Cryptococcus neoformans. Mycopathologia. 128(3) 151-153.

Vogley, S. "Bergamot, anxiety and the elderly," Unpublished dissertation, Hunter, NY: RJ Buckle Associates 2002.

Wagner J, et al. 1998. Beyond benzodiazepines: alternative pharmacologic agents for the treatment of insomnia. Ann Pharmacother. 32(6) 680-691.

Walton SF, McKinnon M, Pizzutto S, Dougall A, Williams E, Currie BJ. Acaricidal activity of Melaleuca alternifolia (tea tree) oil: in vitro sensitivity of sarcoptes scabiei var hominis to terpinen-4-ol." Arch Dermatol. 2004 May;140(5):563-6).

Wan J, et al. 1998. The effect of essential oils of basil on the growth of Aeromonal hydrophila and Pseudomonas fluorescens. J Appl Microbiol. 84(2) 152-158.

Warad SB, et al. "Lemongrass essential oil gel as a local drug delivery agent for the treatment of periodontitis." Anc Sci Life. 2013 Apr;32(4):205-11.

Warnke PH, et al. 2009. The battle against multi-resistant strains: Renaissance of antimicrobial essential oils as a promising force to fight hospital-acquired infections. J Craniomaxillofac Surg;37(7):392-7.

West B, Brockman S, 1994. The calming power of aromatherapy. Journal of Dementia Care. March/April, 20-22.

Weyers W, et al. 1989. Skin absorption of volatile oils. Pharmacokinetics. Pharm Unserer Zeit. 18(3) 82-86.

Wilkinson S, Aldridge J, Salmon I, Cain E, Wilson B. "An evaluation of aromatherapy massage in palliative care." Palliat Med. 1999 Sep;13(5):409-17.

Woelk H, Schläfke S. 2010. A multi-center, double-blind, randomised study of the Lavender oil preparation Silexan in comparison to Lorazepam for generalized anxiety disorder. Phytomedicine. 17(2):94-9.

Woolfson A, Hewitt D, 1992. Intensive aromacare. International Journal of Aromatherapy. 4(2) 12-14.

Worwood V, 2000. Aromatherapy for the Healthy Child. Navato, CA: New World Library.

Worwood, Valierie Ann. (1991) The Complete Book of Essential Oils and Aromatherapy: Over 600 Natural, Non-Toxic and Fragrant Recipes to Create Health — Beauty — a Safe Home Environment. New World Library, Novato, CA.

Yamada K, Mimaki Y, Sashida Y, et al. 1994. Anticonvulsant effects of inhaling lavender oil vapor. Biological Pharmaceutical Bulletin. 17(2) 359-360.

Youdim KA, Deans SG, et al. 1999 Apr 19. Beneficial effects of thyme oil on age-related changes in the phospholipids C20 and C22 polyunsaturated fatty acid composition of various rat tissues. Biochim Biophys Acta. 1438(1) 140-146.

Youdim KA, Deans SG, 1999 Sep 8. Dietary supplementation of thyme (Thymus vulgaris L.) essential oil during the lifetime of the rat: its effects on the antioxidant status in liver, kidney and heart tissues. Mech Aging Dev 109(3) 163-175.

Youdim KA, et al. 2000 Jan. Effect of thyme oil and thymol dietary supplementation on the antioxidant status and fatty acid composition of the aging rat brain. Br J Nutr. 83(1) 87-93.

Yousef R T, and G G, Tawil, 1980. Antimicrobial activity of volatile oils. Pharmazie 35(11) 798-801.

Zakarya D, Fkih-Tetouani S, Hajji F, 1993. Antimicrobial activity of twenty-one Eucalyptus essential oils. Fitoterapia. 64:319-331.

Zanker KS, et al. 1980. Evaluation of surfactant-like effects of commonly used remedies for colds. Respiration. 39(3) 150-157.

Zhang Y, Wu Y, Chen T, Yao L, Liu J, Pan X, Hu Y, Zhao A, Xie G, Jia W. Assessing the metabolic effects of aromatherapy in human volunteers. Evid Based Complement Alternat Med. 2013;2013:35638.

Index

ginger 17, 112, 113, 129, 150, 176, 192, 245, 250, 256, 315, 348, 358

Gingivitis 257

gonorrhea 149, 165, 329

gout 89, 117, 128, 139, 145, 153, 158, 212, 258, 307

Grapefruit 113, 114, 201, 205, 206, 211, 242, 244, 256, 260, 272, 308, 324, 328, 350, 357

Grapeseed oil 47, 55

GRAS 10, 35

Gum 211

H

hair 47, 49, 61, 62, 63, 64, 75, 99, 114, 118, 134, 144, 151, 159, 165, 169, 187, 198, 211, 212, 213, 214, 217, 225, 236, 240, 254, 280, 286, 307, 313, 325, 326, 333, 336, 343

hair loss 99, 144, 211

hands 18, 19, 49, 50, 54, 55, 58, 87, 90, 109, 116, 120, 122, 124, 125, 127, 130, 132, 135, 145, 146, 150, 151, 152, 153, 154, 157, 158, 159, 160, 161, 180, 181, 182, 184, 185, 186, 188, 193, 204, 206, 223, 224, 226, 237, 238, 244, 245, 247, 249, 254, 263, 265, 271, 274, 283, 300, 301, 304, 305, 321, 324, 331, 332, 334, 338, 340, 351, 352

Hashimoto's disease 340

hay fever 47, 106, 189, 191, 192, 196, 203, 209, 227, 231, 260, 261

headache 81, 91, 95, 111, 127, 137, 180, 261, 262, 263, 264, 269, 279, 288, 291, 299, 332, 357, 358

health care professional 2, 61, 204, 206, 208, 209, 212, 213, 214, 215, 216, 220, 221, 222, 225, 226, 233, 237, 240, 241, 242, 243, 246, 248, 249, 250, 251, 252, 253, 254, 255, 256, 257, 258, 260, 261, 262, 264, 265, 266, 267, 268, 270, 271, 272, 273, 274, 275, 276, 277, 279, 280, 282, 283, 284, 285, 286, 287, 288, 289, 290, 291, 292, 298, 299, 300, 301, 302, 304, 306, 307, 309, 310, 311, 312, 314, 317, 321, 322, 323, 324, 325, 326, 327, 329, 331, 332, 335, 336, 338, 339, 340, 341, 343, 344, 346, 347, 348, 352

heart 50, 52, 56, 64, 65, 77, 82, 89, 93, 103, 122, 140, 144, 148, 149, 151, 156, 158, 159, 160, 169, 174, 206, 210, 224, 242, 246, 249, 264, 265, 266, 268, 273, 286, 293, 316, 321, 322, 331, 347, 359

heart attack 224, 265

heartburn 244, 268, 269, 315

Heart Rhythm Disorders 266

heat stroke 269

helichrysum 86, 115, 116, 151, 152, 161, 189, 207, 212, 218, 219, 220, 223, 235, 239, 249, 256, 258, 259, 265, 277, 279, 288, 292, 302, 305, 338, 341, 348

hematoma 115, 218, 219

hemorrhoids 85, 91, 99, 103, 117, 129, 131, 135, 150, 156, 165, 244, 269, 270

hepatitis 22, 189, 227, 244, 270

Herpes simplex 106, 107, 111, 157, 159, 223, 256

Herpes zoster 330

hiccups 271

high blood pressure 99, 120, 123, 125, 145, 167, 169, 267, 364

hives 136, 272

HIV Infection 259

hoarseness 341

honey 85, 94, 112, 113, 115, 137, 190, 193, 205, 208, 213, 225, 226, 228, 229, 230, 232, 236, 238, 252, 257, 260, 263, 268, 275, 278, 285, 289, 290, 291, 292, 304, 311, 323, 325, 332, 335, 340, 348, 349, 350, 352

hormonal 27, 53, 145, 194, 211, 309, 319

hormone 64, 261, 340

hostility 294

Household Uses 72, 94

hydrosol 56, 57

hyperactivity 194

hypertension 127, 131, 161, 167, 169, 243, 267, 357, 358

hyperthyroidism 151, 243

Hypoglycemia 272

Hypotension 267

hypothalamus-pituitary axis 51, 53

Hypothermia 273

hypothyroidism 340

I

immune 51, 53, 62, 75, 100, 109, 114, 120, 127, 129, 133, 145, 146, 156, 176, 186, 190, 191, 192, 196, 197, 198, 204, 207, 208, 209, 215, 217, 218, 221, 222, 231, 232, 235, 239, 241, 248, 255, 259, 272, 279, 285, 286, 287, 289, 290, 291, 310, 340, 343, 346, 359

immune balancing blend 191, 208, 209, 221, 232, 255, 259, 285, 287, 289, 310, 340

immune system 51, 53, 62, 109, 114, 120, 127, 129, 145, 156, 176, 186, 190, 191, 196, 197, 204, 215, 217, 218, 221, 222, 231, 232, 239, 248, 259, 279, 289, 290, 291, 340, 343

immunity 66, 87, 97, 101, 197, 221, 222, 259, 260, 274

impetigo 135, 273, 274

indigestion 94, 111, 112, 113, 122, 123, 136, 142, 267

infants 78, 276, 278

infected wounds 142, 148, 156

infection 62, 63, 67, 70, 72, 81, 85, 89, 96, 102, 105, 107, 109, 117, 118, 127, 132, 134, 135, 136, 140, 146, 148, 150, 156, 158, 160, 177, 178, 179, 205, 206, 209, 212, 213, 214, 215, 216, 217, 221, 222, 225, 235, 238, 239, 243, 246, 247, 248, 256, 257, 259, 270, 272, 274, 276, 277, 279, 280, 283, 284, 285, 289, 290, 291, 299, 304, 306, 312, 318, 322, 323, 324, 325, 326, 331, 332, 333, 335, 339, 341, 342, 343, 344, 345, 346, 348

infectious diseases 17, 93, 105, 107, 112, 113, 120, 123, 129, 133, 140, 169, 231, 358

inflammation 12, 60, 86, 89, 90, 93, 96, 97, 99, 102, 106, 108, 110, 111, 115, 122, 123, 125, 127, 129, 130, 133, 137, 141, 142, 148, 151, 156, 167, 178, 180, 190, 191, 197, 203, 206, 207, 208, 210, 215, 216, 219, 226, 237, 240, 244, 248, 249, 252, 253, 255, 257, 258, 259, 270, 272, 274, 284, 287, 288, 290, 291, 300, 301, 302, 303, 305, 309, 310, 314, 318, 320, 321, 330, 332, 333, 337, 338, 341, 346, 347, 357, 358, 359

inflammation blend 207, 208, 215, 216, 219, 226, 249, 252, 253, 259, 272, 274, 309, 314, 318, 320, 321, 337

influenza 106, 157, 159, 279, 280

ingestion 10, 19, 35, 41, 46, 138, 164, 175, 179, 182, 185, 187, 198, 204, 261, 271, 289, 295, 336

inhalers 64, 67

injuries 158, 215, 218, 219, 223, 239, 300

insect bites 92, 105, 111, 118, 120, 125, 142, 152, 156, 158, 161, 169, 190

insect repellent 93, 97, 100, 103, 105, 107, 118, 119, 123, 141, 144, 152, 156, 159, 160, 161, 165, 281

insomnia 85, 87, 108, 111, 120, 122, 124, 125, 127, 130, 143, 150, 152, 154, 159, 164, 165, 179, 225, 234, 239, 260, 265, 282, 283, 292, 296, 305, 321, 322, 359

memory 9, 64, 100, 104, 147, 153, 157, 169, 196, 291, 328

meningitis 291

menopause 104, 111, 292, 346

menstrual cramps 251, 303, 322, 357

menstruation 96, 99, 103, 108, 109, 111, 117, 119, 127, 128, 137, 142, 145, 161, 164, 165, 167, 272, 292, 321

mental fatigue 116, 138, 145

mental health 295, 296

meridians 50

metabolism 96, 114, 182, 189, 226, 227, 244, 272, 286, 334, 358

methyl salicylate 88, 89, 166, 168

microbes 8, 9, 12, 13, 19, 22, 64, 71, 72, 176, 177, 178, 196, 342, 366

migraine 115, 127, 152, 153, 164, 261, 263, 264, 358

Mind/Body Cleanse 334

minor cuts 184

mites 280, 359

moles 81, 298, 299

Mononucleosis 299

monoterpene 97, 108, 138

monoterpenes 27, 28, 84, 90, 106, 131, 132

monoterpenols 27, 132

mood 12, 59, 87, 150, 169, 182, 185, 186, 194, 286, 292, 296, 357, 358

Morning sickness 303

mosquito bites 281

motion sickness 137, 138, 304, 349

mouth 64, 65, 66, 68, 71, 72, 75, 76, 87, 96, 110, 116, 120, 124, 125, 134, 137, 138, 142, 145, 147, 152, 153, 154, 156, 157, 159, 177, 181, 182, 184, 185, 186, 194, 204, 211, 216, 222, 223, 232, 236, 258, 263, 271, 285, 290, 304, 332, 336, 339, 342, 348, 359, 366

mouthwash 35, 71, 75, 76, 86, 166, 211, 216, 238, 258, 285

"M" technique* 21

mugwort 128, 176

multiple sclerosis 122, 191, 231

muscle aches 92, 93, 99, 105, 112, 115, 119, 139, 141, 153, 158, 161, 340

muscles 55, 56, 58, 59, 75, 76, 85, 86, 87, 90, 91, 94, 96, 100, 102, 103, 105, 107, 108, 110, 112, 114, 115, 125, 127, 133, 137, 152, 153, 154, 158, 164, 165, 167, 169, 180, 183, 184, 185, 188, 212, 217, 219, 234, 238, 251, 282, 287, 296, 300, 301, 302, 303, 304, 305, 309, 315, 316, 317, 318, 324, 327, 330, 339, 345

muscle spasms 12, 94, 127

muscle weakness 269, 287, 340

myrtle 129, 130, 133, 176, 188, 276, 312, 323

N

nails 254, 357

nausea 90, 94, 95, 101, 109, 111, 112, 119, 120, 123, 135, 136, 137, 142, 147, 150, 153, 154, 158, 161, 204, 234, 235, 239, 244, 245, 253, 260, 265, 266, 269, 282, 283, 284, 286, 296, 304, 305, 315, 321, 337, 343, 344, 349, 357, 359

nebulizing diffuser 65, 66, 68, 167, 187, 198

neck pain 59, 137, 287, 305

neroli 110, 112, 113, 120, 121, 122, 127, 131, 141, 143, 161, 169, 235, 265, 317, 326, 330, 332, 334, 344

nervous exhaustion 86, 95, 114, 115, 122, 124, 135, 139, 145, 158, 169

nervous system 29, 53, 87, 114, 123, 131, 145, 148, 159, 164, 212, 263, 307, 323, 339, 357

neuralgia 90, 97, 105, 107, 111, 116, 127, 136, 139, 142, 143, 150, 160, 212, 306, 307

neuritis 143

nosebleed 120, 144

notes 19, 51, 56, 57, 85, 86, 88, 89, 90, 91, 92, 94, 95, 97, 98, 100, 101, 102, 104, 106, 108, 110, 112, 113, 115, 116, 118, 120, 121, 123, 125, 126, 128, 129, 130, 131, 132, 134, 136, 138, 140, 141, 144, 146, 147, 149, 151, 152, 154, 155, 157, 160, 162, 163, 165, 166, 168, 173, 174, 176, 196

nursing 21, 55, 143, 314, 358

O

obesity 114, 120, 125, 126, 132, 148, 149, 158, 308, 350

obsessive-compulsive disorder 233, 319

oil pulling 72, 211, 258

olfactory bulb 63, 64

optical rotation 36

oral 156, 164, 202, 258, 356, 358

orange 33, 40, 71, 74, 86, 97, 103, 108, 112, 130, 131, 132, 154, 173, 184, 189, 192, 200, 213, 228, 234, 239, 245, 248, 260, 266, 282, 283, 296, 305, 308, 324, 333, 350, 357, 358

oregano 5, 18, 29, 47, 55, 60, 70, 72, 79, 80, 81, 132, 133, 134, 144, 157, 158, 159, 163, 166, 174, 176, 177, 188, 192, 205, 222, 244, 254, 255, 289, 314

organic 33, 39, 47, 77, 113, 167

osteoarthritis 88, 158, 188, 207

osteoporosis 215, 309

overeating 261, 334

Oxydes 26

oxygen 9, 28, 29, 162, 204, 255, 262, 263, 312, 318, 358

P

Paget's Disease 309

pain 12, 48, 49, 52, 55, 59, 60, 85, 87, 88, 89, 90, 91, 96, 97, 100, 105, 106, 107, 109, 110, 111, 112, 115, 116, 117, 118, 119, 123, 127, 133, 135, 136, 137, 139, 142, 143, 144, 145, 148, 150, 152, 153, 156, 157, 158, 159, 160, 161, 162, 164, 167, 180, 190, 207, 212, 215, 216, 219, 220, 224, 226, 234, 236, 239, 240, 247, 250, 251, 252, 260, 261, 262, 263, 265, 268, 269, 270, 279, 280, 282, 283, 284, 287, 288, 289, 296, 301, 302, 303, 305, 306, 307, 309, 310, 312, 317, 318, 330, 331, 332, 333, 337, 338, 339, 340, 341, 342, 343, 344, 345, 346, 356, 358

painting 73

palpitations 144, 160

pancreas 52, 117, 122, 242, 310, 334

pancreatitis 244

panic 295

Parasites 310

patchouli 57, 86, 112, 118, 128, 134, 135, 149, 163, 165, 174, 176, 205, 211, 223, 224, 246, 248, 250, 267, 270, 290, 291, 326, 328, 352, 358

Pénoël, Dr. Daniel 4, 6, 10, 12, 20, 26, 48, 76, 202

peppermint 10, 29, 35, 39, 40, 42, 71, 72, 73, 74, 75, 76, 79, 80, 81, 88, 91, 92, 93, 94, 95, 100, 102, 106, 116, 122, 136, 137, 138, 140, 144, 146, 147, 152, 166, 169, 173, 174, 175, 176, 190, 194, 200, 201, 204,

U

V

W

Y

Notes